POLITICS IN THE CORRIDOR OF DYING

POLITICS IN THE CORRIDOR OF DYING

AIDS Activism and Global Health Governance

JENNIFER CHAN

Johns Hopkins University Press
Baltimore

Johns Hopkins University Press
2715 North Charles Street
Baltimore, Maryland 21218-4363
www.press.jhu.edu

Library of Congress Cataloging-in-Publication Data
Chan, Jennifer, author.
Politics in the corridor of dying : AIDS activism and global health governance /
Jennifer Chan.
p. ; cm.
Includes bibliographical references and index.
ISBN 978-1-4214-1597-0 (pbk. : alk. paper) — ISBN 1-4214-1597-6
(pbk. : alk. paper) — ISBN 978-1-4214-1598-7 (electronic) —
ISBN 1-4214-1598-4 (electronic)   I. Title.
[DNLM: 1. HIV Infections.   2. Organizations.   3. Dissent and Disputes.
4. Politics.   5. Social Justice.   6. World Health. WC 503.7]
RC606.5
362.19697′92—dc23
2014014552

A catalog record for this book is available from the British Library.

*Special discounts are available for bulk purchases of this book. For more information,
please contact Special Sales at 410-516-6936 or specialsales@press.jhu.edu.*

Johns Hopkins University Press uses environmentally friendly book materials,
including recycled text paper that is composed of at least 30 percent
post-consumer waste, whenever possible.

To all AIDS activists
—past, current, future—
and to Claire, Paul, and Ian,
for whose generation this book was written

In the world of Herodotus, the only real repository of memory is in the individual. In order to find out that which has been remembered, one must reach this person. If he lives far away, one has to go to him, to set out on a journey. And after finally encountering him, one must sit down and listen to what he has to say—to listen, remember, perhaps write it down. That is how reportage begins; of such circumstances it is born.

A journey, after all, neither begins in the instant we set out, nor ends when we have reached our doorstep once again. It starts much earlier and is really never over, because the film of memory continues running on inside of us long after we have come to a physical standstill.

—*Ryszard Kapuściński*, Travels with Herodotus

CONTENTS

An AIDS researcher gave a talk at my university in 2001 on a topic I cannot recall now. Toward the end of his presentation, he showed us a drawing that he said prevented him from sleeping: an inverted population pyramid that was a result of premature AIDS deaths among people aged 15–49 in one of the hardest hit African countries. The look of disbelief, outrage, guilt, and intellectual helplessness on his face—together with that drawing—left a strong impression on me as a young academic starting my career. I did not imagine that I would be driven by those same feelings in my own circuitous AIDS journey in the ensuing decade, culminating in this book.

I must first and foremost express my heartfelt gratitude to all 107 interviewees who not only gave me their time and insights but also were the very reason I ventured out to different corners of the world to collect their stories. They are mothers and fathers, sisters and brothers, spouses and partners living with HIV and AIDS; visionaries and pioneers; artists and accountants; self-taught lawyers and epidemiologists; lifelong volunteers and bureaucrats; case managers and program directors; peer educators and youth leaders; advocacy officers, press secretaries, consultants, regional coordinators, information managers—and many, many more heroes and underdogs of the epidemic. This research was generously supported by the Social Sciences and Humanities Research Council of Canada.

AIDS remains a sensitive issue in all of the places I visited. A wide network of friends and informants opened up doors and helped me to navigate the difficult sociopolitical terrain of AIDS in each country, region, and sector: Anya Sarang (Central Asia and Russia); Joan Hu, Chen Youding, Odilon Couzin, and Jia Ping (China); Nimit Tienudom, Pascal Tanguay, and Paul Causey (Thailand); Shailly Gupta, Roy Wadia, and Loon Gangte (India); Sergio Souza Costa, Veriano Terto, Renata Reis, and Felipe de Carvalho (Brazil); Apophia Agiresaasi (Uganda);

Sarah Zaidi, Solange Baptiste, Bukelwa Sontshatsha, and Lawrence Mbalati (South Africa); Nadia Rafif, Othoman Mellouk, and Abdo Abu El Ella (Egypt); and Nana Kuo and Kate Thompson (UNAIDS and its co-sponsors). My thanks to you all; you made this journey possible.

Never had I traveled so intensely, with my four-season carry-on luggage and reservation numbers for the next flights and hotels, swinging from city to city, hopping from continent to continent, all the while transcribing the quickly accumulating data whenever and wherever I could. In Moscow, Thibault Crosnier-Leconte, a French expatriate, generously shared his sauna-equipped apartment a stone's throw away from Red Square. In Mumbai, Nargis and Roy Wadia were ideal hosts who introduced the best of the Indian cultural world and the AIDS political world. In Kuala Lumpur, Mona Sheikh Mahmud provided an oasis as well as her deep insights on AIDS in Southeast Asia. Back home in Hong Kong, halfway through the year, I crashed at my sister's place to recuperate. Ian lent his room to his research-crazed aunt; Holly churned out lunch after lunch while I completed fifty interview transcriptions; and Winky, as usual, nourished me with exceeding generosity and fine dishes. No words can express my gratitude for their continuous love and support over the years. In Rio de Janeiro, Elsa Hubert, a French expatriate and a consummate samba artist, opened up her house and walked/danced us through Carnival and everything behind the scenes.

I am blessed with an extraordinary friend, mentor, reader, and editor, Peter Ninnes, who, once again, read through the entire manuscript and gave me the most useful critiques. He is the one to be blamed, or praised, for planting the Foucauldian seeds in me that finally sprouted here. I also want to thank the anonymous peer reviewer, who was generous with his time and critiques and without whose enthusiastic support this book would not have come to fruition in its current form. At Johns Hopkins University Press, Kelley Squazzo and her assistant, Katherine Curran, have been dream editors. They made academic publishing enjoyable, and for this I am tremendously grateful. I also want to thank Juliana McCarthy, the press's managing editor, and Merryl Sloane, an expert copyeditor, for their diligent support during the production process. Will Boase and IRIN generously allowed me to use their beautiful picture as the cover photo.

The contagion of travel is essentially incurable, as Ryszard Kapuściński would argue. I have been away from home for over a quarter of a century. I thank my Mom and Dad for their enduring love and support; they taught me grace and gave me the strength to pursue ideas that I think are worth fighting and living for. I also thank my sisters and brothers—Agnes, Joanne, Tak, Winky, Roy, and Kwai—for being there. The adage that love is not measured by distance but by the fondness of hearts is true. Pik ki, Jolie, Angela, and Kaija continue to provide me with their enduring friendship and companionship.

Pierre, my partner and honorary AIDS advisor, adjusted his own work schedule and came along with me throughout most of my sabbatical year. He introduced me to Central Asia, connected me to a host of experts in the field, helped with travel logistics, and lovingly took up the role of supportive spouse when I buried myself in writing. He was my travel companion, sounding board, reader, and critic all in one. This project would not have been completed without the constant flow of his love, champagne, dark chocolate, and gourmet French meals.

Claire and Paul endured being away from their mother for almost a full year when I was recording these stories. Only these two exceptional children could be so flexible and tolerant of their parent's out-of-the-ordinary schedule. I collected all sorts of mementos from faraway places to share my extraordinary year with them. Midway through, we arranged to meet in Siem Reap to visit the majestic Angkor Wat together. As this book goes to press, I am happy that Claire, almost fifteen, is an avid cellist and shows great interest in being a medical researcher, while Paul, turning twelve, continues his nonchalant existence as a sixth-grader and builds spectacular domino cascades. They continue to give me the greatest joy in my life.

3TC	lamivudine
ABC	Abstinence, Be Faithful, and Condomize
ABIA	Brazilian Interdisciplinary AIDS Association
ACTA	Anti-Counterfeiting Trade Agreement
ACT UP	AIDS Coalition to Unleash Power
AFRICASO	African Council of AIDS Service Organizations
AHRN	Asian Harm Reduction Network
AIDS	acquired immunodeficiency syndrome
ANPUD	Asian Network of People Who Use Drugs
APCOM	Asia Pacific Coalition on Male Sexual Health
API	active pharmaceutical ingredients
ARASA	AIDS and Rights Alliance for Southern Africa
ARV	antiretroviral therapy
ASO	AIDS service organization
AZT	zidovudine
BMS	Bristol-Myers Squibb
CAB	community advisory board
CARAM	Coordination of Action Research on AIDS and Mobility
CBO	community-based organization
CCM	Country Coordinating Mechanism
CDC	Centers for Disease Control
CEWG	Consultative Expert Working Group on Research and Development
CL	compulsory license or licensing
COBI	cobicistat
CSAT	Civil Society Action Team
CSO	civil society organization

ddI	didanosine
DFID	(UK) Department for International Development
DNP+	Delhi Network of Positive People
EAG	expert advisory group
EATG	European AIDS Treatment Group
ECOSOC	(UN) Economic and Social Council
EFV	efavirenz
EMA	European Medicines Agency
EVG	elvitegravir
FDA	Food and Drug Administration
FTA	free trade agreement
FTC	emtricitabine
GAVI	Global Alliance for Vaccines and Immunisation
GIPA	Greater Involvement of People Living with HIV and AIDS
GNP+	Global Network of People Living with HIV/AIDS
GONGO	government-organized nongovernmental organization
GPA	Global Programme on AIDS
GPO	Government Pharmaceutical Organization
GRID	gay-related immunodeficiency
GSK	GlaxoSmithKline
GTPI/REBRIP	Working Group on Intellectual Property of the Brazilian Network for the Integration of Peoples
GYCA	Global Youth Coalition on HIV/AIDS
HBV	hepatitis B virus
Health GAP	Health Global Access Project
IAS	International AIDS Society
ICASO	International Council of AIDS Service Organizations
ICW	International Community of Women Living with HIV/AIDS
IDU	injecting drug user
ILO	International Labour Organization
I-MAK	Initiative for Medicines, Access, and Knowledge
INGO	international nongovernmental organization
IP	intellectual property
ITPC	International Treatment Preparedness Coalition
KEI	Knowledge Ecology International
KETAM	Kenya Treatment Access Movement
LFA	local fund agents
LPV/r	lopinavir/ritonavir

MARA	most-at-risk adolescent
MARP	most-at-risk population
MARYP	most-at-risk young people
MPP	Medicines Patent Pool
MSF	Médecins Sans Frontières (Doctors Without Borders)
MSM	men who have sex with men
NAPWA	National Association of People with AIDS
NGO	nongovernmental organization
NIH	National Institutes of Health
NSWP	Global Network of Sex Work Projects
OSF	Open Society Foundations
OST	opioid substitution therapy
OVC	orphans and vulnerable children
PCB	(UNAIDS) Programme Coordinating Board
PEPFAR	President's Emergency Plan for AIDS Relief
PHM	People's Health Movement
PhRMA	Pharmaceutical Research and Manufacturers of America
PLHIV	people living with HIV
PLWHA	people living with HIV and AIDS
PMTCT	prevention of mother-to-child transmission
pppy	per patient per year
PR	principal recipient
PWA	people living with AIDS
RAL	raltegravir
RedTraSex	Red de Trabajadoras Sexuales de Latinoamérica y El Caribe (Latin American and Caribbean Women Sex Workers Network)
SOGI	Sexual Orientation and Gender Identity strategy
STD	sexually transmitted disease
SWEAT	Sex Workers Education and Advocacy Taskforce
TAC	Treatment Action Campaign
TAG	Treatment Action Group
TASO	The AIDS Support Organization
TDF	tenofovir
TNP+	Thai Network of People Living with HIV/AIDS
TRIPS	Trade-Related Aspects of Intellectual Property Rights
UGANET	Uganda Network on Law, Ethics, and HIV/AIDS
UNAIDS	Joint United Nations Programme on AIDS

UNDP	United Nations Development Programme
UNESCO	United Nations Educational, Scientific and Cultural Organization
UNFPA	United Nations Population Fund
UNGASS	United Nations General Assembly Special Session on HIV/AIDS
UNHCR	United Nations High Commissioner for Refugees
UNICEF	United Nations Children's Fund
UNODC	United Nations Office on Drugs and Crime
USAID	US Agency for International Development
USTR	US trade representative
VL	voluntary license
WAC	World AIDS Campaign
WHA	World Health Assembly
WHO	World Health Organization
WIPO	World Intellectual Property Organization
WTO	World Trade Organization

POLITICS IN THE CORRIDOR OF DYING

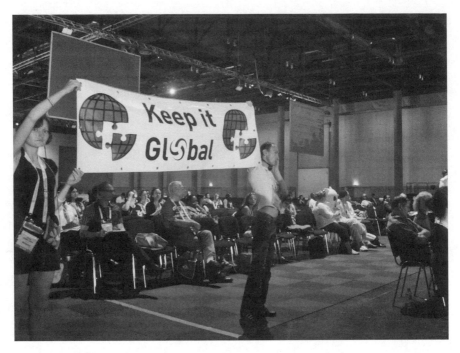

Keep It Global campaign, 2010 International AIDS Conference, Vienna
Photo by author

CHAPTER ONE

Introduction

AIDS Activism and Legitimation Crises

The theme of death became a nexus of protest.
—*Praxis of Necrorealism, an underground*
art movement in late socialist Russia

In October 1988, the AIDS Coalition to Unleash Power (ACT UP) organized a dramatic takeover of the US Food and Drug Administration (FDA) headquarters in Washington, DC, to protest against bureaucratic inaction and long delays in the clinical trials of AIDS drugs.[1] Armed with the slogan "A Drug Trial Is Health Care Too," activists demanded a complete restructuring of the FDA approval process, including more flexible entry so that more patients—in particular, women and people of color—could have access to experimental AIDS treatments through clinical trials.[2] Reported by the media as the largest demonstration since the Vietnam War era, the shutdown of the FDA was followed in September 1989 by another equally colorful action by ACT UP activists, who chained themselves to the banister of the VIP landing at the New York Stock Exchange. Unfurling a banner that declared "Sell Wellcome" and tossing out fake $100 bills imprinted with "We die while you play business," angry protestors accused "Big Pharma" of profiteering from the misery of dying patients by charging $10,000 per person per year for the only approved AIDS drug, AZT.[3] These two events marked the beginning of a long series of dramatic direct actions by ACT UP over the ensuing years, including at St. Patrick's Cathedral in New York, the National Institutes of Health (NIH) headquarters in Bethesda, Maryland, and the peripatetic sites of international AIDS conferences.

In December 1999, 100 members of the Thai Network of People Living with HIV/AIDS (TNP+) and Médecins Sans Frontières (MSF; Doctors Without Borders) set up a "Section 51 Community for ddI Development" three-day camp in front of the Thai Ministry of Public Health to demand the compulsory licensing of didanosine (ddI), the second AIDS drug to be approved after AZT and an important component in antiretroviral therapy (ARV). "Section 51" refers to a provision in the Trade-Related Aspects of Intellectual Property Rights (TRIPS) agreement that allows governments to require compulsory licensing to produce or import generic drugs. In Thailand, ddI sold for about 49 baht ($1.25) per tablet, putting the monthly cost of the two-drug cocktail at 8,000 baht ($205) at a time when the monthly minimum wage was 5,400 baht ($138).[4] One month prior to the sit-in, the Government Pharmaceutical Organization (GPO) in Thailand had submitted a request to the Department of Intellectual Property for a compulsory license to allow the local production of generic ddI to bring the price down to meet the needs of a million HIV-positive Thai patients.[5] In response, Bristol-Myers Squibb (BMS), the patent holder of ddI, threatened the Thai GPO with litigation, while the Pharmaceutical Research and Manufacturers of America asked the US trade representative (USTR) to put Thailand on the "Special 301" Priority Watch List of countries judged to have inadequate intellectual property laws and be subject to sanctions.[6] Activists from ACT UP, MSF, the Consumer Project on Technology, Public Citizen, and other nongovernmental organizations (NGOs) met with the USTR to request that the US government send a letter stating clearly that Thailand would not face pressure from the US government if it issued a compulsory license for ddI. Six months later, in May 2000, the AIDS Access Foundation and two AIDS patients filed a lawsuit against BMS, arguing that the drug was not a new invention and that it had already been widely available before the patent application was submitted in Thailand.[7] The 1999 sit-in was the first large-scale demonstration by HIV-positive Thais, who braved stigmatization to demand affordable treatment. It started a long chain of protests, lawsuits, and diplomatic pressure, which led to the subsequent compulsory licensing of efavirenz (EFV) in November 2006, which provoked more boycotts, court battles, and trade sanctions.

At the end of 2009, Russian activists from the International Treatment Preparedness Coalition (ITPC) gathered other NGOs to start a Keep It Global campaign to protest against new funding eligibility criteria that had been instituted by the Global Fund to Fight AIDS, Tuberculosis, and Malaria based on the World Bank's classification of economies and the World Health Organization's data on disease burden. The new criteria rendered most middle-income countries, including Russia, China, and the majority of Eastern Europe, Latin America, and the Middle East, ineligible. The ITPC campaign targeted the 2010 International AIDS Conference in Vienna, where activists from the Middle East, Latin America, and the Caribbean plastered a plenary session on the future of AIDS funding with Keep It Global placards and flyers. Outside the conference hall, several thousand activists marched to demand "Rights Here, Right Now."[8] Two years later at the 2012 International AIDS Conference in Washington, DC, AIDS activists disrupted the speech of the new general manager of the Global Fund, Gabriel Jaramillo, chanting "End AIDS, no caps on our lives" and carrying signs that read "GF Caps = Death."[9] Before the session ended, the regional coordinator of the Civil Society Action Team for the Middle East and North Africa Region, Nadia Rafif, who was the only civil society representative on the panel, invited the activists back onstage to demand that the panelists sign a pledge: "At the International AIDS Conference on 26th July . . . I will defend the demand-driven Global Fund, and oppose any measure that undermines scale-up, resource mobilization or universal access. In particular, I will oppose proposals to create ceilings or envelopes that cap countries' ambition when applying to the Global Fund." Gabriel Jaramillo, along with Mireille Guigaz, who was the French ambassador for the Fight against HIV and Communicable Diseases, and Rachel Ong, who was the communications focal point for the Communities Delegation on the Global Fund Board, all signed on the spot. Eric Goosby, the US AIDS ambassador, did not.[10]

What do these separate protest actions, spanning three decades and different continents, targeting the scientific establishment, pharmaceutical companies, and the global health governance structure, tell us about AIDS activism? Who are these activists? What claims do they make, and what strategies do they use? Above all, what role have they played in global AIDS governance, and what have been their limitations? Is AIDS activism an exception, or is it a case that teaches us important lessons about social movements and global governance?

Knowledge Makers and Breakers

> Science is nothing without the people. If people themselves cannot own science and translate science for their own health, their own rights, and their own citizenship, then science is meaningless. The law is nothing without the people.
> —*General Secretary, Treatment Action Campaign*[11]

The AIDS social movements that emerged in the 1980s in North America resembled the Necrorealist art movement in Russia in many ways, although on the surface they shared little in common. Using paintings, photographs, and installations, the Necrorealists experimented in novel ways to represent the living death that was everyday life in late socialist Russia. Autodidactic and operating with zero funding, the group started filming and screening in the underground as the only alternative to the official state cinema.[12] What subsequently emerged was a

Necrorealist aesthetics focusing on the exploration of the liminal state between life and death or, in the words of its leading exponent, Vladimir Kustov, the "corridor of dying." For the Necrorealists, "'death' quickly became not only something to be represented on film (both as an event and a condition) but a comprehensive, organizing metaphor for an entire approach to visual representation."[13]

Similarly, death became an instant nexus of protest for AIDS activists. Self-taught, they learned through the tropes of biomedicine, law, economics, and politics as the epidemic unfolded at an alarming speed. In the long corridor of dying—which passed through dilapidated scientific labs, drab government bureaus, the shiny boardrooms of pharmaceutical companies, the grey offices of myriad UN secretariats, and the hustle and bustle of clinics, NGO offices, and local communities—AIDS activists fought hard and made some significant gains. ACT UP protests led to an unprecedented acceleration of clinical trials from the usual seven- to ten-year period down to two or three years and to the expansion of both inclusion criteria and the number of patients eligible for experimental drugs. Above all, they forced scientists to reconceptualize clinical trials and to reassess their assumptions about "risk" in the middle of an epidemic. As one physician put it, "Scientists who run clinical trials are interested in maintaining scientific standards, in doing studies correctly so that they get solid, trustworthy results. People with life-threatening illnesses, on the other hand, are interested in using whatever knowledge is available to make the best treatment decisions they can."[14]

HIV-positive Thai activists, with support from doctors, lawyers, and international NGOs, including ACT UP, the Health Global Access Project (Health GAP), and Oxfam, successfully forced Bristol-Myers Squibb to reduce the price of ddI. International mobilization also led to the inclusion in 2001 of a public health clause in the TRIPS agreement of the World Trade Organization (WTO), which allows governments to issue compulsory licenses on patents for medicines and take other steps to protect public health. AIDS activists in Brazil, South Africa, and India followed the Thai example by organizing large-scale demonstrations, filing oppositions to patent applications, taking Pharma to court, and successfully lobbying their national governments for the compulsory licensing of antiretroviral drugs. In March 2012, China passed a new Compulsory Licensing Regulation that allows the local production of generic medicines in public health emergencies. In October of the same year, Indonesia initiated "the broadest single use of pharmaceutical patent licensing power by a country since the World Trade Organization 1995 Agreement on Trade-Related Aspects of Intellectual Property"[15] by issuing compulsory licenses for seven HIV and hepatitis B drug patents. A month later, Ecuador followed suit and issued its second compulsory license of the combination of abacavir and lamivudine, an important second-line treatment for AIDS. Meanwhile, activists led by the ITPC in Russia convinced the Global Fund Board to create a special targeted funding pool for the "most-at-risk populations" in countries that would no longer be eligible for funding. But activists have learned that the issue of funding is never just about money. It is also about global AIDS governance: who is in charge and how priorities are set. As the coordinator of the US Positive Women's Network, Naina Khanna, puts it, "If you are not at the table, you are on the menu."[16]

This book is a sociopolitical study of AIDS activism since the 1980s. Using a poststructuralist framework that questions the universal truth of metanarratives, I conceptualize AIDS as a series of legitimation crises, in which laypeople have challenged the rules of pure science,[17] the perfect market, and good governance through their own knowledge production. I argue that AIDS activists have played the role of "knowledge breakers"[18] by cracking open the doors of the citadels of science, market, and governance. They have created a new pathway to legitimacy based on credibility, democratic principles and processes, moral acceptability,[19] and human rights. But AIDS activists have done more than learn and appropriate the language of science to be on par with the experts and to keep them accountable, as Epstein argues.[20] They have injected new knowledges and alternative human rights frames into previously tight-knit scientific, market, and governance systems, forcing them to diversify and democratize. Not only are people living with HIV and AIDS (PLWHA) just as credible as the scientists; they have forced science to be open to nonscientific frames of reference based on human rights. They are now included in the design of clinical trials not only because their presence makes better science, but also because of the principle of Greater Involvement of People Living with HIV and AIDS (GIPA). Similarly, the WTO has heeded the public health concerns of the Global South not because it makes better trade, but because it was forced to recognize that intellectual property (IP) protection has negative impacts on access to essential medicines. Various global governance structures have been pushed open not because donors and governments were ready to share power, but because human rights norms have changed the face of business as usual.

To examine only biomedicine, the big pharmaceutical companies, and global governance, however, is to neglect the emergence of the AIDS community as a new regime of power. Along the way in the AIDS corridor, community-based organizations (CBOs) morphed into grantees, delegates, and partners, competing for turf, funding, leadership, and recognition. International AIDS NGOs expanded into multimillion-dollar businesses. AIDS activism has so profoundly changed in identity, focus, strategies, and governance since the heyday of ACT UP that it is important to unmask the power exercised in the name of the community and to see clearly the technologies of the self that activists use to regulate and normalize the AIDS "community expert." In sum, beyond the concrete gains of funding and treatment access, AIDS activism since the 1980s has exposed the fundamental legitimation crises of four contemporary regimes of power—scientific monopoly, market fundamentalism, statist governance, and community control—and transformed them according to new rules of legitimation based on human rights in addition to power.

AIDS research continues to be hampered by false dichotomies constructed by antiquated disciplinary walls and competing ideologies: science versus cultural studies; facts versus representation; political economics versus discourse; theory versus activism; abstinence versus safer sex; prevention versus treatment; horizontal (strengthening health systems) versus vertical (disease-specific funding) orientation; innovation versus access; East versus West; and North versus South. There is concern that engaging in cultural studies means sacrificing a vast body of epidemiological data. Or that focusing on activism is atheoretical.[21] In particular, researchers using a poststructuralist approach risk being charged with ignoring the material effects of power on PLWHA. While I was in the thick of my research, it became more and more clear that the best lens to investigate such a complex topic would be a broad conception of power that would allow me to examine where and how power exerts itself and where and how activism makes a difference.

Two contemporary theorists offer an expansive and mobile definition of power and counterpower that prove useful for a global analysis of AIDS activism. First, Foucault traces a genealogy of power behind the rise of the network of modern institutions. For him, "the notion of repression is quite inadequate for capturing what is precisely the productive aspect of power. In defining the effects of power as repression, one adopts a purely juridical conception of such power, one identifies power with a law which says no, power is taken above all as carrying the force of a prohibition. Now I believe this is a wholly negative, narrow, skeletal conception of power."[22] He argues that power is productive; it creates various knowledge or discursive regimes of power to normalize and control the modern subject.[23] Foucault asks, who has the power to speak? What stories are allowed to circulate? How do some knowledges become legitimated as Truths? Using his power-knowledge-subject nexus, he undertakes arguably the most ambitious and comprehensive study of modern institutions, including sexuality, the family, medicine, demography, law, the factory, pedagogy, the asylum, and the prison. In a groundbreaking study, he deconstructs the power of the modern state in regulating sexuality through a complex organization of four privileged objects of knowledge—the hysterical woman, the masturbating child, the Malthusian couple, and the perverse adult.[24] Given the diffused nature of power, he argues, "points of resistance are present everywhere in the power network. Hence there is no single locus of great Refusal, no soul of revolt, source of all rebellions, or pure law of the revolutionary. Instead there is a plurality of resistances, each of them a special case."[25]

Second, Castells focuses on the development of resistance culture and identity as "the process of construction of meaning" in his extensive study of social movement networks and globalization in the twenty-first century.[26] He argues, "If power is exercised by programming and switching networks, then counterpower, the deliberate attempt to change power relationships, is enacted by reprogramming networks around alternative interests and values, and/or disrupting the dominant switches while switching networks of resistance and social change."[27] Social movements throughout history, he claims, are "the producers of new values and goals around which the institutions of society are transformed to represent these values by creating new norms to organize social life. Social movements exercise counterpower by constructing themselves in the first place through a process of autonomous communication, free from the control of those holding institutional power."[28]

Despite their theoretical insistence on networks of power, however, postcolonial, feminist, and queer scholars are quick to reveal the racial, gendered, and sexual assumptions of these two abstract theories of power. Postcolonial scholar Stoler rightfully asks, "Why, for Foucault, [do] colonial bodies never figure as a possible site of the articulation of nineteenth century European sexuality? And given this omission, what are the consequences for his treatment of racism in the making of the European bourgeois self?"[29] Meanwhile, between the lines of Foucault's dense prose, feminists have discovered that what he describes as disciplinary surveillance techniques are gendered and that the resultant docile bodies are more often than not feminine. According to Bartky, such "self-surveillance is a form of obedience to patriarchy."[30] Queer theorists further argue that Foucault's "perverse adult" is widely imagined to be a homosexual. Hence, any study of modern sexuality that does not deconstruct the dual regimes of heterosexuality and homophobia is incomplete.[31] Ultimately, when we ask whom his discourse is about, we discover that Foucault's epistemological subject is a White, European, heterosexual, masculine body. The question then becomes: What would an "off center court"[32] rereading of the history of sexuality and of AIDS reveal?

A poststructuralist and postcolonial "off center court" approach to AIDS takes us back to the racialized sexualities and sexualized racial bodies in colonial Congo français. According to the French Canadian historian Jacques Pepin, AIDS began with the mass population movements inaugurated by the French colonial administration in order to construct the Congo-Océan railway in the 1920s. He explains: "The type of sex trade that existed during the colonial era corresponded to what is currently referred to as concomitant partnerships or semi-prostitution. . . . If that woman got infected with HIV-1, she could only transmit the virus to one of her other steady clients, who might eventually infect another free woman." AIDS spread as a result of colonial public health policies, civil war, and greed:

> For a long time, starting in the early 1930s, free women were forced to attend the Dispensaire Antivenerien in Leo-Est for regular STD [sexually transmitted disease] screening. Those with a positive syphilis serology . . . were treated with injectable drugs, most often administered IV. In 1953, more than 150,000 injections were administered just in this one institution, which treated up to 1,000 patients each day. Documentary evidence reveals that syringes and needles were not sterilised but only rinsed between patients, with the result that many cases of iatrogenic hepatitis B acquired in this STD clinic were recognized by a clinician at the main hospital of Leopoldville, even in a setting where only a small minority of adults was susceptible to infection with HBV [hepatitis B virus]. This situation created an extraordinary opportunity for the spread of HIV-1: the women infected iatrogenically were semi-prostitutes, who could in turn transmit the infection, now sexually, to some of their regular clients. And then a perfect storm developed.[33]

In particular, during the civil war in the 1960s, thousands of refugees poured from all parts of Congo into the capital; the spread of high-risk prostitution led to a generalized AIDS epidemic between 1970 and 1980. From Congo, HIV traveled to Rwanda and Burundi; to other countries in southern, western, and eastern Africa via different routes; and then to Haiti after the repatriation of 4,500 Haitian technical assistants who had been sent to Congo between 1960 and 1966 for postwar reconstruction.[34] Contrary to the common belief about the primary role of American gay tourists, the breeding ground for HIV in Haiti seemed to have been the Hemo-Caribbean plasmapheresis center, a lucrative business operated by Luckner Cambronne, the "vampire of the Caribbean," that was exporting up to 6,000 liters of plasma to the United States each month in 1972. The "plasma farming" center was eventually closed by President Jean-Claude Duvalier, but a "geography of blaming," which focused on all Haitians, could not be undone.[35]

By the time the first American cases were reported in the June 5, 1981, Morbidity and Mortality Weekly Report of the CDC, AIDS had already been raging in Africa and Haiti.

Location matters in the study of AIDS; where you stand in terms of geopolitics, global economics, gender, race, ethnicity, age, sexuality, indigeneity, disability, and migrant status determine your access to treatment. As I argue in the ensuing chapters, the major achievement of AIDS activists in the corridor of dying has been to infiltrate a vast network of localized epistemological centers of science (including the NIH, the FDA, and the International AIDS Conference), the market (patent laws and trade rules enshrined in the WTO and in bilateral and regional trade agreements), governance (the G8, WHO, the Joint United Nations Programme on AIDS, the Global Fund, the President's Emergency Plan for AIDS Relief, and the Bill and Melinda Gates Foundation), and community (large international, regional, and national NGO networks) with alternative knowledges based on human rights frames. Against science, gay activists and queer theorists have debunked the homophobic and heterosexist assumptions behind the classification of "risks" early in the AIDS epidemic.[36] As transmission routes changed and expanded, it did not take long for other most-at-risk populations (MARPs), including drug users, sex workers, transgender people, migrants and truckers, women, youth, children, and prisoners, to be assessed against the supposedly objective epidemiological yardstick of "risk." Against Pharma, AIDS activists have deconstructed an IP regime protected by the WTO that makes treatment inaccessible and have challenged the predominant market narrative in which your life depends on your location in the global political economy.[37] Against governance, NGOs and CBOs have criticized a state-based intergovernmental structure and have demanded their place in AIDS decision making. Against community, AIDS activists have confronted each other with questions about power and representation. In short, what AIDS activists have been fighting since the 1980s is an overlapping governing logic and the cultural hegemony of science, market, governance, and community.

Cultural theorists, including Patton, Treichler, Crimp, and Epstein, have blazed a trail in the study of representation and the signification of AIDS.[38] They show us how the dominant AIDS narratives exist as a "technology of social repression."[39] Further, a cultural turn in social movement studies and international law in the 1990s has given us new understandings about the dialectical relationship between social movement learning, meaning-making, and cultural production.[40] According to Conway, "[S]ocial movements produce knowledges through their everyday practices of survival, resistance, organizing and solidarity. . . . Pedagogy in this sense is a kind of cultural politics—a purposeful intervention in the shaping of knowledges and identities for a political project, and constitutive of a permanent process of ongoing cultural transformation."[41] The international legal scholar Rajagopal asks, how do social movements write resistance into international law? He posits that social movements, as cultural politics with struggles over meanings and values, pose radical theoretical and epistemological challenges to the liberal model of international law. By demanding the right to democratic governance—but without aspiring for state power as an end itself—social movements forward alternative understandings of rights, development, and modernity.[42] Medical anthropologists and activist scholars highlight the importance of a social inequality approach focusing on the history of structural violence, human rights, and citizenship. Farmer reminds us that "violence, poverty, and inequality are the fault lines along which HIV spreads" and that AIDS cannot be studied in isolation from the long history of structural violence of colonialism and economic exploitation.[43] He argues that poverty is the most daunting barrier to effective treatment and care and that AIDS "risks" are structured by economic and political forces.[44] In their study of a cholera outbreak in eastern Venezuela in 1992–1993, Briggs and Mantini-Briggs argue that access to treatment was based on medical profiling, separating the sanitary citizens from the unsanitary indigenous residents in the delta, and that the major limitation to prevention was the "austerity conditions imposed by international lenders, the World Bank, and the International Monetary Fund," which capped infrastructural investments in potable water, sewage disposal, and waste treatment.[45] Activist AIDS scholars remind us that being gay, injecting drugs, or engaging in sex work does not necessarily make us vulnerable to HIV; but being arbitrarily arrested and detained and being deprived economically, socially, medically, and politically do.[46]

In this book, I use a Foucauldian lens to conceptualize AIDS as legitimation crises of four contemporary systems of power—science, market, governance, and community—and I use a Castellian notion of counterpower to investigate how AIDS activists have produced alternative cultural meanings. What we find in the corridor of dying is not only scientific dominance, as Epstein argues, but also unfair trade rules in a neo-imperialist global political economy, an outdated Westphalian state structure in global governance that continues to marginalize the people most affected by AIDS, and an increasingly expert-dominated AIDS community that is not always accountable. The complex reality of AIDS forces us to look simultaneously at all of these angles where power exerts itself.

Necrotexts: Deconstruction and AIDS Activism

To deconstruct the opposition, first of all, would be to overturn the
hierarchy at a given moment.

—*Jacques Derrida, "Interview with*
Julia Kristeva"[47]

My encounter with AIDS activism began with MSF's Access to Essential Medicines campaign at the WTO ministerial meeting in Cancun in 2003. The community gathering outside the conference halls looked like a country fair except
for the heavy barricades that separated the hotel strip from the rest of town and
the serious demands for reparation for colonialism, debt relief, and trade justice.
MSF had the biggest installation, a five-meter-high platform from which succes-
sive activists, at one-minute intervals, dived to an inflatable mattress below while
trying to grab a white capsule, in vain. "Too Poor to Treat" was the slogan on the
banner dangling from the platform.

I had traveled to Cancun with a colleague in law to research the General Agreement on Trade in Services (GATS), which has had a huge impact on the deregula-
tion of education and cultural industries. My colleague had just finished writing a
book on offshore call centers in India, while I was working on the global justice
movement. I knew nothing about the IP controversy in AIDS treatment, which
was already raging in Thailand, South Africa, Brazil, and India. I too had uncon-
sciously relegated concerns about TRIPS to lawyers and legal researchers. It was
my colleague who opened the AIDS Pandora's box for me: "Intellectual property
does not belong to the WTO. TRIPS should not have existed in the first place."

This serendipitous moment turned into a decade-long journey that included
an unforgettable encounter in 2004 with Paul Farmer in his public health seminar at Harvard University—where he debunked the treatment-versus-prevention
myth—and his awe-inspiring organization, Partners in Health. An intellectual
leap of faith took me to the International Congress on AIDS in Asia and the Pacific in Kobe in 2005; to the WTO ministerial meeting in my native city, Hong
Kong, in that same year; to the International AIDS Conference in Mexico in 2008
and Vienna in 2010; and to countless workshops, teach-ins, and events on AIDS.

Between December 2010 and March 2013, in noisy cafés or at their homes, I
met with AIDS activists in their varying capacities as founders, executive directors, general secretaries, board members, advocacy officers, program managers,
finance staff, regional coordinators, team leaders, communications assistants, and

focal points. In the opulent luxury of the Oberoi hotel in New Delhi, over chai and pakoras, I met with the secretary-general of the Indian Pharmaceutical Alliance to talk about the future of treatment access, before flying to Mumbai to meet with one of the true heroes of the epidemic, Yusuf Hamied, the CEO of Cipla, who slashed ARV prices from $12,000 per patient per year (pppy) to $300 pppy in 2001, turning the treatment revolution from a dream to reality.

I continued on, from AIDS service organizations (ASOs) in Uganda to business coalitions in Russia, passing through an Indian hospital where a doctor was examining an AIDS patient with a CD4 count of four. The hot streets of Rio de Janeiro were plastered with safer sex messages during Carnival. In beautiful St. Petersburg, a young HIV-positive mother showed me a box of medication that she was sending to her friend as part of the vast underground network of the patient control movement, because either the drugs from the local AIDS center were expired or they were absent. In sleepy Dushanbe, I chatted with four HIV-positive women who were under the care of an activist Muslim doctor. In Beijing, the national project director of MSF showed me on his calculator the amount of money the Chinese government would save if it issued a compulsory license for tenofovir, an important first-line drug for both AIDS and hepatitis B treatment: US$5 million a year, two-thirds of the current price tag, for AIDS patients alone. I retrieved my long-forgotten Mandarin ("How do you say 'stigma' again in Chinese?") to speak with an AIDS activist who had been tortured and imprisoned for his work in Henan. We met in the comfortably neutral space of a McDonald's in downtown Beijing before I braved the brand-new bullet train to Shanghai to talk to the flamboyant male chief of probably the largest sex worker advocacy network in the world, in the equally anonymous environment of a Starbucks.

In the security of a hotel room in downtown Bangkok, three veteran Asian drug user activists deconstructed for me the hypocrisy of global drug conventions. In Khayelitsha, a poor township outside Cape Town, where MSF teamed up with the local health department to roll out ARV treatment in 2000, the young HIV-positive general secretary of the Treatment Action Campaign was living proof of MSF's uncompromising motto: treatment scale-up is possible even in resource-poor settings. On the day of the verdict in the trial of Hosni Mubarak, Egyptian AIDS activists took me to the center of their revolution, Tahrir Square, and told me that the fight for treatment also had been part of their revolution. In Tel Aviv, my interview was interrupted when the young executive director of the Israel AIDS Task Force had to step out to communicate with an elderly woman about her HIV test results. Whether in China, India, Brazil, South Africa, Uganda, or

Canada, I met with more lawyers than doctors, and they opened up cans of AIDS-related legal worms.

By June 2012, my children were reminding me that my sabbatical was running out, but the UN division of labor on AIDS meant that Geneva and New York were both *passages obligés*. The Global Fund was having its own revolution from within after the contentious High-Level Independent Review Panel report was published in September 2011 in which wholesale changes were proposed. All of the contacts I had cultivated over the years were "restructured" out; my only consolation was that former staff actually had more freedom to speak. I could not interview people from UNAIDS without also crossing the street to the WHO, given, or despite, the age-old animosities between them. And there were the UN Development Programme (UNDP) and the UN Population Fund (UNFPA), both claiming to be in charge of MSM (men who have sex with men) and other gender-related HIV issues; the International Labour Organization (ILO) because it too was in the division-of-labor chart; UNITAID because I had contributed to it directly through the airline tax; and the Medicines Patent Pool, which has caused so much bad feeling among AIDS activists. And I could not study AIDS without looking at its dwarfed twin sisters: malaria and tuberculosis. Is AIDS activism a stand-alone case in global health governance? Or can we draw lessons to apply to other diseases? By the time my passport pages were filled to the last corner, I had collected more than a hundred stories in eighteen countries across seven regions: Africa (South Africa, Kenya, Uganda); Asia (China, India, Thailand, Malaysia); Central Europe and Asia (Russia, Kyrgyzstan, Tajikistan); the Middle East (Egypt, Israel); Latin America (Brazil, Argentina); North America (United States, Canada); and Europe (Switzerland, Belgium).

I draw on earlier analyses of AIDS service organizations and NGOs,[48] but choose to focus on advocacy networks in part to reflect the shift to treatment-focused activism after 1996, when antiretroviral therapy became available. In order to make a historical comparison of focus, strategies, and governance structures, I sampled organizations and movements from each of the past three decades. I grouped the nongovernmental AIDS organizations, networks, coalitions, and partnerships into six overlapping categories: (1) global, national, and local HIV-positive networks, along with patient-control movements; (2) issue-focused groups (e.g., men who have sex with men; injecting drug use; commercial sex work; gender and prevention of mother-to-child transmission; migration; children affected by AIDS; youth; transgender people) and one cross-issue coalition; (3) treatment access, literacy, and advocacy networks; (4) medical and legal networks; (5) AIDS prevention and treatment research groups; and (6) others, including AIDS service organizations, watchdogs, information clearinghouses, AIDS and human rights education groups, and health networks and movements (table 1; for a full list of interviewees, see the appendix).

The first decade of AIDS activism, the 1980s, saw the founding of organizations that would become household names, like ACT UP and the Lawyers Collective, and the emergence of the first Global Network of People Living with HIV/ AIDS (GNP+). This period was marked by pioneering ASOs and CBOs in North America and Europe that focused primarily on service provision and prevention education. There were also ASOs in other countries, such as The AIDS Support Organization (TASO) in Uganda, the Israel AIDS Task Force, the Jerusalem AIDS Project, and the Freedom Project in Egypt, and a few exceptional advocacy groups, such as the Brazilian Interdisciplinary AIDS Association (ABIA).

The second period, the 1990s, was characterized by the rise of professional legal, medical, and AIDS research networks first in North America and Europe and then elsewhere; the growth of global and national networks of people living with HIV/AIDS; the rapid expansion of local and national NGOs across Asia, Latin America, Africa, and the Middle East; pioneering treatment advocacy groups post-1996; and the emergence of regional networks of affected populations.

The last period I cover in this book, the 2000s, saw the increasing sophistication of the AIDS movement in a well-funded environment marked by more treatment advocacy and IP-focused networks; a stronger emphasis on human rights; new networks concerned about the "late" issues, including mother-to-child transmission, youth and children affected by AIDS, and drug policy; the proliferation of CBOs and NGOs in low- and middle-income countries supported by the Global Fund, PEPFAR, Open Society Foundations, and UNAIDS; and the appearance of watchdog NGOs.

Given the contention over representation, I included various networks of people living with HIV and AIDS, significant issue areas and populations, and geographical areas outside the familiar contours of North America and Europe as best I could. I was less concerned about the disease burden per se in a particular country or region than I was about the advocacy issues taken up by activists. Hence, I chose groups that dealt with stigmatization and human rights in the Middle East and with access to treatment and the criminalization of HIV transmission in Africa. My overall focus in this book on treatment advocacy rather than prevention reflects to a large extent the bias in AIDS activism at large.

The interview data are supplemented with secondary materials, including publications by all the co-sponsors of UNAIDS, by PEPFAR, and by the foundations

TABLE 1
AIDS Advocacy Groups and Organizations Interviewed

Year	Nongovernmental Groups	Intergovernmental Organizations and Foundations
1985	Israel AIDS Task Force	
1986	ABIA	
	GNP+	
1987	ACT UP	
	TASO	
	Jerusalem AIDS Project	
1989	Freedom Project, Egypt	
1991	AIDS Access Foundation, Thailand	
1992	Canadian HIV/AIDS Legal Network	
	Egyptian AIDS Society	
	EATG	
	ICW	
	National Community of Women Living with HIV/AIDS in Uganda	
	TAG	
1994	Asia Pacific Network of Sex Workers	
1995	UGANET	Open Society Foundations, International Harm Reduction Development Program
1996	SWEAT	UNAIDS
1997	CARAM	
	RedTraSex	
1998	TAC	
	Global Campaign for Microbicides	
	Health and Development Network	
	Lawyers Collective, HIV/AIDS Unit	
1999	Chi Heng Foundation	Roll Back Malaria Partnership
	Health GAP	
	MSF Access Campaign	
	TNP+	
	AHRN	
2000	Al Shehab Foundation, Egypt	
	DNP+	
	PHM	
2001	Global Business Coalition for Health	ILO, Programme on HIV/AIDS and the World of Work
	Health Rights Action Group, Uganda	
	M2M	Stop TB Partnership
		WHO, HIV/AIDS Department
2002	ARASA	Global Fund
	Egyptian Initiative for Personal Rights	
	KETAM	
	7 Sisters	
2003	Action Group on Health, Human Rights, and HIV/AIDS, Uganda	Avahan, Gates Foundation
	Chain, China	
	ITPC	
	NEPHAK	
	GTPI/REBRIP	

(*continued*)

TABLE 1 *(continued)*

Year	Nongovernmental Groups	Intergovernmental Organizations and Foundations
2004	GYCA	
	Russian Harm Reduction Network	
	WAC	
2005	AIDS Accountability International	
	Coalition for Children Affected by AIDS	
2006	Center on Mental Health and HIV/AIDS, Tajikistan	Global Health Workforce Alliance
	KEI	UNITAID
2007	APCOM	
	Astra Women's Foundation, Russia	
	Access to Medicines Research Group, China	
	Global Fund Watch, China	
	International Drug Policy Consortium	
	Shanghai AIDS Prevention Center	
	Friends of Life, Egypt	
	Andrey Rylkov Foundation, Russia	
2008	Asia-Pacific Transgender Network	
2009	China Sex Worker Organization Network Forum	
	Dongzhen Center for Human Rights Education and Action	
	Tamkin Project	
	ANPUD	
2010	Patient-Control Movement, Russia	Medicines Patent Pool
	Youth Lead	
	Malaysian Network of People Who Use Drugs	
2011	Tajik Network of Women Living with HIV/AIDS	

and NGOs whose staff members I interviewed for this research. I have used the methodologies of deconstruction and discourse analysis. Deconstruction requires the researcher to pay attention to the hidden hierarchy in a text (broadly defined to include any discourse, policy, law, or agreement), to how different texts are related to each other, and to how normality is constructed.[49] In discourse analysis, the researcher traces how certain narratives become dominant and investigates the techniques of power behind the emergence of a particular regime.[50] Using deconstruction and discourse analysis, I cross-read WHO's technical guidelines and queer theory; compared the bland UNAIDS epidemiological data to colorful activist tales; analyzed dense legal depositions and even denser patent rules; labored through the agreement between the Medicines Patent Pool and Gilead with the help of the *Intellectual Property Handbook* published by the World Intellectual Property Organization (WIPO) and the equally authoritative *Untangling the Web of Antiretroviral Price Reductions* published by the MSF; and studied the threatening website of the USTR next to the more relaxing Brazilian posters of safer sex. Despite the grim statistics, AIDS is a field filled with promising slogans: universal access, Treatment 2.0, 15×15, the Millennium Development Goals, Countdown to Zero, Born HIV-Free, and AIDS-Free Generation. Declarations, agreements, plans for action, frameworks, agendas, memorandums of understanding, consultations, meeting summaries, time-bound targets, goals, indexes, (no) progress reports, and reviews—internal, external, independent, and not-so-independent—overflowed from my bedroom into the bathroom. Next to these were cartons of scientific abstracts, NGO shadow reports, press releases, presentations, submissions to the special rapporteur on the right to health, investigative research papers, annual reports, governance reviews, manuals, toolkits, flyers, booklets, and publications of all sizes. I also explored online discussions on listservs, blogs, and the websites of advocacy networks and international organizations. And I learned about ARV drugs (3TC, ABC, ATV, d4T, ddI, DRV, EFV, FPV, FTC, IDV, LPV/r, MVC, NFV, NVP, RAL, RTV, SQV, TPV, and, very important, TDF) and their combinations (ABC/3TC, 3TC/d4T, 3TC/d4T/NVP, 3TC/d4T+EFV, TDF/FTC, TDF/FTC/EFV). I slotted these voluminous AIDS materials and my 1,030 pages of transcribed interview data into five compartments: the ecology of AIDS activism: its emergence, activities, strategies, organizations, governance, and evaluation; stigmatization, discrimination, and human rights; access to treatment; global health governance; and representation, collaboration, and competition in the AIDS social movement.

I see AIDS activism as an encompassing concept that includes advocacy—the conscious attempt to achieve a political aim— by a wide range of actors in CBOs, NGOs, nonprofit organizations, civil society organizations (CSOs), nongovernmental networks, coalitions, movements, and partnerships. As soon as I started fieldwork in Central Asia and Russia, I learned to discard the false dichotomy between service and advocacy. The reality is that chronically resource-starved community-based groups have to fulfill both functions on the ground. "If you do not know, how do you advocate?" the president of the Delhi Network of Positive People reminded me.[51] The executive director of the Israel AIDS Task Force, a pioneering ASO founded in 1985 by a US-trained Israeli psychologist, said it well:

> We are somewhere in the middle between the extreme of a service NGO and the other extreme of an advocacy group. We see ourselves as a leader in social change, but on the way to social change, we cannot ignore supplying the needs. Sometimes supplying the needs is the strategy to change when nobody even recognizes the needs. Social change is about targeting a vacuum [in] advocacy, but there are many

tory, every seat gained in Geneva, every extra dollar raised for service or treatment, and every new drug approved and made accessible, what does AIDS activism mean, and what is its legacy? Despite important national and regional case studies, until now there has not been any book-length examination of the global impact of AIDS activism.[62] It is one thing to study Brazil, China, South Africa, Uganda, or Kenya in their individual historical, sociopolitical, and cultural contexts; and it is another to see how activists from those countries and others relate to each other individually, organizationally, ideologically, and strategically in an epidemic that has forced them to respond together. It is with this aim in mind that this book was written.

My focus on four regimes of power—science, market, governance, and community—is deliberate. This is where AIDS advocacy work has been most important, I argue. Other studies have rightfully focused on media, religion, or state (in)action.[63] By focusing on scientific disputes, trade wars, political turf battles, and community infighting, my objective in this book is not only to document AIDS activism in order to give credit where credit is due, but also to critically examine the roles and pitfalls of community mobilization in complex scientific, legal, economic, political, and social environments and, in turn, the effects of activism on democracy, citizenship, and global justice.

The rest of this book is structured in five chapters. Each chapter focuses on one main sector and follows a rough nexus of power-knowledge-subject-resistance in which I ask, "What is said and done in HIV and AIDS and with what effects in the name of science, market, governance, and community?"

Chapter 2 looks at the scientific construction of AIDS risks and the regulation of ten stereotyped "at-risk" bodies: the promiscuous gay, criminal junkie, dirty whore, innocent mother and child, AIDS orphan, hormone-charged youth, *Homo sexualis africanus*, suspicious foreigner or migrant, transgender pervert, and dangerous outlaw. I use the recent wave of HIV/AIDS laws as a case study to look at how the scientific construction of AIDS risks plays out in courtrooms. I end by examining activists' mobilization against science through the application of a human rights framework.

Chapter 3 first discusses the myriad technologies of power employed by Pharma to enforce an intellectual property regime worldwide. Through stories of the compulsory licensing of four ARV drugs—efavirenz (EFV), tenofovir (TDF), lamivudine (3TC), and lopinavir/ritonavir (LPV/r)—in Brazil, Thailand, South Africa, China, and India, I analyze activist mobilization against Pharma and the intellectual propertization of life. I take the 2011 Medicines Patent Pool's agreements with Gilead as an example of activists' engagement with Pharma and examine the ideological, class, and tactical divisions among activists over the agreements.

Chapter 4 begins with a history of multilateral cooperation on AIDS, the politics of the division of labor among UN agencies, and the emergence of an AIDS-funding oligopoly involving PEPFAR, the Gates Foundation, and the Global Fund. I then examine AIDS activists' battles for inclusion in global AIDS governance based on the principle of GIPA. I end by discussing activists' reform proposals in five areas of the global AIDS architecture: donor coordination; governance harmonization; health system integration and national leadership; IP and the private sector; and civil society engagement and capacity building.

Chapter 5 looks at the organization, politics, and role of the AIDS community itself. I begin with snapshots of different kinds of community organizations, including their governance and funding, and a typology of four different advocacy models. I analyze power struggles in the AIDS community through the framework of external and internal techniques of power. I end by evaluating the roles and limits of AIDS activism in community organizing and empowerment, voice and advocacy, and knowledge building.

Finally, I conclude by summarizing the key activist interventions in each of the four regimes of power and by proposing policy recommendations for each: diversifying global governance, operationalizing human rights standards, moving beyond the existing IP regime, and decolonizing community development.

Welcome to the corridor of dying . . .

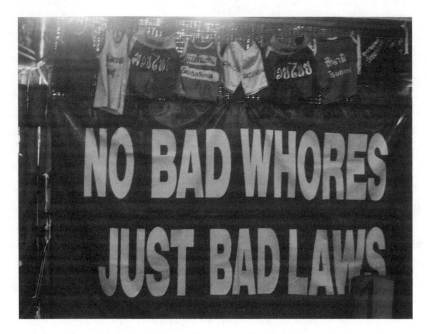

Photo by author

CHAPTER TWO

Against Science and the Stigmatization
of the "At-Risk" Body

In all infectious disease control programmes, the first step is to
identify high-risk groups and focus efforts on these.
    —*Jacques Pepin*, The Origins of AIDS

Whose body stands as the model of social order, and whose social
order is anatomized as a normal body?
    —*Catherine Waldby*, AIDS and the Body Politic

Science does not exist in a vacuum. It exists in a world of money
and votes, a world of media enquiry and lobbyists, of pharmaceutical manufacturing and environmental activism and religions and
political ideologies and all other complexities of human life.
    —*Elizabeth Pisani*, The Wisdom of Whores

Every disease has its own metaphors, which "giv[e] the thing a name that belongs
to something else": the sinful leper, the consumed tubercular patient, and the battle against cancer.[1] Few diseases have been given as many names and provoked
as wild imaginings as AIDS: anal pleasures with 10,000 partners; dirty needles
in dark alleys; sexual initiation with whores; mothers killing their infants by transmitting HIV; wiped-out African villages and AIDS orphans; the black death; continents in peril; testosterone-filled youth; the AIDS-infected foreigner or migrant;
men dressed as women who have sex with men and women; and HIV-positive
prisoners released back to their communities.[2] Scientific researchers, epidemiologists, physicians, public health officials, bioethicists, anthropologists, and economists measure, classify, and define AIDS risks. Journalists, religious zealots,
vote-conscious politicians, and educators instrumentalize and popularize their
own theories of risk. Parliamentarians debate and pass laws to codify scientific and not-so-scientific claims of AIDS risks, which are enforced by police.

International organizations, with the help of highly paid consultants, provide regular updates and technical guidelines on "minimum," "standard," and "extended" packages of interventions according to a detailed taxonomy of HIV risk. "Know your epidemic," they say.

What has arisen since the 1980s is a vast network of institutions that continually speak about the at-risk AIDS body in the name of science. By singling out already marginalized and stigmatized sections of society—variously called "vulnerable populations," "subpopulations," "at-risk groups," "most-at-risk populations (MARPs)," "key populations," and "key affected populations"—this type of risk taxonomy replaces "a scientific problem (what factors are causally responsible?) with a moral and political one (who is accountable?)"[3] that legitimizes the control of the AIDS body.

In this chapter, I discuss the ten most common stereotypes about objects of knowledge in AIDS: the promiscuous gay, criminal junkie, dirty whore, innocent mother and child, AIDS orphan, hormone-charged youth, *Homo sexualis africanus*, suspicious foreigner or migrant, transgender pervert, and dangerous outlaw. I then focus on recent HIV-criminalizing laws as the legal sanction of the scientific regulation of the at-risk body. Finally, I examine how activists have been pushing to move beyond an epidemiological model of AIDS and toward a human rights framework in five nonnegotiable areas: nondiscrimination and decriminalization, treatment, funding, GIPA, and rights-based shared governance.

The Panopticon of Risk and a Taxonomy of Blame

We know what works and what needs to be done.
—*UNICEF, UNAIDS, and WHO,* Young People
and HIV/AIDS: Opportunity in Crisis[4]

Applying classical epidemiological methods to HIV/AIDS ensures, even predetermines, that "risk" will be defined in terms of individual determinants and individual behavior. Epidemiology has thus far failed to develop models and methods suited to discovering the societal dimensions that strongly influence and constrain individual behavior.
—*Jonathan Mann, "Human Rights and AIDS:*
The Future of the Epidemic"[5]

Promiscuous Gay

As soon as the term GRID (gay-related immunodeficiency) started circulating un-officially among CDC scientists after the June 1981 Morbidity and Mortality Weekly Report, the search began to ascertain the connections between gay sex and Kaposi's sarcoma and *Pneumocystis carinii*.[6] Medical researchers immediately descended on examining rooms in New York to gather data:

> During grueling sixteen-hour days, CDC doctors interviewed 75 percent of the living patients in the United States. The task force had spent the summer piecing together the form, sixty-two questions on twenty-two pages, that covered every conceivable behavior and exposure that might be involved in the epidemic, right down to what plants, pets, cleaning compounds, and photo chemicals were around the house. In an effort to cross-match for every aspect of the cases' lives, four controls were selected for each patient. One was a heterosexual of comparable age and background; another was a gay man from a private doctor's practice; and still another gay control would be a patient's friend with whom he had not had sex. This last category proved the most difficult to fill since it seemed that just about every friend of a patient was also somebody the patient had once made love to. . . . The CDC staffers could tell gay from straight controls by the way they reacted to the questions about every aspect of their intimate sexual lives. Heterosexuals seemed offended at queries about the[ir] preferred sexual techniques, while gay interviewees chatted endlessly about them. One gay man flipped out a pocket calculator to estimate his lifetime sexual contacts.[7]

A lifestyle hypothesis of AIDS was soon expounded despite confirmed cases among injecting drug users (IDUs), hemophiliacs, pregnant women, and Haitians: "Although the cause of the acquired immune deficiency syndrome (AIDS) in homosexual men remains unknown, the study presented here and in the companion paper has identified a distinctive lifestyle as an important risk factor."[8] In an interview by the *Journal of the American Medical Women's Association* in 1982, Joyce Wallace, an AIDS researcher, said, "During the last year we have become aware of an unusual number of infections and cancers in formerly healthy homosexuals who admit to a promiscuous lifestyle."[9] Selma Dritz of the San Francisco Department of Public Health began to look into the closure of public bathhouses, a symbol of gay liberation that overnight became the epicenter of the storm.[10]

Even after a viral theory was confirmed in 1983, the image of the "promiscuous gay" remained the dominant representation through which Americans came to know about AIDS. Patton calls this the "queer paradigm": the equation of AIDS with homosexual perversion regardless of the route of transmission. The genie was already out of the bottle. "Scientific" knowledge of AIDS gave ammunition to conservative doctors and politicians in the Reagan administration, who rationalized their own "God's curse" theory: "AIDS is God's way of weeding his garden."[11] The Reverend Greg Dixon said, "If homosexuals are not stopped, they will in time infect the entire nation, and America will be destroyed."[12] Homophobia drove AIDS hysteria in the national calls for compulsory antibody testing, the tattooing of infected people, and quarantining.

Criminal Junkie

Like it encouraged homophobia, AIDS "gave new fuel to old prejudices"[13] against drug users. Narcologists and psychiatrists define addiction as a disorder in the *Diagnostic and Statistical Manual of Mental Disorders*. Academic experts tell us that drug addicts are compulsive, suffer from other psychiatric illnesses, and chronically relapse.[14] Drug rehabilitation professionals advise a treatment matrix consisting of relationship therapy, cognitive restructuring, aversive conditioning, and sensitivity training.[15] Criminologists develop profiles of drug addicts' behavior, which are fodder for law enforcement officers to carry out their duty.

At the international level, drug regulation had received early attention. In May 1931, a conference was held in Geneva to discuss the banning of opium, coca, and derivatives such as morphine, heroin, and cocaine, which led to the signing of the Convention for Limiting the Manufacture and Regulating the Distribution of Narcotic Drugs two months later. This and other early treaties were subsequently replaced by the comprehensive 1961 Single Convention on Narcotic Drugs: "all nonmedical use of narcotic drugs, such as opium smoking, opium eating, consumption of cannabis (hashish, marijuana) and chewing of coca leaves, will be outlawed everywhere . . . a goal which workers in international narcotics control all over the world have striven to achieve for half a century."[16] These treaties were further supplemented by the 1971 Convention on Psychotropic Substances, which prohibited newly discovered drugs, such as amphetamines, barbiturates, benzodiazepines, and psychedelics. When AIDS exploded among injecting drug users, their bodies instantly became a site of competing ideologies and bureaucratic control between the Commission on Narcotic Drugs (CND) and the UN Office on Drugs and Crime (UNODC), on the one hand, and UNAIDS and WHO, on the other. The junkie is at once a criminal to be eradicated and an at-risk person to be controlled, depending on which side of the UN corridor you stand, and in both instances, IDUs are under the heavy surveillance of "zero tolerance" or "comprehensive intervention." The effect of the "sphinxization" of drug users—with a criminalized head and a medicalized body—is best described by Bijay Pandey, the leader of a Nepalese IDU organization: "[T]he Ministry of Health distributes needles and syringes but then the Ministry of Home Affairs arrests us for carrying them."[17] Most countries today continue to rely on a "war on drugs" approach that criminalizes drug possession and use, and thirty-two retain the death penalty for drug offenses.[18]

Dirty Whore

So much has been said and done about the "courtesan," "call girl," "slut," "whore," "free woman," "dangerous woman," and "sexually available woman" in modern science. She is the preferred Petri dish for biomedical scientists to study sexually transmitted diseases (STDs) and the subject of perennial fascination for anthropologists, demographers, sexologists, sociologists, feminists, and criminologists. Outside the ivory tower, she is the targeted site of reforms by vote-hungry politicians; the object of crusades by social conservatives, religious zealots, antitraffickers, and abolitionists; and the prey of police harassment, blackmail, and brutality.[19]

When AIDS arose, narratives about this "extremely efficient" "vector" of transmission spread as quickly as the virus itself. Some scientists claimed that prostitutes in Central Africa around 1960 were the "culprits" behind the heterosexual transmission of AIDS, which produced a global epidemic: "As documented by several observers, high-risk prostitution appeared, with sex workers providing sexual service to a few men every day, potentially more than 1,000 per year, in downmarket brothels which were little more than glorified shacks."[20] Between 1970 and 1980, just before CDC scientists reported the first cases in the United States, the prevalence of HIV infection in mothers in Kinshasa shot from 0.25% to 3%. Prostitutes had infected men, who then infected their wives; the rest is AIDS history. The acknowledgment of heterosexually transmitted AIDS was a watershed moment; politicians, the media, public health officials, teachers, and the general public were being told: it could be any of us. In Thailand, although junkies had been dying by the scores in the late 1980s and early 1990s, it was heterosexual AIDS fueled by prostitution that spurred the government into action. "We'd seen HIV storm through the sex trade in Thailand in the first few years of the 1990s," an epidemiologist writes, "but the government there had acted quickly and comprehensively to bring things under control."[21]

The highly sexed bodies of prostitutes were also the preferred laboratories for Western scientists. In 2004, as part of a large NIH-funded international study on 2,000 sex workers in Cambodia, Ghana, Cameroon, Nigeria, and Malawi, researchers from the University of California in San Francisco and the University of New South Wales were ready to fly into Phnom Penh to meet with the Cambodian Ministry of Health. They wanted to test the effects of an ARV, Viread (tenofovir), on 960 sex workers in Cambodia, but the trial never went ahead. Cambodian sex workers, who grew up with the fear of Agent Orange, walked out when their request for health insurance for thirty years to treat possible side effects caused by the drug was turned down.[22]

AIDS epidemiology has exposed many inconvenient truths, one of which is that buying sex is a lot more normal than most people would like to admit. Nice married men looking for an outlet for forbidden desires, business travelers flush with company money, young boys looking for their first initiation, aroused police officers, lonesome migrants, and troops stationed far from home—all make good use of cheap sexual labor. Referring to Thailand, an AIDS medical researcher writes, "Once HIV entered this vulnerable population, however, it became clear that the majority of Thai men, married and unmarried, patronized sex workers, and the sexual behaviors of these men became an issue for all Thais . . . to see beyond their fixed assumptions of what constitutes 'normal' sexual behavior."[23] Prostitution helps to preserve the family institution and social order.

Moral crusaders, however, managed to legitimize their "sinful victim" narrative through international development aid. In February 2002 in his National Security Presidential Directive, President George W. Bush explains his belief: "The United States opposes prostitution and any related activities, including pimping, pandering, and/or maintaining brothels as contributing to the phenomenon of trafficking in persons. These activities are inherently harmful and dehumanizing."[24] The US Agency for International Development (USAID), the NIH, and the CDC became anti-vice police after the infamous anti-prostitution pledge in the President's Emergency Plan for AIDS Relief (PEPFAR) was passed in 2003, which prohibited funding to any organizations, inside and outside the United States, involved in prostitution or sex trafficking. In one of the greatest tales of AIDS hypocrisy, Bush's first global AIDS coordinator and anti-prostitution czar, Randall Tobias, resigned suddenly in 2007 over a link with a "DC madam." His name was on a list of clients given to a US news outlet, ABC, by the owner of the escort company in the capital city. Tobias insisted that there was "no sex" during the women's visits to his condo.[25]

Innocent Mother and Child

The narratives flooding the sex worker body stand in great contrast to those surrounding the expectant HIV-positive woman. If the whore is surrounded by the competing discourses of epidemiological urgency, clinical interest, social functionality, and moral sanction, there is only one thing to say about the innocent mother: we must save her. For once, moral conservatives seemed to agree with scientists. The high prevalence rates among mothers in antenatal clinics—the proxy measure used by epidemiologists to understand the general epidemic—rang an alarm bell for everyone. This was about saving not the promiscuous gay, the criminal junkie, or the dirty whore, but the "womb of the nation." After ACTG 076 (a phase III, randomized, double-blind, placebo-controlled clinical trial) confirmed in 1996 that oral AZT for the mother in the last three months of pregnancy, intravenous AZT during labor, and oral AZT for the infant for six weeks after birth reduced the HIV infection rate among babies from 25% in the placebo group to 7%,[26] the prevention of mother-to-child transmission (PMTCT) became the best angle to "sell" AIDS to reluctant donors. A UNAIDS epidemiologist confesses:

> All the evidence also suggested that governments don't like spending money on sex workers, gay men or drug addicts. . . . There are no votes in being nice to a drug addict. We had to find a way to translate the truth into something that governments might care about. We came up with two options: money and babies. Politicians could save both, we argued, by paying more attention to HIV while it was still low. . . . As a lobbying tool, the "buy needles now, save on hospital costs later" argument rests on the assumption that politicians give a damn about what happens "later." So in fact, the money argument often isn't enough to make politicians do nice things for junkies. . . . We argued quite truthfully that men who inject, men who have sex with one another and men who buy sex are likely to pass HIV on to their innocent wives. And then came the sleight of hand. Once innocent wives were infected, we implied, HIV would blaze through the "general population." . . . We weren't making anything up. But once we got the numbers, we were certainly presenting them in their worst light. We did it consciously. I think all of us at that time thought that the beat-ups were more than justified, they were necessary. We were pretty certain that neither donors nor governments would care about HIV unless we could show that it threatened the "general population."[27]

The innocent mother and child are often embodied as African. While an AZT regimen became the standard of care in the Global North, and HIV transmission to children has practically disappeared there, many HIV-positive pregnant mothers in developing countries remain too poor to treat.[28] In 2004, President Thabo Mbeki discontinued AZT clinical trials in South Africa because it was too expensive to provide treatment for all HIV-positive mothers.[29] Over a decade after ACTG 076, donors, funding agencies, and celebrities finally heard the drumbeat of PMTCT. In 2008, the former First Lady of France, Carla Bruni-Sarkozy, was named as the Global Fund's first AIDS ambassador. Heading the Born HIV-Free campaign, she was to be the "voice for mothers and children infected with or affected by HIV/AIDS":

> AIDS is actually not an indiscriminate killer. . . . I decided to focus on the most vulnerable of all: babies in the developing world. . . . Women are the heart of society—earners, caregivers, nurturers, drivers of change. It is our shared responsibility to help ensure that our sisters in developing countries also have access to the basic rights and services that most of us have the luxury to take for granted. By investing in women, we are investing in the health and development of families, of communities and ultimately of entire countries.[30]

In 2011, UNAIDS adopted the five-year Global Plan towards the Elimination of New HIV Infections among Children by 2015 and Keeping Their Mothers Alive. In December 2012, the US secretary of state, Hillary Clinton, announced a call to action for an "AIDS-free generation" through scaling up the treatment of HIV-positive people, preventing mother-to-child transmission, and expanding voluntary medical male circumcision. The slogan of the CDC, a partner in this initiative, is "Proven science, smart investments, and shared responsibility."[31] AIDS science is never far away from business and politics.

AIDS Orphan

Consider this narrative: "A 13-year-old Kenyan AIDS orphan gave away her virginity in exchange for an apple. Asked why, she replied, 'No one's ever given me anything before.' The tragedy of AIDS does not end with the death of the sufferer. It continues through the lives of the children who are orphaned. In Africa, where the epidemic is at its worst, a whole generation of children is growing without parents."[32]

The logics behind the predominant discourses on "innocent mothers and children" and "AIDS orphans" are similar: they are vulnerable and should be saved. But somehow, noble aspirations have failed to materialize into concrete actions. For the first twenty years of the epidemic, no one was talking about children affected by HIV and AIDS. While the highly educated White gay men of New York

and San Francisco were busy protesting, while IDUs were demanding clean needles, while sex workers were boycotting clinical trials, and while activists and experts in the Geneva AIDS orbit were churning out glossy reports, millions of children were orphaned and affected by the epidemic. Until the Durban conference
in 2001, when the articulate 12-year-old HIV-positive Nkosi Johnson spoke,
nobody—scientists, UN bureaucrats, governments, donors, or activists—thought
it was strange that children had never spoken at an international AIDS conference plenary. When OVC (orphans and vulnerable children) finally made it to the
international AIDS agenda in the early 2000s, everyone started talking about
AIDS orphans, but at the expense of a great number of other children affected
by the epidemic. Since then, they have been abundantly spoken to, and on behalf
of, by a range of experts: doctors, psychologists, social workers, economists, consultants, journalists, and self-made AIDS pundits. The first Global Partners Forum on children and AIDS, a joint effort of UNAIDS and the United Nations Children's Fund (UNICEF), was held in 2003 to monitor the progress of promises
made for children in the 2001 Declaration of Commitment on HIV/AIDS. In
2005, the "Unite for Children, Unite against AIDS" campaign was launched to
"put the face of children at the center of the global, regional, and national HIV
and AIDS agenda."[33] This face too is African:

> Why is there an AIDS orphan crisis in Africa? Apart from the obvious answer that
> AIDS has killed large numbers of adults of parenting age, most African families
> like to have big families. . . . Many African parents are no longer living long enough
> to see their children reach maturity. Weakened by malnutrition, HIV-positive Af-
> ricans tend to sicken and die faster than HIV-positive Westerners. They can't afford
> enough food, clean drinking water and the drugs to treat opportunistic infec-
> tions, let alone the cocktails of antiretroviral drugs that keep HIV-positive North
> Americans and Europeans alive for years. . . . African countries face a stark
> choice. If they do not find ways to care for the growing multitude of AIDS orphans,
> they could soon find their streets crowded with angry, intoxicated adolescents. Be-
> sides being a human tragedy, this could aggravate the continent's already high
> levels of crime.[34]

This typical AIDS orphan narrative tells us many things about Africa: its culture, society, and economic development. But despite what the author says, the
real answers are far from obvious. Where in Africa is the author talking about?
Why is antiretroviral therapy not available to African parents? Why are Africans
too poor to treat? Which children have been most affected? Above all, when will
we hear the children speak?

Hormone-Charged Youth

In AIDS, the innocent mother, vulnerable child, and reckless youth are often read as a continuum along a social axis as targets of prevention among the "general population" in contrast to the traditional high-risk groups of gays, addicts, and prostitutes. If mothers are to be protected and children saved, youth must be educated. UNAIDS, WHO, and UNICEF write:

> There is a way to halt the spread of HIV/AIDS. We must focus on young people. More than half of those newly infected with HIV today are between 15 and 24 years old. Yet the needs of the world's 1 billion young people are routinely disregarded when strategies on HIV/AIDS are drafted, policies made and budgets allocated. This is especially tragic as young people are more likely than adults to adopt and maintain safe behaviours. Each day, nearly 6,000 young people between the ages of 15 and 24 become infected with HIV. Yet only a fraction of them know they are infected. . . . Young people are our greatest opportunity to defeat HIV/AIDS.[35]

The reasons given for youth intervention are many. Young people have sex; young people lack information; girls are very vulnerable; many young people are at especially high risk, including for addiction and violence.[36] Even when they do have information, youth may "lack the skills to negotiate abstinence or condom use. They may be fearful or embarrassed to talk with their partner about sex. Still others may not adopt safe behaviours because they perceive their individual risk to be low."[37] Adolescents "often have a sense of immortality and find it difficult to think about future consequences of today's actions. With an emerging sense of autonomy they challenge authority, and it is normal during this phase of development for them to seek new experiences, some involving risks."[38]

Since the 1990s, uninformed, disempowered, irresponsible, hormone-charged youth have been one of the preferred objects of AIDS discourse, not unlike Foucault's masturbating child except that they are, once again, African. A Harvard professor of anthropology concludes, "The main behavioral changes that occurred in Uganda in its earlier epidemic phase (1986–1991) were partner reduction, followed by delay of sexual debut as well as increased abstinence practiced at later ages." These behaviors, according to him, are "indigenous":

> As an anthropologist, it is glaringly clear to me that AIDS prevention programs designed by Western experts have been to a large extent incompatible with the cultures of Africa and other resource-poor parts of the world. Why have more Africans and other recipients of donor assistance not complained about this? . . . It reflects

ethnocentrism and technological arrogance. After all, who can know more about how to influence the behavior of Ugandans and Senegalese than Ugandans and Senegalese themselves? In any case, the export of Western models of behavior change has not had much impact on the ultimate measure—national HIV prevalence. Meanwhile, AIDS prevention and behavior change responses that have been to a large extent indigenous seem to have had significant impact on national HIV prevalence.[39]

This American behavior-change expert turned his knowledge into action. He testified before the US Congress in March 2003, helping to spur a multimillion-dollar ABC (Abstinence, Be Faithful, and Condomize) business officially sponsored by PEPFAR.[40] Just in case "zero grazing" did not work, the US surgeon general, Joycelyn Elders, when asked if "masturbation might be taught as a way to prevent AIDS" at the 1994 World AIDS Day Conference at the United Nations, replied, "Masturbation is something that is a part of human sexuality, and is a part of something that perhaps should be taught," but added later, "masturbation is really something you don't have to teach."[41] The United States might have been aggressively funding behavior change, but this was a different story. Elders was fired by President Bill Clinton one week later for "values contrary to the administration."[42] Eighteen years later, the business of behavior change finally reached China. To celebrate World AIDS Day 2012, a sex toy manufacturer, Aihuirun, organized the first masturbation contest in China. In the company of scantily clad female models dancing with blow-up sex dolls, ten excited male contestants wore masks and hid their genitals with orange buckets in the name of "HIV-risk-free sexual freedom."[43]

Homo Sexualis Africanus

In AIDS, science slips easily into culture and vice versa. What is said and done in the name of science becomes also what is said and done in the name of culture. The innocent mother and child, the AIDS orphan, and the hormone-charged youth also appear on another continuum, this time along a cultural and racial axis with the *Homo sexualis africanus*, as part of the ongoing construction of "African AIDS."[44]

Social scientists have a lot to say about the hypersexualized African body: "[m]ost traditional African societies are promiscuous by Western standards"; "[a]s elsewhere, African men (who make condom use decisions) have shown great reluctance to use condoms with spouses or regular partners"; and Africans have "extended, overlapping networks" and "surprisingly modern attitudes towards sexuality" and are the least inclined toward "sexual restraints" compared to Caucasians and Mongoloids.[45] From a political point of view, Fassin warns, "the invention of an '*Homo sexualis africanus*' goes hand in hand with a '*cultura sexualis africana*' . . . and has produced an image of Africa and its inhabitants mixing an imaginary representation of sexuality and decontextualized data on sexual behavior, a vulgate that has spread to Europe and North America."[46]

This predominant narrative of the oversexed African rarely circulates alone. The second part of the African AIDS story is that treatment is not for Africans:

> If only drugs were a solution for Africa's AIDS crisis. Drugs are part of the solution, but they are far from the whole solution. My reservations, expressed in this book's original Introduction, which follows, remain the same. . . . If South Africa's government were to provide all five million HIV-positive South Africans with anti-retroviral drugs, it could cost a seventh of all state spending each year. If families were to have to pay all or part of the cost, it would be all too easy to fall into debt. Parents might live a little longer, but their orphans might end up worse off. One of the drug industry's fears has always been that charging lower prices in developing countries would create a black market. This fear is far from absurd.[47]

An AIDS historian continues:

> Even infinite amounts of money would not completely solve the problem, however. The drugs remained highly toxic, commonly causing diarrhea, nausea, liver failure, and pancreatic damage. As many as 20 percent of patients who began the drug treatment plan found that they could not tolerate it. Compliance with the treatment plan was probably no higher than 80 percent, and that was in wealthy developed nations where patients could easily refrigerate the drugs and take them on schedule with appropriate doses of food and drink. New resistan[t] strains of the virus were constantly evolving, and the expected lower compliance rates in Africa would only accelerate this process. And distribution in a continent that measured its paved roads by the hundreds of miles, rather than by the thousands, in which railroads, modern highways, private automobiles, and electric power were all scarce or nonexistent, and in which cultural and linguistic norms were inconsistent with modern medicine, was sure to be difficult.[48]

Instead of asking why Africans are not receiving treatment, the bulk of the scientific and not-so-scientific energy on African AIDS since the mid-1980s has gone to sexual network mapping, identifying African hot spots name by name. An American epidemiologist, John Potterat, formerly with the US Centers for Disease Control, asks, "Why is HIV/AIDS striking hard in certain populations in

Africa? . . . Why is it concentrated in the eastern and southern part of the continent? Network mapping can help us find answers to questions like these—then take steps to stop infection."[49] AIDS epidemiology so often slides into a politics of blaming.

Suspicious Foreigner or Migrant

Fifty-nine countries continue to impose restrictions on the entry, stay, and residence of people living with HIV based on their status.[50] Of these, twenty-seven countries deport individuals when their HIV-positive status is discovered.[51] In Singapore, entry is denied to HIV-positive people and to foreigners diagnosed with AIDS. An HIV test is mandatory for stays beyond thirty days. Foreign nationals with AIDS or who are HIV-positive are expelled (the HIV-positive foreign spouses of Singaporeans are exempt). Entering Singapore with ARVs for personal use requires approval by authorities, and doctors are required to report anyone found to be HIV-positive.[52] These measures are usually justified in the name of public health science. A Singaporean Health Ministry spokesperson said, after nine HIV-positive women were deported from Singapore in 2000, that the repatriation of HIV-positive foreigners is "necessary to ensure that they will not pose a threat to the public health in Singapore" and is part of the country's attempt to "further strengthen the control of communicable diseases like HIV infection."[53] The suspicious foreigner is also considered to be a possible "treatment tourist," who will burden the national health system.[54] The same Singaporean Health Ministry spokesperson adds that treatment is also "expensive. It is better to channel our subsidies to more cost-effective treatments for the benefit of the majority of our patients."[55] Science meets economics and stigma to produce some of the most draconian measures to regulate the AIDS at-risk body. In Singapore, all deceased people with HIV are double-bagged and incinerated within twenty-four hours. Singapore's authorities claim that the HIV virus remains active for several days in the body of the deceased; thus, "embalming . . . minimise[s] the risk of transmission. Without embalming, a body decomposes rapidly in Singapore's tropical heat, thus justifying the 24-hour cremation ruling."[56]

The foreign migrant is always suspect. She may not speak the language. He may be living on the political, economic, and social margins of the host society. She may be undocumented. He may not have health insurance. She may carry the virus. He may not know his rights. For the sending countries, she is a source of remittances. For the host countries, he is disposable labor.[57] Since September 11, 2001, the foreign migrant is even more suspect—a security threat—whether he is in North American, ASEAN (Association of Southeast Asian Nations),

SAARC (South Asian Association for Regional Cooperation), or GCC (Gulf Co-operation Council) countries.[58]

Transgender Pervert

Another of the many inconvenient truths that AIDS has revealed is that human sexuality is diverse and may not fit neatly in scientific categories. Those who do not fit into the duality of male or female are simultaneously layered with sexual and orientalist fantasies *and* rendered invisible in scientific research: "Thai men like *katoey* [a local term for a transgender person, sometimes spelled *kathoey*] for several reasons. In purely erotic terms, they will do things, like oral sex, that Thai women, especially social equals like wives, are taught to think of as dirty. They are described as 'tight' and 'dry,' references to the muscular anal sphincter."[59] At the same time, the "pervasive stigmatization, denial and the hidden nature of some transgender people have led to the exclusion of transgender people from much research."[60]

Whether they are called *kathoey* in the Mekong region, *waria* in Indonesia, *hijra* in India, Pakistan, and Bangladesh, or *fa'afafine* in the Pacific, transgender people defy the imaginations of AIDS scientists and their categorization of the at-risk body. For them, a man who dresses like a woman who has sex with a man is categorized as MSM (men who have sex with men), which is defined in a UN-AIDS document: "While we use the term 'men who have sex with men' here it is within the context of understanding that the word 'man'/'men' is socially constructed. . . . Within the framework of male-to-male sex, there is a range of masculinities, along with diverse sexual and gender identities, communities, networks and collectives, as well as just behaviors without any sense of affiliation to an identity or community."[61]

Lumping together transgender people and MSM in AIDS prevention efforts, however, continues to mask the different sexual practices and needs of a third gender. In one AIDS study on Thai soldiers having sex with men, researchers got a surprisingly low response rate, which doubled when the question was rephrased from "Have you ever had sex with another man?" to "Have you ever had sex with another man, or with a *katoey*?"[62] In another study in Laos, the researchers spoke at length to ninety-three men who included "men who are overtly effeminate a majority of the time (long-hair[ed] *kathoeys*)"; "men who act effeminately, but who depending on circumstances, may also choose not to do so (short-haired *kathoeys*"; "men who identify as gay, but not *kathoey*"; "single men who have sex with men on occasion, but who do not identify as gay or *kathoey* (partners of *kathoeys* or gay men); and "married men who have sex with men." The researchers conclude:

> MSM is an awkward typology and not a local term. It is meaningless in everyday conversation. Kathoey is the local vernacular catch-all term. It depicts a gender identity (somewhat feminine), a sexual orientation (towards men) and [a] social category (somewhat valorized in very specific situations, but more broadly stigmatized when placed against normative male-female identities) with a long history in local Thai, Cambodian and Lao cultures.[63]

There is also a pervasive stereotype of transgender people as sex workers, which again masks the diversity in the transgender community.[64] Having been subsumed under the umbrella of MSM, transgender people's sexual practices and specific health needs, such as hormone treatment and plastic surgery, and way of life still remain to be addressed.

Dangerous Outlaw

HIV-positive prisoners have been subject to a security regime of prison management and crime control. Criminologists have written extensively on the industrialization and privatization of penal control in the United States, based on the rhetoric of retribution and deterrence:

> The complex organization of punitive state control formally commences with the processes of surveillance, designation, arrest, and criminalization. . . . The Resurrection of the "Dangerous Classes" [is] a product of the shift from social welfare to punitive criminal justice state policy as an industrialized crime-control response to the threats to capitalist social order posed by a growing surplus of labor group composed of the marginalized and disenfranchised. . . . "Slaves of the State" . . . [refers to] the prison-industrial complex's growing interest in the utilization of these carceral commodities as an organized industrial workforce producing Third World–style products (e.g., textiles) at sweatshop prices. The importance of race, class, and gender to the actual workings of criminal justice is borne out in the composition of prison populations, where the poor and people of color are significantly overrepresented.[65]

At the Eleventh UN Crime Congress in 2005, governments note that "the physical and social conditions associated with imprisonment may facilitate the spread of HIV in pre-trial and correctional facilities and thus in society, thereby presenting a critical prison management problem."[66] There is also concern about the effect of HIV-positive prisoners once they are released: "There is a constant flow of people between the community and prisons. With 30 million prisoners released back to the community each year, increased rates of illness in prison have serious consequences for society as a whole."[67]

Structural factors are recognized as fueling HIV transmission in prison settings: "often condoms are not available. When drugs are injected, needles and syringes—being scarce, illegal and difficult to hide—are almost always shared, carrying with them a high risk of transmission of infectious diseases."[68] Yet most prisons worldwide still do not provide HIV-prevention measures. Instead of adopting scientifically recognized harm reduction approaches that aim at minimizing the harms related to drug use, the reduction of the drug supply remains the predominant goal in prisons. A 2008 WHO, UNAIDS, and UNODC toolkit for policymakers, program managers, prison officers, and healthcare providers in prison settings reiterates, "Taking drugs inside prison is obviously unlawful and in many countries strenuous efforts are made to keep prisons drug-free. These include preventive measures such as regular searching of prisoners, staff and visitors, the use of specifically trained dogs and other security checks. They also include strict punishments for those who take drugs in prison and those who smuggle them in."[69]

Risks and the AIDS Straw Man

In a hurry to hunt down the drivers of the AIDS epidemic, a network of power over the body—which is "approached not directly in its biological dimension, but as an object to be manipulated and controlled"—has arisen to build an elaborate confessional apparatus of desire: "With whom did you last have sex? When? Where? How?"[70] Through medical examinations, clinical trials, NIH-funded studies, scientific presentations, pedagogical interventions, international development policies and programs, monitoring and evaluation, and an expansive system of "nationally representative, population-based surveys; behavioural surveillance surveys; specially-designed surveys and questionnaires; patient tracking systems; sentinel surveillance; and the National Commitments and Policy Instrument questionnaire,"[71] AIDS professionals in diverse local centers of power have dedicated themselves to examining the "at-risk" body ad infinitum.

The assumptions behind this predominant taxonomy of risk is that "[w]e know what works and what needs to be done."[72] Is it not true that gay men, drug addicts, prostitutes, mothers, orphans, youth, migrants, transgender people, prisoners, and all Africans are at risk? Let us compare this taxonomy of risks with the ten

"Targets and Elimination Commitments" promised by world leaders in the 2011 UN General Assembly Political Declaration on HIV/AIDS:[73]

Target 1. Reduce sexual transmission of HIV by 50% by 2015.

Target 2. Reduce transmission of HIV among people who inject drugs by 50% by 2015.

Target 3. Eliminate new HIV infections among children by 2015 and substantially reduce AIDS-related maternal deaths.

Target 4. Reach 15 million people living with HIV with life-saving antiretroviral treatment.

Target 5. Reduce tuberculosis deaths in people living with HIV by 50% by 2015.

Target 6. Close the global AIDS resource gap and reach annual investment of US$22–$24 billion in low- and middle-income countries.

Target 7. Eliminate gender inequalities and gender-based abuse and violence and increase the capacity of women and girls to protect themselves from HIV.

Target 8. Eliminate stigma and discrimination against people living with and affected by HIV through promotion of laws and policies that ensure the full realization of all human rights and fundamental freedoms.

Target 9. Eliminate HIV-related restrictions on entry, stay, and residence.

Target 10. Eliminate parallel systems for HIV-related services to strengthen integration of the AIDS response in global health and development efforts.

Of the ten targets, only two (2 and 3) mention specific groups: people who inject drugs, children, and mothers. The eight other targets look at access to treatment, TB co-infection, funding gaps, and a range of critical enablers, including human rights and health system strengthening, pharmaceutical companies charging inaccessible prices for ARV drugs, national laws that discriminate, institutions and practices that stigmatize and prevent access to treatment and services, and donors who do not meet their funding commitments. None of these critical groups has ever been labeled a "key population" even though AIDS science tells us that they stand in the way of universal access.[74]

When we look deeper into the indicators for targets 2 and 3, we realize that what scientists have been asking governments to track are the *individual behaviors and contextual factors that put people at risk*—consistent condom use, clean needles, testing, HIV knowledge, access to prevention services, and availability of treatment—rather than any particular at-risk *group* as such.[75] Similarly, the bulk of the fourteen indicators for target 1 (reducing the sexual transmission of HIV) measure risk factors such as prevalence rate, condom use, the reach of HIV programs, and testing, and these concerns matter whether we are discussing the general population, sex workers, men who have sex with men, heterosexual adults, or youth. None of the ten targets and thirty indicators singles out any particular race or culture, nor do any of them focus on the number of sexual partners people have, why people take drugs or sell sex, whether a child affected by HIV fits the definition of an "AIDS orphan," or whether an adolescent has recently masturbated or changed partner.

The juxtaposition of the ten stereotypes of the AIDS at-risk body and the thirty UNAIDS indicators of risk reveals a glaring gap between the dominant narratives (perpetuated in the name of science) and the key actions (demanded also in the name of science). The two taxonomies do not match up: one singles out specific populations, many of which had already been marginalized and stigmatized before AIDS, and the other focuses on the specific factors that are the root causes of HIV infection. Why has there been such an investment of discursive energy on MARPs, and what has been the effect?

Since the 1980s, the science of locating the AIDS at-risk body has turned into the politics of locating blame. AIDS science has helped to construct, reinforce, and legitimize a normative order of sexuality and lifestyle through the regulation of a wide range of at-risk subjects. As Patton observes early in the epidemic, "All of the discourse of AIDS has encoded the homosexual Other."[76] The same is true for the other most-at-risk populations, who are pitted against the law-abiding, normalized, heterosexual, Western general population.

The persistent use of at-risk labeling essentializes and perpetuates AIDS mythologies: gay sex is always risky; drug use is dangerous; prostitution is to blame; only AIDS orphans are vulnerable; all Africans are oversexed; puberty is an inherent bag of risks; and migrants carry viruses. It also contributes to the stigmatization—a " 'significantly discrediting' attribute possessed by a person with an 'undesired difference' "[77]—of already marginalized populations. Discrimination and fear create barriers for people living with HIV and make it difficult to access prevention and treatment services. Singling out specific marginalized populations masks the reality of a complex epidemic: "Clients of sex workers make up the largest key population at higher risk in Asia: depending on the country, between 0.5% and 15% of adult men in the region are believed to buy sex"[78]—and yet heterosexual men have never been labeled as a MARP.

What are the effects of the continuous underrepresentation, overrepresentation, and misrepresentation of the so-called at-risk body? AIDS scientists tell us that "[o]rphaning is not the only way that children may be affected by HIV/AIDS. Other children made vulnerable by HIV/AIDS include those who have an ill parent, are in poor households that have taken in orphans, are discriminated against because of a family member's HIV status, or who have HIV themselves."[79] Pitying children affected by AIDS, however noble the intention, can only bring us so far when "less than one quarter of the children eligible for treatment are accessing antiretroviral therapy."[80]

Risk labels also fuel government denial and discourage accurate reporting. In a 2009 consultation by UNICEF, a number of countries (mainly in Africa) reported that indicators for IDUs were not relevant to their national context.[81] The concept of MARPs also pits one marginalized group against another ("We really need to get over this love affair with the fetus and start worrying about children").[82] In 2011, the Global Fund changed its eligibility criteria, creating a new category called the Targeted Funding Pool with a cap of US$12.5 million per application only for the most-at-risk populations in middle-income countries that would not otherwise be eligible. The result is that people living with AIDS (PWA) are now subject to the Global Fund's at-risk governmentality, and there is increased competition among MARPs for the limited funds.[83]

UNAIDS itself is inconsistent in its risk science. On the one hand, it groups its key action indicators under five non-population-specific categories—behavioral outcome, disease impact, infrastructure, policy, and program/service at the community, facility, global, national, and provincial levels[84]—and warns against the use of certain labels in its 2011 *Terminology Guidelines*. On the other, it retains the use of the concept of "key populations" despite its stigmatizing effects (emphases mine):

Key Populations at Higher Risk of HIV Exposure

The term "key populations" or "key populations at higher risk of HIV exposure" refers to those most likely to be exposed to HIV or to transmit it—their engagement is critical to a successful HIV response, i.e., they are key to the epidemic and key to the response. In all countries, key populations include people living with HIV. In most settings, men who have sex with men, transgender persons, people who inject drugs, sex workers and their clients, and seronegative partners in serodiscordant couples are at higher risk of exposure to HIV than other people. There is a strong link between various kinds of mobility and heightened risk of HIV exposure, depending on the reason for mobility and the extent to which people are outside their social context and norms.

Group

The term "high-risk group" should be avoided because *it implies that the risk is contained within the group, whereas, in fact, all social groups are interrelated.* The use of the term "high-risk group" may create a false sense of security in people who have risk behaviours but do not identify with such groups. It can also increase stigma and discrimination. Membership of groups does not place individuals at risk, behaviours may. In the case of married and cohabiting people, particularly women, the risk behaviour of the sexual partner may place them in a "situation of risk."

Bridging Population (Don't Use)

The term "bridging population" (or "bridge population") describes a population at higher risk of HIV exposure whose members may have unprotected sexual relations with individuals who are otherwise at low risk of HIV exposure. Because *HIV is transmitted by individual behaviours and not by groups,* avoid using the term bridging population (or bridge population) and describe the behaviour instead.

Most at Risk (Don't Use)

Terms such as "most-at-risk adolescents" (MARAs), "most-at-risk young people" (MARYP), and "most-at-risk populations" (MARPs) should be avoided because communities view them as stigmatising. *It is more appropriate and precise to describe the behaviour each population is engaged in that places individuals at risk of HIV exposure,* for example unprotected sex among stable serodiscordant couples, sex work with low condom use, young people who use drugs and lack access to sterile injecting equipment, etc. In specific projects where such expressions continue to be used, it is important never to refer to a person (directly or indirectly) as a MARA, MARYP, or MARP.

High-Burden Country

The term "high-burden country" describes a country with a high HIV prevalence and is sometimes also used in reference to high tuberculosis prevalence. Such expressions should be used with caution in order to avoid stigmatisation.

Gay

The term "gay" can refer to same-sex sexual attraction, same-sex sexual behaviour, and same-sex cultural identity. The expression "men who have sex with men" should be used unless individuals or groups self-identify as gay.[85]

The World Bank defines vulnerability as "a high probability of a negative outcome" or "an expected welfare loss above a socially accepted norm . . . shaped by risk and stress characteristics such as magnitude, frequency, duration, and scope, to which individuals, households and communities are exposed."[86] UNAIDS looks at structural factors that shape "unequal opportunities, social exclusion, unemployment, or precarious employment and other social, cultural, political, and economic factors that make a person more susceptible to HIV infection and to developing AIDS. . . . These factors, alone or in combination, may create or exacerbate individual and collective vulnerability to HIV."[87]

A key-population approach, in contrast to a vulnerability framework, slots people into stigmatizing categories. It ignores their multiple identities; masks the social, economic, cultural, and political bases of risk; and keeps political energy away from the real crises. For example, in 2011, among 107 reporting countries, only 42 had needle and syringe programs, and only 37 offered opioid substitution therapy.[88] It is not drug use per se but the absence of access to effective prevention and treatment in the majority of countries worldwide that fuels AIDS. "The world is now faced with a multitude of AIDS epidemics, differing in their timing, their scale and the populations they affect—and often differing even in the factors fuelling them," according to UNICEF in 2002.[89] Shorthand labels are stigmatizing and stand in the way of universal access.

Battle over the Science of Risk: Criminalizing HIV Transmission

Tragically, it is stigma that lies primarily behind the drive to criminalization. It is stigma, rooted in the moralism that arises from sexual transmission of HIV, that too often provides the main impulse behind the enactment of these laws. Even more tragically, such laws and prosecutions in turn only add fuel to the fires of stigma. Prosecutions for HIV transmission and exposure, and the chilling content of the enactments themselves, reinforce the idea of HIV as a shameful, disgraceful, unworthy condition.

—*Edwin Cameron, Scott Burris, and*
Michaela Clayton, "HIV Is a Virus, Not a
Crime: Ten Reasons against Criminal
Statutes and Criminal Prosecutions"[90]

The risk to our societies lies not only in HIV infection. It lies also in the way in which our societies respond to that infection and the pandemic which it threatens.

—*Michael Kirby, "The New AIDS Virus—*
Ineffective and Unjust Laws"[91]

At the 1988 International AIDS Conference in Stockholm, Justice Michael Kirby cautioned about the advent of a new mutant of the AIDS virus: what he called "highly ineffective laws." As soon as the epidemic started, public alarm created the demand for drastic laws, including mandatory testing of the entire population or "vulnerable groups," compulsory disclosure of HIV status, and criminalization of HIV transmission exposure and transmission. In the twenty-first century, the control over the HIV at-risk body has intensified in courtrooms and legislatures. Existing criminal laws are increasingly being used to prosecute HIV exposure and transmission in Europe and North America, while new HIV-specific laws have spread in Africa, Asia, Latin America, and the Caribbean.[92] At the center of these debates are political contestations over the meaning of HIV risk, often layered with gendered, racial, and cultural overtones: How risky exactly is an HIV-positive person? When is the risk of transmission "real" or "significant"? Who determines what is a "significant level of risk" and how? Can an HIV-positive person be held responsible for infecting others if she is unaware of her status? Is risk reduced by safer sex measures such as condom use? What if the viral load of an HIV-positive person is low or undetectable? How about oral sex or other sexual practices that are scientifically considered to be less risky in terms of HIV transmission? If an HIV-positive person discloses his status, can he still be prosecuted? Are women more likely to learn of their status first in maternity checkups, and are they vulnerable to violence when they disclose it? Does HIV nondisclosure equal rape?[93] How do we measure intent in cases of "willful transmission"? What if a woman consents to unprotected sex despite knowledge of her partner's status? Under what circumstances, if any, are compulsory testing and disclosure justified? When does protection for someone become discrimination against another? Do such laws or prosecutions advance public health, or do they criminalize and stigmatize people living with HIV? Is there an "African Immigrant Damnation Syndrome" where Black men are disproportionately prosecuted for HIV transmission?[94]

In Canada, judges at different levels continue to debate the scientific evidence of HIV risk. In 1993, a Ugandan living in Ontario was charged with aggravated assault for failing to disclose his HIV status in three sexual encounters, but he died before his verdict was rendered. In 1998 in *R. v. Cuerrier*, the Supreme Court of Canada had the opportunity for the first time to rule based on the notion of "significant risk" in the context of HIV. The question at hand, involving a British Columbian man who tested positive for HIV in 1992 and subsequently had sexual relationships with two women, was whether nondisclosure constituted fraud that in effect nullified consent for unprotected sexual activity. The majority decided that "an HIV positive person can be convicted of aggravated assault even if there is no actual transmission of HIV. Fraud is established where failure to disclose HIV status had the effect to expose the consenting partner to a significant risk of serious bodily harm."[95] Hence, "a person only has a legal duty to disclose his or her HIV-positive status to sexual partners before having sex that poses a 'significant risk' of HIV transmission." In other words, "an HIV-positive person who practices safer sex does not necessarily have a legal responsibility to disclose his or her status."[96] What remains open to interpretation, however, is the definition of "significant risk of serious bodily harm." Richard Elliott of the Canadian HIV/AIDS Legal Network writes, "The science around HIV has also greatly evolved since *Cuerrier* in 1998. It became increasingly clear that an undetectable viral load dramatically reduces the risk of HIV transmission, but what this means for the legal duty of people living with HIV to disclose is not yet clear."[97] Since *Cuerrier*, people who are not informed that a sexual partner is HIV-positive cannot truly give consent to sex. As a result, any subsequent death due to HIV exposure is automatically considered to be murder. In 2009, Johnson Aziga, who was diagnosed with HIV in 1996 and had unprotected sex with eleven women (two of whom had died) without disclosing his HIV status, became the first Canadian to be convicted of first-degree murder for HIV nondisclosure.[98]

In 2012 in *R. v. Mabior*, a man from Manitoba was convicted on six counts of aggravated sexual assault for HIV nondisclosure. The trial judge considered that "even when a condom is used there is a significant risk of HIV transmission for the purpose of the criminal law. She also reached the same conclusion for an undetectable viral load. According to the trial judge, the risk would only be sufficiently reduced when a person has both an undetectable viral load *and* uses a condom."[99] The Manitoba Court of Appeal was asked to determine whether the trial judge erred in her interpretation of "significant risk," and it decided that when a condom was carefully used *or* when the accused's viral load was undetectable, there was no significant risk of HIV transmission. The accused was subsequently acquitted of four counts of aggravated sexual assault "with respect to those sexual encounters in which he carefully used a condom (even though his viral load was detectable) *or* did not use a condom but had an undetectable viral load."[100] The Court of Appeal made it clear that "[l]egal assessments of risk in this area should be consistent with the available medical studies" and acknowledged that "[t]he application of the legal test in *Cuerrier* must evolve to account appropriately for the development in the science of HIV treatment."[101]

The *Mabior* decision was considered by advocates of people living with HIV to be a step in the right direction "by recognizing that—based on science—people should not be convicted when they carefully use a condom or have an undetectable viral load." However, in October 2012, the Supreme Court of Canada ruled in *R. v. Mabior* and *R. v. D.C.* that "people living with HIV have a legal duty, under the criminal law, to disclose their HIV-positive status to sexual partners before having sex that poses a *'realistic possibility' of HIV transmission*" (emphasis mine).[102] The Court recognized penile-vaginal sex when a condom is used *and* when the person living with HIV has a low or an undetectable viral load as not posing a realistic possibility of HIV transmission. If both of these conditions are met, then there is no obligation under the criminal law to disclose one's HIV status. Otherwise, not disclosing means a person with diagnosed HIV could be convicted of aggravated sexual assault.[103]

Based on these two decisions, people living with HIV can be prosecuted even if they have no intent to harm. An HIV-positive person has a legal duty to disclose "before having vaginal or anal sex without a condom (regardless of your viral load), or before having vaginal or anal sex with anything higher than a 'low' viral load (even if you use a condom)."[104] In the ruling, Chief Justice Beverley McLachlin writes, "The only 'evidence' was studies presented by interveners [a coalition of AIDS organizations] suggesting that criminalization 'probably' acts as a deterrent to HIV testing. . . . The conclusions in these studies are tentative and the studies were not placed in evidence and not tested by cross-examination. They fail to provide an adequate basis to justify judicial reversal of the accepted place of the criminal law in this domain." Widely criticized by AIDS advocates as "a major step backwards for public health and human rights," these decisions "went as far as they could have gone in the direction of criminalization."[105]

HIV Model Law

Meanwhile, in other parts of the world, a wave of HIV-specific laws has been enacted. In western Africa alone, twelve countries have passed laws to criminalize HIV infection since 2005: Guinea and Togo (2005); Benin and Mali (2006); Guinea-Bissau, Mauritania, Niger, and Sierra Leone (2007); Burkina Faso, Cape Verde, and Liberia (2008); and Senegal (2010). Two Nigerian states—Enugu (2005) and Lagos (2007)—have also passed such laws, while similar proposals are being discussed in Ivory Coast and Gambia.[106] If we add the six countries in eastern Africa with similar laws —Burundi (2005), Djibouti (2007), Kenya (2006), Madagascar (2005), Mozambique (2009), and Tanzania (2008)—it is clear that Africa is the most heavily legislated continent in terms of HIV. Mauritius is the only East African country to decide against criminalizing HIV exposure or transmission due to "concern about detrimental impacts on public health and the conviction that it would not serve any preventive purposes."[107]

Most of these laws were based on the African Model Law, a template created in September 2004 at a workshop in N'Djamena, the capital of Chad, which was organized by Action for West Africa Region–HIV/AIDS (AWARE-HIV/AIDS), funded by USAID, and implemented by Family Health International.[108] Supposedly designed to address the human rights needs of those infected by and exposed to HIV through provisions on counseling, services, and antidiscrimination, these laws are built on a three-pronged duty doctrine: the duty to test, the duty to warn, and the duty to protect. The most disquieting elements in these laws are compulsory testing, mandatory disclosure, and an offense of "willful transmission." In Guinea, for example, HIV testing before marriage is mandatory. In Togo, sex workers have to go through periodic mandatory testing for HIV and sexually transmitted diseases; HIV-positive people are prohibited from having unprotected sex, regardless of whether they have disclosed their status to their partner; and people who fail to use male or female condoms in "all risky sexual relations" are liable to criminal charges. In Benin, Guinea, Mali, and Niger, an HIV-positive woman can be criminally charged with not taking the steps necessary to prevent transmission to her unborn child, such as taking ARV drugs during pregnancy.[109] In every single western African country except Togo, the laws establish the specific offense of willful HIV transmission without defining "willful."[110]

In Uganda, the HIV and AIDS Prevention and Control Bill was proposed in 2009 on the heels of the controversial Anti-Homosexuality Bill, which includes the death penalty for "aggravated homosexuality" or life imprisonment for "the offence of homosexuality." While the HIV bill has a number of good provisions on treatment and antidiscrimination, it includes mandatory testing for HIV, forces the disclosure of HIV status, and criminalizes the willful transmission of HIV. Testing is mandatory for any person convicted of drug abuse or the possession of paraphernalia, a sexual offense, or prostitution. Routine testing is required for the victim of a sexual offense, a pregnant woman, and her partner. The result of an HIV test may be released to the sexual partner(s) of the person tested. Disclosure may also be authorized to a physician, nurse, or paramedical staff; the parent or guardian of a minor; the legal guardian of a person of unsound mind; and any person authorized by the act, any other law, or a court. The most alarming provision pertains to "intentional transmission": President Yoweri Museveni had advocated the death penalty for the offense in the original bill.[111] Under Section 40, a person who intentionally transmits or attempts to transmit HIV to another person commits an offense of "intentional transmission of HIV."[112]

A broad-based coalition of almost twenty Ugandan AIDS advocacy organizations, formed in 2010, is not opposed to the idea of a law on HIV per se but wants to see one that is informed by an evidence-based "balance between human rights . . . and public health."[113] According to the coalition, mandatory testing perpetuates the marginalization of vulnerable groups, such as injecting drug users and sex workers; compulsory disclosure "creates a disincentive to test" and "oppress[es] women, who are likely to know their status earlier than men because of contact with health services during pregnancy"; and criminalizing HIV transmission does not reduce the spread of the virus but distracts from more important issues that the bill should have addressed, such as social structures that hinder the access of people living with HIV to care, treatment, and prevention.[114] The coalition points to the East Africa HIV Prevention and Management Law, adopted by the five members of the East African Community (Burundi, Kenya, Rwanda, Tanzania, and Uganda) in April 2012, as a model in which there are no punitive measures for willful transmission.[115]

HIV-specific laws have created a false debate between public health and human rights, a "red herring that diverts us from addressing the real problems with prevention and care," according to Stephen Gendin, the former vice president of *Poz*, a magazine that focuses on the lives of people living with and affected by HIV and AIDS.[116] Proponents of stringent HIV-specific legislation argue that criminalization controls risk and serves the public health. Opponents debunk the scientifically unsubstantiated link between criminalization and risk reduction. In a ten-point argument, forty-three AIDS NGOs and networks summarize their position against such ineffective and unjust laws:

1. Criminalizing HIV transmission is justified only when individuals purposely or maliciously transmit HIV with the intent to harm others. In these rare cases, existing criminal laws can and should be used, rather than passing HIV-specific laws.
2. There is little evidence that applying criminal law to HIV exposure or transmission reduces the spread of HIV.
3. A criminal law approach undermines HIV prevention efforts by creating a false sense of security and creating distrust in relationships between HIV-positive people and their healthcare providers.
4. These laws promote fear and stigma.
5. They endanger and further oppress women, who may be prone to violence in disclosure.
6. Such laws are drafted and applied too broadly.

7. They are often applied unfairly, selectively, and ineffectively.

8. These laws effectively shift the total burden of HIV prevention onto people living with HIV rather than using proven methods to empower them to avoid the onward transmission of HIV and to empower others to protect themselves from infection.

9. Punitive approaches to drug use, sex work, and homosexuality fuel stigma and hatred against these socially marginalized groups, pushing them further into hiding and away from services to prevent, treat, and mitigate the impact of HIV and AIDS.

10. The most effective responses to HIV are based on human rights.[117]

The arbitrary definition of "risk" poses more human rights issues than it solves.

Can the Subaltern Speak? Human Rights Approaches to HIV

Punitive laws and human rights abuses are costing lives, wasting money and stifling the global AIDS response.
—*Global Commission on HIV and the Law,*
HIV and the Law: Risks, Rights, and Health[118]

Vulnerability to HIV reflects the extent to which people are, or are not, capable of making and effecting free and informed decisions about their health.
—*Jonathan Mann, "Human Rights and AIDS:*
The Future of the Epidemic"[119]

The terror is not that of HIV and AIDS, but that of stone walls we've built around our consciences, the cement fortress that we built in our minds, and the silence and ignorance slowly turning into a bomb that . . . slaughters everyone, not only [people living with HIV/AIDS].
—*Khaled Montasser, Forum to Fight Stigma*
and Discrimination against People Living
with HIV/AIDS, Egypt[120]

Can the stigmatized and criminalized at-risk body speak? People living with AIDS, rather than doctors, biomedical scientists, epidemiologists, politicians, or international bureaucrats, were the first to fight against their objectification and regulation. The insistence of the AIDS body to be heard marked a human rights turn in the epidemic. Looking back at the global response to AIDS in the 1980s,

Jonathan Mann, the indefatigable physician who headed the Global Programme on AIDS (GPA) at the WHO between 1987 and 1990, observed that early HIV prevention efforts took three approaches, all of which failed to bring the epidemic under control: uncertainty and urgency (1981–1984), individual risk reduction (1985–1988), and vulnerability analysis (1988–early 1990s).[121] The early years were characterized by confusing messages and an absence of any particular guiding concept. Subsequent efforts focused on behavioral changes, and a public health rationale was used to legitimize work on discrimination against those infected with HIV. Such an individualistic and instrumental approach did not go far, however. After 1988, a broader vulnerability framework was adopted that looked at barriers to individual control over health. But "public health has had great difficulty going beyond the stage of simply listing a broad range of contextual factors and influence."[122] Mann laments that even the latest approach to "the societal determinants of HIV vulnerability is essentially tactical, rather than strategic. There is no common understanding, let alone consensus, about the ways in which the societal factors should change to better promote and protect health."[123] Hence, although nongovernmental organizations have identified the most common political, sociocultural, and economic factors, including government inaction, taboos about sexuality, and a lack of resources for HIV programs, "this work lacks a coherent conceptual framework to describe and analyze the nature of the societal factors."[124]

What then does a human rights strategy entail? Mann argues, "It would mean that in addition to everything we already do, we would identify *the specific rights whose violation contributes to HIV vulnerability in our particular community or country*. . . . This brings us to the threshold of empowerment [which] rests on two pillars. One is knowledge. . . . The second pillar is . . . the possibility of change" (emphasis mine).[125] With this broad definition, Mann lays out the vast program entailed in a right-to-health approach to AIDS: nondiscrimination and equality before the law, women's rights, children's rights, the right to marry and found a family, privacy, education, freedom of expression and information, freedom of assembly and association, the right to work, enjoyment of the benefits of scientific progress, freedom of movement, an adequate standard of living and social security, participation in political and cultural life, asylum, liberty and security, and freedom from degrading treatment.[126]

Addressing vulnerability, discrimination, recognition, and equitable participation is the foundation of a human rights approach to HIV. Vulnerability refers to "groups and sub-populations that experience disempowerment and marginalisation because they are dispossessed of rights or are unable to exercise them [becoming] vulnerable to contracting HIV."[127] Discrimination occurs when "HIV has become a ground for denying people their rights. People living with HIV frequently face denial, discrimination and rights violations in public and private institutions—health care settings, employment, educational institutions, family and community, on the sole ground of their HIV status."[128]

The 1996 International Guidelines on HIV/AIDS and Human Rights was the first global document to lay out a comprehensive human rights strategy, including an effective national framework; political and financial support for community strengthening; public health, criminal, and human rights law reforms; access to prevention, treatment, and care; legal support to educate people about their rights; enabling a strong community environment; antidiscrimination and antistigmatization education; codes of conduct in professional settings; monitoring and enforcement; and international cooperation and knowledge sharing. In 2011, the UNAIDS Reference Group on HIV and Human Rights summarizes a human rights framework in five "nonnegotiables": (1) laws, policies, practices, stigma, and discrimination that block effective responses to AIDS should be eliminated; (2) HIV treatment should be available to all who need it, which requires the "maximum use of flexibilities under the TRIPS agreement to ensure the competition needed to lower the price of second-line and third-line treatments and their production in generic form"; (3) there should be funding commitments for appropriate HIV response until the achievement of the Millennium Development Goals in 2015; (4) people living with HIV should be at the center of the response; and (5) there should be a rights-based, shared AIDS governance.[129] When we look back at the global response to AIDS in the past three decades, these are precisely the five key areas where AIDS activists have intervened.

Nondiscrimination and Decriminalization

One of the most significant gains of AIDS activism has been "protecting the rights of [not only] those affected by HIV/AIDS but also those who are vulnerable to HIV/AIDS, including sex workers, injecting drug users, gays, lesbians, trans-gendered communities and other sexual minorities whose vulnerability is exacerbated due to non-recognition of their rights."[130] Marginalized communities affected by AIDS have been at the forefront of the global movement for decriminalization and nondiscrimination. ACT UP activism "transformed biomedicine, the whole drug regulation process, the notion of privacy, health care, medical research, confidentiality, and the rights of patients."[131]

Networks organized by gay men succeeded in disassociating AIDS from the "gay plague" concept by institutionalizing the term "men who have sex with men" (MSM), which describes this type of sexual behavior "regardless of gender identity, motivation for engaging in sex or identification with any or no particular 'community.' The words 'man' and 'sex' are interpreted differently in diverse cultures and societies as well as by the individuals involved. As a result, the term MSM covers a large variety of settings and contexts in which male to male sex takes place."[132] A founding member of the Asia Pacific Coalition on Male Sexual Health (APCOM) explains, "Using a human rights language has allowed doors to open that wouldn't have opened before. Back then, it was just about epidemiology. We had a president who didn't even say the bloody word for four years. Reagan didn't do anything. The community formed organizations, and transmission immediately dropped to very low levels within ten years."[133]

Similarly, networks of drug users and advocacy organizations, including the International Harm Reduction Program, the International Network of People Who Use Drugs, the Eurasian Harm Reduction Network, and the International Drug Policy Consortium, can be credited with the introduction of the concept of harm reduction as "policies, programmes and practices that aim to reduce the harms associated with the use of psychoactive drugs in people unable or unwilling to stop. The defining features are the focus on the prevention of harm, rather than on the prevention of drug use itself, and the focus on people who continue to use drugs."[134] This has replaced the traditional biomedical model of rehabilitation in some countries. Needle and syringe programs, opioid substitution therapy, and other drug dependence treatments are now part of a comprehensive package for the prevention, treatment, and care of HIV among people who use drugs as defined by UNAIDS, WHO, and UNODC.

Along the same lines, sex workers radically reframed prostitution as sex work and took up the agenda of decriminalization. The Global Network of Sex Work Projects (NSWP) states:

> More than mere political correctness, this shift in language had the important effect of moving global understandings of sex work toward a labour framework which signposts solutions to many of the problems faced by sex workers. It also questions the stigma of sex work and represents [a] greater recognition of sex workers as rights bearers, with the capacity to make a difference. As a result of NSWP advocacy, female, male and transgender sex workers have presented the case for protection of their human rights at international forums such as international and regional conferences on AIDS, the Fourth World Conference on Women in Beijing 1995, UNGASS, the UNAIDS Programme Co-ordinating Board and the Global Fund consultations.[135]

Working closely with various marginalized communities are AIDS legal networks, which have sprung up worldwide.[136] They pursue a three-pronged strategy of legal activism through litigation, advocacy, and research. In India, the Lawyers Collective fought the first antidiscrimination lawsuit for a person living with HIV. In *Lucy D'Souza v. State of Goa* (1989), a man was incarcerated in a TB hospital upon the discovery of his serostatus after a blood transfusion under the amended Goa Public Health Act, which authorized the state to mandatorily test and isolate persons found to be HIV-positive. In 1998, the Lawyers Collective set up an HIV/AIDS Unit and has since fought many cases concerning employment, the right to marry, confidentiality, negligence in blood transfusion, quack AIDS cures, and access to health care.[137]

In 2001, the Lawyers Collective petitioned on behalf of the Naz Foundation India in the Delhi High Court, challenging the constitutionality of Section 377 of the Indian Penal Code, which criminalizes "carnal intercourse against the order of nature," on the grounds that it violates the right to privacy, dignity, and health; the equal protection of law and nondiscrimination; and freedom of expression under the Indian Constitution. In 2009, the Delhi High Court issued a landmark judgment, striking down the colonial sodomy law and decriminalizing homosexual acts, but this was reversed by an Indian Supreme Court decision in 2013.[138] In yet another unprecedented decision, in 2011, in response to a petition filed by the Indian Harm Reduction Network and argued by the Lawyers Collective, the Bombay High Court struck down the mandatory death penalty for drug offenses.[139] The Lawyers Collective has also drafted a comprehensive HIV/AIDS bill, which was submitted in 2006 but has yet to be considered by the parliament. The proposed bill specifically prohibits HIV-related discrimination; requires free and informed consent for HIV-related testing, treatment, and research; guarantees the confidentiality of HIV-related information; provides for the right to access treatment; imposes an obligation on healthcare institutions to provide necessary universal precautions; decriminalizes risk reduction strategies, such as the provision of clean needles; obligates the state to institute information, education, and communication programs that are evidence-based, age-appropriate, gender-sensitive, nonstigmatizing, and nondiscriminatory; provides for health ombudsmen as a redress mechanism; and recognizes certain rights for women, children, and prisoners who, due to social, economic, legal, and other factors, are more vulnerable to HIV and are disproportionately affected by the epidemic.[140] According to its co-founder, the success of the Lawyers Collective lies in its ability to put "human rights at the center in all cases and advocacy work. . . . Learning is a very important part of the process. Going to court forces you to be critical and [to] recognize reality from the lived experiences of marginalized communities."[141]

Since 1992, the Canadian HIV/AIDS Legal Network has established a good track record in litigation in drug policy, prison health, sex workers' rights, criminal HIV nondisclosure, and access to treatment; it has also done advocacy work at both the national and international levels.[142] In 2005, together with other AIDS advocacy networks, the Canadian HIV/AID Legal Network used the upcoming 2006 International AIDS Conference in Toronto as an opportunity to successfully change Canadian immigration policy, eliminating the HIV-disclosure requirement for short-term visitors.[143] It also played an instrumental role in the 2011 Supreme Court of Canada decision in favor of Vancouver's safe injection site, InSite. In addition, it is one of only a few advocacy networks worldwide that focuses on AIDS in prisons. In 2012, it supported a lawsuit filed by Steven Simons, a former federal prisoner, and several organizations (Prisoners with HIV/AIDS Support Action Network, CATIE, the Canadian Aboriginal AIDS Network) against the government of Canada over its failure to implement clean needle and syringe programs to prevent the spread of HIV and hepatitis C in federal institutions; the rates of HIV and hepatitis C among Canadian prisoners are ten to thirty times higher than the rates of infection in the overall population.[144] "People do not surrender their human rights when they enter prison, including their right to access health services equivalent to those outside prisons. Society should not sentence people to a higher risk of infection with HIV or hepatitis. . . . Prison health is public health," says Sandra Ka Hon Chu, a senior policy analyst with the Canadian HIV/AIDS Legal Network.[145]

The Canadian HIV/AIDS Legal Network also has intervened in an ongoing constitutional challenge launched by a former sex worker, Sheryl Kiselbach, and an organization run by and for street-based sex workers, Sex Workers United against Violence, against four specific sections in the Canadian Criminal Code—Sections 210 and 211 on "common bawdy-houses," 212 on "procuring" prostitution, and 213 on "communicating for the purposes of prostitution"—which make it very difficult for sex workers to engage in prostitution without risking criminal charges despite the fact that sex work is legal in Canada.[146]

At the international level, the Canadian HIV/AIDS Legal Network has done extensive analyses of HIV criminalization issues, including model laws, for organizations such as UNAIDS that have helped to push for revisions in some countries.[147] Contrary to Jonathan Mann's concern about the absence of a human rights framework, the executive director of the legal network argues:

Human rights have been part of the AIDS agenda from the very beginning, even before ACT UP. Civil society fought for health care [for] positive people who were sick and [for] the visitation rights of their partners. Those were clearly human rights issues. The initial framing was the most obvious: this was about discrimination against gay people and people living with HIV. Their claims were more easily understandable for a community coming off the struggles of gay liberation. The discrimination was seen as an attack against them, and their response was an added layer to flex their political muscle. A human rights concept for sex workers and drug users, however, was less developed. The struggles for human rights evolved over time; it is more fleshed out thirty years on. It is not surprising because what we started to see as well is violence against women and poverty as drivers of the epidemic. We also started to see horrible violence against sex workers and people who use drugs. So our human rights response has grown, but it has always been there. Civil society has taken a lot longer to get various international institutions to look at AIDS from a human rights perspective, however. The purchase of human rights in global institutions overall is still tenuous; often it is just rhetorical commitment. We've had big fights, for example, at UNGASS [the UN General Assembly Special Session on HIV/AIDS, 2001], about whether we could name certain populations and how strong the human rights language could be. Those things that had to be fought for are now implanted in world AIDS response[s]. Bits and pieces get more attention. Certain groups are ignored. Some governments don't want to hear about human rights. But the idea that human rights have a key role to play is there. Of course, it doesn't mean that it can't be removed or there won't be backlash.[148]

Treatment Literacy and Access to Treatment

AIDS activism in the legal arena has created a large body of research, documentation, and jurisprudence based on the lived experiences of the marginalized and stigmatized at-risk body.[149] It has also played an instrumental role in access to treatment by increasing reach, quality, affordability, and sustainability. Access issues touch on counseling, testing, diagnosing, pricing, funding, procurement, stocking, delivery, quality, health workforce and community mobilization, research, R&D (research and development) funding, and the removal of barriers so that marginalized and disenfranchised groups can access treatment. Treatment advocacy also centers on a three-pronged strategy: treatment literacy, legal activism, and medical activism.

The fight for treatment in the United States was initiated by people living with HIV and AIDS, who educated themselves as lay experts and successfully lobbied for access, especially for women and people of color, to experimental drugs, such as AZT and ddI, through clinical trials. They were able to change the criteria for clinical trials, change the definition of AIDS, and accelerate drug approval. As Epstein notes:

> Over the course of the epidemic, members of the AIDS movement have taught themselves the details of virology, immunology, and epidemiology. They have criticized scientific research that seemed to be fuelled by antigay assumptions, defended speculation about alternative theories of AIDS causations, asserted that community-based AIDS organizations have the expertise to define public health constructs such as "safe sex," demanded scientific investigation of potentially useful treatments, established a grassroots base of knowledge about treatments, conducted their own "underground" drug trials, and criticized the methodologies employed in AIDS clinical research. They have established their credibility as people who might legitimately speak in the language of medical science, in particular with regard to the design, conduct, and interpretation of clinical trials used to test the safety and efficacy of AIDS drugs.[150]

Activists' self-education, or what one ACT UP member calls the "leveraging [of] science and evidence by nonscientists,"[151] forms the basis of treatment literacy, which has transformed AIDS advocacy worldwide. A direct legacy of ACT UP, says one member, is that "many people are trained. The treatment literacy model came directly from the Treatment Data Committee and then became more widespread. We did the training for TAC [Treatment Action Campaign]. . . . Their model became the face of treatment literacy in the developing world. People were not going to New York to train; they [would] go to South Africa to get trained."[152]

In the 1990s and 2000s, a whole new generation of treatment literacy activists sprang up worldwide. In Russia, Frontaids, an access-to-treatment movement active in the 1990s, was inspired by ACT UP.[153] The executive director of the Kenya Treatment Access Movement (KETAM) emphasizes, "You can't treat what you are not aware of. We make people treatment literate to demand treatment."[154] In 2007, the Access to Medicines Research Group, China, was formed by local lawyers to fill a crucial gap in treatment research and literacy in China. Its co-founder explains, "MSF did a great job in building the access debate and knowledge, but the majority of the data and cases we used were from other countries. My friends and I found that local treatment research was the part most lacking in China. Few Chinese NGOs do research and we wanted to fill this gap."[155] The legal network collaborates with Beautiful Life, an HIV-positive network in Shanghai, to provide treatment literacy training:

They are a peer group and know what patients need while we know the technical stuff. They designed a peer education tool, starting with basic information about AIDS, and then gradually talking about how to take drugs and how to identify your drugs. From there, they talk about access issues, about which foreign company owns which drugs and why we don't have access. Access is a small portion in the manual, but their intention is that you need to have a group of informed patients. If they don't have the right info about their disease, how can they jump to advocacy and policy?[156]

In Thailand, Youth Lead, a new network that focuses on building the capacity of young affected populations in Asia, credits ACT UP for its empowerment model: "Thirty years ago, there was ACT UP. Now the action is in Asia."[157] In India, the Delhi Network of Positive People runs a treatment literacy advocacy program in the neigborhood of Neb Sarai. Its president explains the treatment turn of his activism:

Initially, everywhere I went, I would say my name is so-and-so, [and] I am HIV-positive, blah blah blah. . . . I was dealing mostly with stigma and discrimination. Since 2003, I have mainly focused on access-to-treatment issues because it helps me with my previous work. Each week I had to bury two to three people despite the best care. I realized the viral load replication in the body had to be stopped; everything else came second. It couldn't be stopped by counseling or good work or giving people good nutrition. The medicine was there, but it was too expensive. This is the first thing that needs to be stopped. After that, you can deal with the socioeconomic situation, stigma, and discrimination, family, children, and food. . . . Everything else comes second.[158]

In southern Africa, the AIDS and Rights Alliance for Southern Africa (ARASA) runs a twelve-month treatment literacy program that has been training twenty to thirty trainers in each country in the region. Upon completing the program, a new trainer can apply for a grant of about US$10,000–$20,000. The idea is that "you have learned all this stuff. Here is the funding to support you to do this work in the community."[159] South Africa's TAC has garnered worldwide attention for its outstanding advocacy work; it cajoled the government out of denial, and ARV treatment was finally rolled out in 2004. There is a difference between TAC members and members of other social movements, according to TAC's general secretary:

A TAC member is able to articulate, using actual facts. We are taught and trained on how to use the knowledge. That really gave me a new identity. When I came out of that clinic in 2001, my identity changed. I became an HIV-positive young woman with no future, no self-esteem. I had given up on life. I was waiting for my death. The knowledge gave so much to the construction of my new identity. I can give back to my society. I can fight. And if I can fight and mobilize others to fight with me, then the course of my destiny is changed. Once we got treatment, then we decided on what was going to be the next struggle. Now we can live until our eighties, like other people. HIV, yes it lives amongst us, but we need to look for other things. Other things for me were the fact that we learned about this science, about this complicated law stuff. Why are we not going back to school? Why are we not taking back our voices? Why are we not formally affirming ourselves? People are not patients. We are people. As a result, I went back to school because I was diagnosed early. Many were diagnosed early. I went back to school because of treatment literacy. My brain was able to take up so much knowledge.[160]

While access remains an issue of life and death in the Global South, treatment literacy in the North means something quite different. "Treatment literacy has been on our agenda from early days," a researcher from the European AIDS Treatment Group (EATG) says:

> In the early days, it was telling people how to better survive. Then the focus was changed to how to cope with drugs and side effects. Now it has been changed to how to cope with lifelong treatment in the long run. Being an HIV patient has changed over the years. When I got infected, it was a deadly disease. In the late 1990s, we understood we had treatment to probably survive with. Now we have treatment to survive rather well with. If you have a diagnosis today, you don't have to become an activist any more. We have excellent physicians and good regimens. In most countries, you can trust them and leave it there. But still, as you are living with a lifelong disease, adherence can be an issue. There are certain things you can learn as a patient in order to be successful with your treatment. The challenge is reaching all patients [to help them learn] what they need to know.[161]

Treatment literacy created the demand for treatment. But once antiretroviral therapy became available after 1996, it became immediately apparent that the supply in the South was heavily constrained by two things: a global patent system that priced drugs completely out of reach, and a prevailing ideology among Western donors and international AIDS bureaucrats that prevention, not treatment, was the most effective intervention for patients in the South. Treatment advocacy networks such as the International Treatment Preparedness Coalition (ITPC) work with legal networks such as the Lawyers Collective and medical NGOs such as

MSF to keep up the pressure both on Pharma to drop ARV drug prices and on international organizations to commit to universal access.

Since 1996, an enormous amount of treatment activism has been going on in Brazil, Thailand, India, South Africa, and China, with varying degrees of success. It has involved litigation, political lobbying at the WTO, and legal activism to re-form domestic patent laws. In Brazil, "AIDS activists were the first group to ef-fectively equate the constitutional right to health [with] drug access" in what Biehl calls the "judicialization of the right to health."[162] Brazilians living with AIDS first filed lawsuits in 1988 to demand treatment for AIDS-related opportunistic infec-tions and then in 1996 to claim ARV therapies as part of their right to health care and right to life.[163] "Community advocates recognized that opposing HIV-related stigma and discrimination on human rights grounds was imperative," according to Safreed-Harmon. "They also asserted that the right to health implies the right to treatment with the best available drugs. While civil society representatives en-gaged in dialogue with government agencies, they also pursued their rights-based goals through the legal system."[164]

At the same time, at the global level, a coalition of treatment advocates led by MSF, ACT UP, Health GAP, the Consumer Project on Technology, and Oxfam suc-cessfully lobbied for a public health clause in the TRIPS agreement that would affirm governments' right to use the agreement's flexibilities to protect public health. The Doha Declaration sets two specific tasks: "The TRIPS Council has to find a solution to the problems countries may face in making use of compul-sory licensing if they have too little or no pharmaceutical manufacturing capac-ity. . . . The declaration also extends the deadline for least-developed countries to apply provisions on pharmaceutical patents until 1 January 2016."[165] The Doha Declaration opened up a legal and political opportunity to challenge the interna-tional patent system. But the footwork—educating and lobbying governments to amend their national patent laws to take full advantage of TRIPS flexibilities, fight-ing Big Pharma when it takes or threatens to take national governments to court for issuing compulsory licensing, and filing pre-grant oppositions against new patent applications for old ARV drugs—had to be done country by country, min-istry by ministry, and NGO by NGO to mobilize not only AIDS groups but a broad range of public health organizations that see access to essential medicines as a basic human right. Once the patent hurdle was cleared at the international level, treatment advocates lobbied the activist-oriented Jim Kim, the head of the Global Programme on AIDS in the WHO, to adopt the 3 by 5 Initiative to treat 3 million people in the South by 2005. The target was missed, but treatment scale-up increased tenfold from 400,000 in 2003 to close to 4 million in 2009, and 9 million in 2012. Although 2005 came and went, activists kept up the access-to-treatment campaign and lobbied for universal access in both the 2006 and 2011 Political Declarations on HIV/AIDS.

On the ground in the Global South, where AIDS was in effect a death sentence, it was medical activist groups, such as Partners in Health and MSF, that went into resource-poor settings to provide treatment and, in showing by doing, debunked the prevailing treatment skepticism of donors and international bureaucrats. MSF began treating people living with HIV in the 1990s and started antiretroviral treatment programs in Cameroon, Thailand, and South Africa in 2000. It now operates HIV/AIDS programs in thirty-two countries and provides ARV treatment to more than 100,000 HIV-positive patients—including 7,000 children.[166] MSF has also relentlessly fought against Pharma on the patent bottleneck. "*Untangling the Web of Antiretroviral Price Reductions,* [which is] a very strong systematic analysis of ARV pricing, reviewed and updated every year, is an amazing resource for everyone," says a former staff member of MSF–Hong Kong. "It didn't necessarily change the patent governance structure, but it certainly forced people to make that a priority. By showing that lowest price equals access, it put the patent issue front and center on everyone's plate. Obviously, people are not getting treatment because of the price. MSF has definitely been at the front of the pack in patent activism."[167]

As frontline doctors, MSF has also persistently spoken out on the problems of HIV co-infections; the lack of new drugs in extremely resistant TB, malaria, and hepatitis, which are the major causes of death for HIV-positive adults and children; and the expensive, suboptimal pediatric ARV treatments for children. Above all, MSF programs are testimony to local and national governments that quality treatment is possible, and, when partnered with local AIDS groups, they build demand for treatment from the ground up. According to the national project director of MSF-Beijing, "The biggest impact of the two MSF projects in Nanning, Guangxi, and Xiangfan [now Xiangyang], Hubei, is that patients now know what good treatment is. Give them a model of good, comprehensive, high-quality care, and they can compare it with the government model. In 2008, the MSF model became replicated in forty-five other sites."[168] MSF worked closely with AIDS Care China, a UN Red Ribbon Award–winning, community-based organization that grew from a shelter service for HIV/AIDS patients to a multisite HIV/AIDS care program with Red Ribbon Centers in four Chinese provinces. "AIDS Care China benefited from [the] MSF project," a former staff member of MSF–Hong Kong explains:

All the MSF patients would go to the Red Ribbon Center next to MSF for counseling, follow-up, and peer support. After MSF passed on its program to the government, AIDS Care China moved into the MSF building. Part of what makes people respect Thomas [Cai, the founder of AIDS Care China] is that the Red Ribbon Centers had access to MSF resources, not so much money but pediatric medicines that all of us were smuggling into China by literally carrying them in backpacks from Hong Kong to the MSF clinic. Thomas's focus is very different from the previous generation of AIDS activists. He has been building up the base by educating people about treatment.[169]

Sustainable Funding

The same activists who built the global access-to-treatment movement saw AIDS funding as an integral part of a human rights response to AIDS. In 1992, the Treatment Action Group, which split off from ACT UP, exposed the US government's inadequate funding of AIDS research in the pioneering study *AIDS Research at the NIH: A Critical Review*, which led to the NIH Revitalization Act of 1993.[170]

In the late 1990s, an advocacy alliance led by the Global AIDS Alliance, Health GAP, MSF, the African Advocacy Network, and RESULTS was formed to pursue an agenda beyond improving bilateral programs.[171] Specifically, these groups "demanded the creation of multilateral global AIDS mechanisms, dramatic reform of intellectual property laws, and sweeping international debt relief as essential elements of effective global AIDS policy. . . . These groups . . . insist[ed] that funding should be driven by global need rather than U.S. budget constraints ('need versus supply-based demand')."[172] The alliance successfully lobbied for the creation of the Global Fund to Fight AIDS, Tuberculosis, and Malaria in 2002. According to a Health GAP activist:

We were going to get cheap drugs, but who was going to pay for it? There was no money. This whole treatment-versus-prevention thing seemed to me to say that Africans had been used to dying; they should keep on doing that. We just couldn't find any way to get money. So we cooked up from scratch a whole new thing. We built it out of lots of pieces that were lying around. Congresswoman Barbara Lee had passed something called the World Bank AIDS Trust Fund. It was passed into law in the US but had not been funded. The mechanisms had been set up in the World Bank for donors to do something about AIDS somehow. UNICEF had a system in place to do distribution [of] medicines. There was a [group] of people gathered around Jeffrey Sachs in the WHO that got a bit of momentum on some kind of AIDS fund thing that subsequently became the Global Fund. Jim Kim had something called the TD Green Committee that would approve medicines and ship them around. When 1999 turned into 2000, a whole bunch of things had to be put in place before the Global Fund could be created. Clinton felt that this AIDS thing was giving him a lot of trouble and wanted Kofi [Annan] to do something. He put some White Iowa kid, probably a political favor, who knew nothing to be in charge of the AIDS thing in Kofi's office. Whom did he call? He called the protestors, who said you have to put together this Global Fund thing. We wrote Kofi Annan's speech for him that he gave in Abuja that called for the creation of the Global Fund. It's like verbatim, cut and paste. It's me and my colleague from Health GAP. We drafted the talking points that became the [director-general]'s speech.[173]

The same advocacy alliance also pushed for a "complete reversal of [the US] position that antiretroviral (ARV) treatment was unaffordable, unwarranted, and unfeasible to administer in developing countries" through the establishment in 2003 of PEPFAR, a $15 billion initiative on AIDS in fourteen African and Caribbean countries:

> The Global AIDS Roundtable, which is comprised of approximately 100 organizations and staffed by the Global Health Council, was actively involved in most aspects of the U.S. global HIV/AIDS policy debate. In fact, the chief executive officers of two of the roundtable groups were included in private White House discussions that preceded the president's State of the Union announcement. The Roundtable then employed a substantial advocacy campaign to modify and pass the United States Leadership Against HIV/AIDS, Tuberculosis, and Malaria Act of 2003. Among their priorities were: substantial increases in overall funding for global AIDS programs; ensuring that global HIV/AIDS funding was new money, rather than shifting funds from other global health and development accounts; strong U.S. funding for the Global Fund; and programs that target orphans and vulnerable children (OVC) as well as mother-to-child transmission (MTCT).[174]

Between 2003 and 2008, the US Congress appropriated $19 billion for PEPFAR, and another $48 billion was committed till 2013 through the US Global Leadership against HIV/AIDS, Tuberculosis, and Malaria Reauthorization Act of 2008, sponsored by Tom Lantos and Henry Hyde.[175] Since 2002, the Global Fund has committed $30 billion for prevention and treatment programs in 151 countries.[176] The total funding commitment to AIDS is unparalleled in the history of any disease. The executive director of the Canadian HIV/AIDS Legal Network remarks:

One of the most significant impacts of AIDS activism is the money [that] has been mobilized for the AIDS response. The money wouldn't have existed. That is a huge achievement of civil society. I think civil society has also most often been the source of work that shifted the paradigm and exploded the notion of what is acceptable and feasible. It's because civil society didn't just accept [that] millions of people in the South [were] not going to get treatment because it's too costly. . . . Things have been changed extraordinarily. . . . And they happened only because civil society has been constantly pressuring. There [would have been] no Global Fund without civil society pressure. There were Kofi Annan and some governments, but without civil society, it wouldn't be there.[177]

GIPA: Greater Involvement of People Living with HIV and AIDS

AIDS activists not only fought for nondiscrimination, access to drugs, and sustainable funding, but also insisted from the very beginning that they be at the center of the AIDS response. The idea of having people living with HIV participate in all aspects of policymaking and programming did not originate from a legal scholar or from the UN's High Commissioner for Human Rights. It came out of AIDS activists' early protests against government indifference and scientific control, and culminated in the historic Denver Principles, which were formulated at a gay and lesbian health conference in 1983: "We condemn attempts to label us as 'victims,' a term which implies defeat, and we are only occasionally 'patients,' a term which implies passivity, helplessness, and dependence upon the care of others. We are 'People With AIDS.' "[178] The basic human rights principles of nondiscrimination, right to health, right to work and housing, right to privacy and sexuality, and participation in treatment and decision making were clearly articulated.[179] The GIPA principle—"a greater involvement of people living with HIV/AIDS through an initiative to strengthen the capacity and coordination of networks of people living with HIV/AIDS and community-based organizations"[180]—was finally recognized by some governments at the Paris AIDS Summit in 1994 and was formally adopted by UNAIDS in 1997.

One of the first steps taken by AIDS activism to ensure the implementation of GIPA as meaningful involvement rather than token participation was the creation of alliances of people living with HIV and AIDS. The Global Network of People Living with HIV/AIDS (GNP+) was created in 1986 to focus on access to treatment, care, and prevention; opposition to stigma and discrimination; and greater involvement of people living with HIV.[181] According to a technical support officer, GNP+ has been most effective in giving voice, increasing representation, and advocacy.[182] It helped to found six independent regional networks of people living with AIDS in Africa, Asia and the Pacific, the Caribbean, Europe, Latin America, and North America. One of the most recent initiatives, the HIV Leadership through Accountability program (2009–2014), involves national networks of PWAs in fifteen countries that are developing and implementing reporting tools to monitor the implementation of GIPA—the Stigma Index, the GIPA Report Card, the Global Criminalization Scan, and Human Rights Count!—and a guidance package for sexual and reproductive health and rights.[183] A large body of qualitative and quantitative evidence of human rights violations has been generated for PWAs to use for advocacy purpose.[184] GNP+ has also been instrumental in ensuring community input into the WHO's antiretroviral guidelines.[185]

The International Community of Women Living with HIV/AIDS (ICW) was created in 1992 out of frustration that an international meeting of GNP+ the year before "was a gathering of and for men: their reality, the issues they faced were discussed. It was also them who made all decisions."[186] Its Twelve Statements clearly include the human rights principles of nondiscrimination and women's rights, and emphasize, in particular, the omission of women in science and governance; the need for the inclusion of symptoms and clinical manifestations specific to women in any definition of AIDS; and decision-making power at all levels of policy and programs.[187] According to a Steering Committee member:

> Even the very existence of ICW—the fact that we have [the] membership of positive women around the world—should be considered as a success. We have brought so much to the table. At the beginning, anything said about women was only lip service. Then the talk was all about pregnant women and how to save the children. . . . We had to fight to get women on clinical trials. Then we looked at the determinants of health for women, lobbied for more funding, and we ended up trying to infiltrate into UNAIDS and WHO. We fought very hard for women, successfully to a degree. The most important was getting references to women in the Declaration of Commitment on HIV/AIDS in UNGASS.[188]

The ICW and GNP+ have joined hands numerous times to advocate for policy changes based on GIPA. Along with networks of people who use drugs, they successfully lobbied the WHO to include methadone on its Model List of Essential Medicines and to add a new section for medicines used for substance dependence after the historic meeting in 2004 with Lee Jong-wook, the first of its kind between the director-general of WHO and people living with HIV.[189] The following year, they issued the joint "Position Statement: Injecting Drug Users and Access to HIV Treatment," which advocated for harm reduction strategies.[190]

Between 2010 and 2011, GNP+ and ICW held a series of consultations with people living with HIV that influenced the strategic framework of the Interagency Task Team on Prevention of HIV Infection in Pregnant Women, Mothers, and Their Children.[191] The GIPA principle has now been widely recognized and adopted by various marginalized groups, including injecting drug users and sex workers.[192]

Shared, Rights-Based Governance

People living with AIDS did not ask to be at the center of only their local community's response; meaningful participation means having a seat at the science, Pharma, and governance tables too. More than any other social movement—the environment, women's rights, children's rights, LGBT rights, torture and arbitrary detention, migrants' rights, indigenous people's rights, and disability, all the subjects of UN human rights conferences in the past three decades—the AIDS movement has made unprecedented headway in a closed global health governance system defined by a postwar regime of international cooperation based on nation-states.[193] People living with AIDS are represented on the Programme Coordinating Board of UNAIDS (without voting rights) and the board of the Global Fund (with voting rights). The Country Coordinating Mechanism (CCM) mandated by the Global Fund also requires the representation of civil society and of people living with the three diseases (TB, malaria, and AIDS). And there are a number of consultative mechanisms, such as the UNAIDS Advisory Group on HIV and Sex Work and the Interagency Task Teams on HIV, which work with young people and children.

Participation is not the same as equality, however. Global AIDS governance structures vary in their receptivity to civil society participation and influence. UNODC does not recognize activists' role in the same way as UNAIDS does. WHO might be open to the inclusion of methadone in its Model List of Essential Medicines but is nonetheless firmly entrenched in a member-state structure. Above all, despite a rhetoric of engagement, most NGOs and CBOs, with the exception of big international ones, lack the capacity to participate meaningfully. In 2005, GNP+ published a guide on tools for strengthening PLHIV involvement in the Global Fund's Country Coordinating Mechanisms based on the contributions of 400 people living with AIDS in thirty countries.[194] Despite the limits and pitfalls of constructing a shared, rights-based governance structure, a subject to which I return in chapter 5, we can conclude that AIDS activism has been "hugely influential in driving accountability. Now it is hard to imagine not . . . includ[ing] civil society [representatives] on board structures. It doesn't mean it wasn't lip service. But pluralism has been created by civil society involvement, by bringing different players together."[195]

Human Rights Challenges

It is much easier to blame a certain "key population" than to pinpoint the failures of donors, governments, or international organizations. The challenges of a human rights approach to AIDS are myriad. The boundaries of an AIDS response stretch beyond public health to include trade, finance, public order, security, immigration, labor, and education. For most people, the AIDS–human rights links are far from obvious. Justifications constantly need to be made for the invocation of a specific right in defense of people living with AIDS, whether in court or at a scientific debate. Politically, rights-based claims attract government objections as domestic interference, Western imperialism, anti-government activities, or irrelevant. As the special rapporteur on the right to health laments, governments have used different ways to criticize his outspoken reports on the diverse issues of discrimination experienced by people living with AIDS:

> They say it's outside my mandate. They say certain issues such as decriminalizing homosexuality are not internationally accepted human rights standards and hence discrimination could not be said to exist. I say criminalization stigmatizes and discriminates and therefore impedes access. Some accept that these are issues but say that I should prioritize other issues, e.g., HIV. They ask, why should I talk about gay rights? But in the same report, I talk about HIV. These criticisms do not carry weight; they lack substance. They cannot say that abortion is not a health issue; it doesn't make sense. . . . Another issue is that it [is] easy to accuse developing countries of human rights violations. When you start to attack developed countries, you rock the boat. The West is right; what is wrong with the West? For me, it makes no difference whether it's developed or developing countries. Human rights mean[s] upholding certain standards.[196]

Human rights activists are subject to arrest and harassment. The Health and Discrimination Project manager of the Egyptian Initiative for Personal Rights says: "The difficulties of being human rights defenders in a repressive regime are that sometimes we get calls from state security, now national security. They are not open threats. But there is [a] risk of government repression. There are all kinds of harassment and troubles. You go to a hotel and reserve a room, but it gets canceled all of a sudden. You are denied [the right to] travel . . . abroad."[197] Moralistic and sociopolitical forces continue to impede the basic rights of marginalized populations, for example, the anti-prostitution pledge under PEPFAR, the continuous war on drugs, and the archaic anti-sodomy laws still in effect in over forty former British colonies. Economically, efficiency arguments have been made time and again "against national and international human rights obligations to meet the rights to health and non-discrimination; the[re is a] feeling that AIDS advocacy has resulted in disproportionate funding for HIV compared to other health threats and that it is unjust or unethical to spend resources on AIDS treatment."[198] Meanwhile, human rights are assumed only for certain categories of social groups, and the Holy See and a handful of Middle Eastern countries have systematically blocked effective AIDS prevention strategies, such as condom use.[199]

A human rights framework also demands a painstaking process of education, so that people know and can demand their rights. Unfortunately, human rights advocacy work is often the first target of budget austerity. In 2012, the Canadian HIV/AIDS Legal Network had two-thirds of its funding cut by Health Canada and the Public Health Agency of Canada because "[i]t was unclear from the details provided in the proposal whether the resource would be used for advocacy purposes, which is ineligible for funding."[200] Many NGOs experience a "real capacity gap between responding to human rights violations and finding lawyers to assist."[201]

Tactically, AIDS activists continue to struggle with whether and how to use a rights framework. The executive director of the Asia Pacific Network of Sex Workers finds that "a labor rights framework is more useful. . . . There is no use for us to fight for human rights because human rights only apply to people with status as equal humans. Sex workers are not treated as equal before the law."[202] In China, human rights and AIDS activists tread a fine line:

> There is a lot you can do, for example, on gender, children, environment, and labor. . . . But there is also a lot you can't do, like [concerning] Falun Gong and Tibet, etc. We don't know whether we will face problems, but we know which areas are particularly sensitive. Our approach is to talk about human rights problems in China, and through television and magazines introduce human rights concepts. We also introduce international human rights law. . . . Human rights are universal, but often Chinese tend to divide them into two groups. On the one end, for the Chinese government, human rights are politicized by the US. On the other, Chinese liberals think the US is a human rights paradise. For us, both are wrong: there are lots of human rights issues in China as well as in the US. We criticize both. If we criticize only China, we will be accused of [the wrong] political inclination. So we use examples from both China and the US. . . . When it comes to human rights issues, it is easier to work through international NGOs [INGOs]. Once, we invited

someone from [the] AIDS Law Project in South Africa to come to China. Through his meeting with the representatives of the Chinese government, we could raise some rights issues. So sometimes we . . . organize activities with IN-GOs or UN agencies and use those as a platform to raise some issues.[203]

When human rights approaches are used, activists have to search for locally acceptable language. The executive director of the Russian Harm Reduction Network explains:

> The problem is that if we try to have dialogue with the government, we should not use the word "harm reduction" too much, as of now. . . . In this context, we have to use the terminology that is accepted in the country and that is understandable and clear to decision makers. That's why we try not to focus on the two words of harm reduction, but on the content [of] what we are doing: this is voluntary counseling and testing, provision of sterile equipment and condoms, referral to treatment; this is legal help; this is shelter; this is drop-in centers. We focus on the type of services we provide.[204]

Scientists might have been happy to keep AIDS narrowly contained in a disease model where the at-risk body is a subject of surveillance and control. But from ACT UP to ITPC, from the Lawyers Collective to MSF, AIDS activists' insertion of a human rights approach into science has radically transformed the understanding of HIV, which has moved from an epidemiological model based on individual behavior to an emphasis on human rights violations that increase vulnerability, including discriminatory laws, barriers to access to treatment, funding shortages, lack of genuine participation, and closed governance structures. As the seminal 2012 report of the Global Commission on HIV and the Law, *HIV and the Law: Risks, Rights, and Health,* concludes, the end of the global AIDS epidemic is within reach, but that goal will only be possible if science is accompanied by a tangible commitment to human rights.[205]

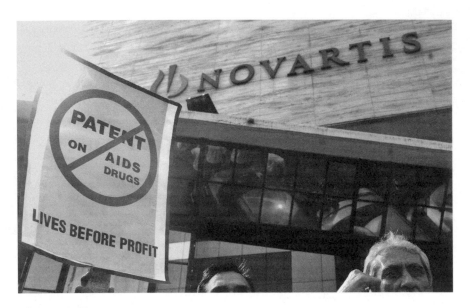

Photo © Guddu

CHAPTER THREE

Against Pharma and the Intellectual Propertization of Life

There is an economic war going on. This is a great opportunity
for the Indian . . . generic companies to conquer the world. If
they could just get rid of our patents then the whole developing
world would open up to them. So this is an economic war.
There are a couple of pirate companies who want to undermine
the patent system. . . . This is the first time there is a genuine
risk that intellectual property would disappear in the
developing world.
　　—Jean-Pierre Garnier, CEO, GlaxoSmithKline

Can you even begin to imagine how a doctor feels when he knows
there is treatment for a merciless disease but no way to get it to your
patients simply because of its cost?
　　—Peter Mugenyi, who runs an AIDS clinic
　　　　　　in Kampala, Uganda

There is a crime being committed here! You cannot have 42 million
people dying and have the issue be about money!
　　—Chatinkha Nkhoma, AIDS Activist, Malawi

In 2002, more than twenty years into the AIDS epidemic, only 300,000 people
in low- and middle-income countries were receiving ARV therapy. By the end of
that decade, the figure had risen to 6.5 million, an increase of more than twenty-
fold, but 9 million people were still waiting in line for treatment.[1] This chapter focuses on the AIDS activists' battles that produced this dramatic treatment
scale-up. We travel from the campaign trails of US presidential elections, to national ministries of health and trade, to patent offices in Thailand, Brazil, South
Africa, India, and China, and to the boardrooms of Big Pharma and the WTO,

in the tumultuous decade and a half between 1996, when ARV therapy proved to be effective in controlling HIV, and 2010, when the retreat of donors translated into decreases in funding for treatment.[2]

Like the circulation of the various at-risk narratives examined in chapter 2, I look at the treatment-access battle as competing "property stories" by different regimes of power and at the activists' fight against the market and the intellectual propertization of life.[3] Has Pharma been committing a crime, killing people through its IP monopoly, as the activists claim? Is generic competition a global economic and trade war, as the pharmaceutical companies claim to the media and the WTO? Squeezed in the middle of this David versus Goliath fight, how have international organizations, such as UNAIDS, WHO, and UNITAID, and national governments been navigating the access issue? What were the conditions and decisions that made it possible for essential medicines to be turned into intellectual property? What contests for meaning arise when activists and governments position themselves as knowledge owners against the monopolistic control of Pharma, and how have these contests been resolved?

According to McSherry, intellectual property stories "both speak to and constitute moral communities by setting up shared principles and assumptions that make origin stories seem like common sense. For this common sense to be maintained, property stories must be continually retold, and that retelling must assume and construct an audience."[4] I look at the construction and circulation of property stories at three different levels. First, I examine the emergence of a global IP regime through the WTO TRIPS agreement and other TRIPS-plus measures that Pharma has been pushing through a variety of carrot-and-stick measures. Then I analyze the access battles in the Big Five countries—Thailand, Brazil, South Africa, India, and China—focusing on four key ARV drugs: efavirenz (EFV), tenofovir (TDF), lamivudine (3TC), and lopinavir/ritonavir (LPV/r). Finally, I look at the creation and the effects of the Medicines Patent Pool, a compromise between a private property rights regime and public health interests. At the center of these analyses are broad questions of knowledge control and legitimation: Who holds the power to define patentability and innovation, and on what terms? Do innovation versus access and profits versus public health represent false dichotomies? How can the rights of the "public" be continually argued for, and do they need to be justified in the shadow of the market?

Trade Fetishization: Neo-Imperialism,
Third World Pirates, or Mass Murderers?

There is nothing in the WTO intellectual property agreement
which prevents or discourages the use of generic drugs. . . . Parallel
importing (and compulsory licensing) are clearly allowed under the
WTO's intellectual property agreement, particularly in national
emergencies. South Africa has cited these rules.
        —*World Trade Organization*[5]

A growing body of international trade law and the over-reach of
intellectual property (IP) protections are impeding the production
and distribution of low-cost generic drugs. IP protection is
supposed to provide an incentive for innovation but experience has
shown that the current laws are failing to promote innovation that
serves the medical needs of the poor.
    —*Global Commission on HIV and the Law*, HIV
        and the Law: Risks, Rights, and Health[6]

Scratch the surface and the AIDS access battle reveals a single, ugly
motive: profit.
    —*Anne-Christine D'Adesky*, Moving Mountains:
        The Race to Treat Global AIDS[7]

The World Trade Organization, created in 1995, replaced the General Agreement on Tariffs and Trade, as "the international organization whose primary purpose is to open trade for the benefit of all" through a system of various agreements
and a forum for trade negotiations and dispute settlements.[8] Its founding and
guiding principles are "the pursuit of open borders, . . . non-discriminatory treatment by and among members, and a commitment to transparency . . . [that]
contribute to sustainable development, raise people's welfare, reduce poverty,
and foster peace and stability."[9] According to the former director-general, Mike
Moore, the WTO represents the deepening institutionalization of a specific
economic and trade regime:

The "trade" agenda . . . has grown inexorably since 1980. In an initial stage, trade
negotiations moved from addressing border measures that represented obstacles to
trade in goods to behind-the-border measures such as non-tariff barriers or technical barriers to trade. The Uruguay Round took this development one stage further by taking up issues such as trade in services and intellectual property rights

(TRIPS) and opening the door on foreign direct investment (FDI). The Doha Declaration may extend this process even further to include competition.[10]

WTO critics, however, argue that the free trade doctrine based on a "gains from trade" assumption is "more about religion than science."[11] They object to the colonialist development mentality espoused in the WTO:

> The development problem of the less developed countries is one of converting a "traditional" society predominantly based on subsistence or near-subsistence agriculture and/or the bulk export of a few primary commodities, in which per capita income grows slowly or may even be declining as a result of population pressure, into a "modern" society in which growth per capita income is internalized in the social and economic system through automatic mechanisms promoting accumulation of capital, improvement of technology, and growth of skill of the labor force.[12]

For the majority of the developing countries that are members of the WTO (117 out of 157), market expansion through the removal of trade obstacles has sidestepped their poverty concerns. They ask the legitimate question, whose WTO is it? They challenge the continually expanding trade agenda that focuses on the interests and existing rules of high-income countries, the trade barriers whose removal would stimulate growth that would help the poor in low-income countries, and the complex rules and negotiations that are often beyond the capacity of low-income countries.[13]

In response to the Seattle generation of activists, who deconstruct its "free trade *über alles*" ideology, the WTO launched a development round at its fourth ministerial meeting in Doha, Qatar, in 2001 to demonstrate to the world that "the WTO is not just about opening markets, and in some circumstances its rules support maintaining trade barriers—for example, to protect consumers or prevent the spread of disease." The organization promised to be "more beneficial for less developed countries" by "permit[ting] members to take measures to protect not only the environment but also public health."[14]

While the WTO had originally focused on the liberalization of trade in goods and services, a global intellectual property regime became integrated and normalized when twelve men representing the pharmaceutical, entertainment, and software industries on the US-based ad hoc Intellectual Property Committee, together with their European and Japanese counterparts, crafted a proposal based on industrialized countries' existing patent laws and presented it to the secretariat of the General Agreement on Tariffs and Trade in 1988. Six years later, these "twelve incredibly efficacious individuals . . . succeeded in getting most of what they wanted from a global IP agreement, which now has the status of public international law."[15]

The TRIPS agreement, by granting a monopoly to a patent holder for a period of twenty years, "represents a harmonisation of patent laws. The industry had been pushing for this kind of move for decades. It's a one-size-fits-all policy that aims at extending the stricter patenting laws previously used in industrialised countries to developing countries, regardless of their radically different social and economic conditions."[16] TRIPS was based on two assumptions for improving incentives, first, "for companies to develop technologies," and second, for "licensing those technologies in countries that have weak IP protection."[17]

In AIDS, however, these assumptions do not hold. Countries such as India, South Africa, Thailand, Brazil, and China have developed indigenous technological capabilities to develop generic versions of ARV drugs and do not require foreign direct investment to license Western technologies. On the contrary, being TRIPS-compliant since 2005 (2016 for the least-developed countries) has forced these and other countries to amend their laws to observe global patent laws, which has had a "considerable impact on access to medicines and public health [b]y limiting competition and local manufacturing."[18]

Above all, as negotiations for the Doha development round stalled, the United States and the European Union pushed for stricter patenting measures, known as TRIPS-plus provisions, in bilateral and regional free trade agreements (FTAs). Common examples include more stringent restrictions on compulsory licensing and parallel importing, patent extensions beyond the twenty-year minimum, data exclusivity, and patent linkage. While TRIPS leaves it to each WTO member to determine when and for what reasons it needs to grant a compulsory license, US-initiated free trade agreements "may limit the situations in which a compulsory license can be issued to three: government use, national emergency or circumstances of extreme urgency, and to correct practices found to be anti-competitive."[19] TRIPS allows a country to import a patented medicine from another country where it is cheaper. In bilateral FTAs, however, "countries may be pressured to effectively stop parallel importation."[20]

Two TRIPS-plus measures have attracted a great deal of criticism among AIDS activists. Data exclusivity, which grants exclusive rights over the test data submitted by companies to drug regulatory authorities for market authorization, is considered by MSF to be "a backdoor way of preventing competition, so that even when a medicine is not protected by a patent, a pharmaceutical company will receive a minimum period of market monopoly when artificially high prices can be charged."[21] When a generic manufacturer wants to register a drug in a country, "it must either sit out the exclusivity period, or take the route of repeating lengthy clinical trials to demonstrate the safety and efficacy of the drug—trials that have already been undertaken. This happens even when the originator product is not patented."[22] Meanwhile, patent linkage, which requires that the approval of a drug's registration be linked to its patent status, "would mean that a generic medicine imported or manufactured under compulsory license may not be able to be registered until the patent has expired."[23] In the Thai-EU FTA negotiations, for example, the European Union pushed for five years of data exclusivity, a provision accepted by the Thai Department of Trade Negotiation despite AIDS activists' contention that data exclusivity is a life-and-death issue. By delaying a generic medicine's entry into the market and inflating drug costs, essential medicines become inaccessible.[24] The WHO and UNAIDS have recommended that developing countries not incorporate data exclusivity into their national laws due to its detrimental impact on access. For example, a 2007 study by Oxfam found that out of 103 medicines registered in Jordan since 2001 that had no patent protection, at least 79% had no competition from a generic equivalent because Jordan had implemented data exclusivity as part of the US-Jordan FTA. The study also confirmed that the prices of medicines under data exclusivity were up to eight times higher in Jordan than in neighboring Egypt.[25]

In addition to TRIPS and TRIPS-plus, Pharma has used a wide range of carrot-and-stick measures to publicize its "goodwill" toward public health, on the one hand, and its readiness to punish those who challenge the overall IP hegemony, on the other. After the Seattle demonstrations and the Drop the Debt Jubilee Campaign in 2000, five pharmaceutical companies partnered with five UN organizations in the Accelerating Access Initiative to provide deeply discounted drugs to the least-developed countries, while "that same month they backed a WTO complaint to prevent Brazil from acquiring and making generics, and two months later revived their lawsuit against South Africa."[26] When lawsuits or WTO complaints were dropped due to public pressure, as in the case of South Africa, Brazil, and Thailand, the US trade representative threatened trade sanctions to ensure compliance. So far, few countries have moved to adopt Brazil's model of generic production, probably due to fear.[27] As a preemptive measure to maintain market dominance, a number of pharmaceutical companies have also been aggressively buying out or merging with local companies, notably in India.[28] Further, Pharma increasingly has entered into voluntary licensing agreements with local generic producers in its bid to expand access while still controlling the market. Since 2006, Gilead, for example, has signed agreements with various Indian partners, pushing the lowest available price of a Gilead antiretroviral to $74 pppy, which is comparable to generic prices.[29] The devil of such agreements, however, is in the details. When he approached Johnson and Johnson in 2011 for a voluntary license to manufacture rilpivirine, the CEO of Cipla, Yusuf Hamied, notes:

> They [were] willing to give me a license on their terms, not my terms. My terms are, I will manufacture the API [active pharmaceutical ingredients]. I will pay them a royalty on sales in those countries where they have valid patents. If they don't have valid patents in those countries, I won't pay them [a] royalty. In India if they have a valid patent I am willing to pay them a royalty on my raw material that I am exporting to Uganda. But Uganda has no patents on the drug, so I can't pay them a royalty there. I'm paying them a royalty on my bulk in India. I will not encroach, until the patents expire, in the regulated markets of the US, Canada, Europe, Japan, or Australia. But they cannot stop me from doing it in select countries of Latin America, Southeast Asia, or Africa. They gave me a list of the least developed countries and sa[id], "These are the 90 countries where we will give you permission." No Brazil, no Argentina, and no Chile on the list. So what are they giving me? I do not need their permission to set up in the least developed countries.[30]

Pharma has also pursued global IP protection through a different door in the form of the Anti-Counterfeiting Trade Agreement (ACTA). This "secret treaty" was negotiated with little public input, and the treaty draft was "properly classified in the interest of national security" by the US trade representative's Freedom of Information Office.[31] It was signed by eight countries (Australia, Canada, Japan, Morocco, New Zealand, Singapore, South Korea, and the United States) in 2011 and by Mexico and the European Union in 2012 despite its massive rejection by the European Parliament the summer before (478 against, 39 in favor, and 165 abstaining).[32] Proponents of ACTA argue that it provides "a more effective legal framework to address the problem of counterfeiting and piracy."[33] AIDS activists, however, see ACTA as a blank check for the pharmaceutical companies, allowing overly broad enforcement measures to impede access to qualified generic medicines. By authorizing the border detention of in-transit medicines destined for developing countries, ACTA, according to MSF, is "putting third parties that use medicines at the heart of an enforcement dispute—like distributors and even nongovernmental organisations like MSF, or public health authorities—at risk of severe penalties."[34] It also acts as a deterrent to the production of and trade in generic medicines, since it shifts the risks entirely onto the generic manufacturer and undermines the ability of developing countries to apply the Doha Declaration to protect public health.[35]

In April 2012, the High Court of Kenya ruled in favor of Patricia Asero Ochieng and two other HIV-positive patients that Section 2 (definition of counterfeiting), Section 32 (offenses), and Section 34 (powers of the commissioner to seize suspected counterfeit goods) of Kenya's 2008 Anti-Counterfeit Act are unconstitutional: "There can be no room for ambiguity where the right to health and life of the petitioners and the many other Kenyans who are affected by HIV/AIDS are at stake."[36] As forms of IP protection have proliferated globally, the fight for access to medicines has played out in mass protests and battles in clinics and courtrooms.

Emperor with No Clothes: Evergreening, Frivolous Patenting, and Compulsory Licensing

The ability of many persons with HIV to purchase and take medicines that treat HIV and its attendant illnesses, has a profound and inseparable bearing on the constitutional rights to human dignity and life, and access to health care. In this respect people with HIV are directly dependent on the State's ability to fulfill its constitutional duty to bring about the progressive realization of their rights to health care services.

—*Treatment Action Campaign, affidavit in* Pharmaceutical Manufacturers Association of South Africa v. Government of South Africa[37]

How much is my life worth?

—*Executive Director, ITPC*[38]

If India falls, everyone falls.

—*Advocacy Officer, MSF–New Delhi*[39]

The long battle for AIDS treatment began with ACT UP protesting against Burroughs Wellcome at the New York Stock Exchange in 1989, forcing it to reduce the price of AZT from $10,000 to $6,400 pppy, although that price was still prohibitive for the majority of HIV-positive patients worldwide. "Every death from 1990 and 2000 you can attribute to the patenting of AZT," says Yusuf Hamied, the CEO of Cipla, who marketed AZT in 1993 for under $700 pppy, one-fifth of the prevailing international price.[40] Even after ARV therapy became widely available in the Global North in 1996, little happened concerning treatment in the South. In 1997, French president Jacques Chirac was the first state leader to highlight the global treatment gap by launching the International Therapeutic Solidarity Fund to fund pilot treatment projects in francophone Africa.[41] Two years later, at the Conference on Increasing Access to Essential Drugs in a Globalized Economy, MSF, the Consumer Project on Technology, and Health Action International issued the Amsterdam Statement on Access to Medicines, which framed the access problem as a market failure, which remains true today:

> In the developing world, a lucrative or "viable" market for lifesaving drugs simply does not exist. But clearly what does exist is need. The market has failed both to provide equitably priced medicines and to ensure research and development for infectious diseases. This lack of affordable medicines, and research and development for neglected diseases is causing avoidable human suffering. Market forces alone will not address this need: political action is demanded.[42]

Conference participants called for the creation of a Standing Working Group on Access to Medicines in the upcoming negotiations at the WTO's Seattle meeting later that year and demanded a balance between the rights of patent holders and the rights of citizens in intellectual property rights regulations.[43] The proposals in the Amsterdam Statement on TRIPS flexibilities included compulsory licensing, parallel importing, and differential rules for essential medicines, and they became the blueprint for the subsequent public health clause adopted in Doha in 2001: TRIPS "can and should be interpreted and implemented in a manner supportive of WTO members' right to protect public health, and in particular, to promote access to medicines to all."[44] That same year, MSF launched its Access to Essential Medicines campaign, working with a range of international nongovernmental groups and foundations, including the Third World Network, Health Action International, and the Clinton Foundation, as well as local AIDS advocacy groups in Thailand, India, Brazil, South Africa, and China.

Two months before the 2000 International AIDS Conference in Durban, South Africa, UNAIDS announced that five pharmaceutical companies—Bristol-Myers Squibb, Glaxo Wellcome, Merck, Boehringer Ingelheim, and Roche—had pledged to sell their drugs in Africa "for as little as pennies above manufacturing costs. Some are considering prices as much as 85% or 90% below the prices Americans pay," a move considered by activists to be a preemptive public-relations effort to pacify the angry protestors who were expected to demand drug company concessions.[45] Several companies said that they agreed to take part in this effort only after the WHO director-general, Gro Harlem Brundtland, reassured them in a January speech that intellectual property rights would be protected to stimulate innovation.[46] Despite the dramatic discounts, however, little treatment expansion occurred because of the existing patent structure. Glaxo, for example, said it was willing to offer Combivir, a mixture of AZT and 3TC, for only $2 a day, one-eighth of its US price of $16.50 a day. But long-term AIDS therapy required the addition of at least one other drug, often owned by a competitor, which could drive the treatment price up to $5–$7 a day.[47]

It was Cipla, the Indian generic producer, that ushered in the Global South's treatment era in 2001 by selling the world's first triple-drug cocktail, Triomune, at a price of $350 pppy, that is, less than $1 per patient per day, only 3% of the prevailing international price of $12,000 pppy.[48] According to Anand Grover of the Lawyers Collective, "What Cipla did was show everyone that the emperor had no clothes. . . . For years the multinationals claimed it cost so much to make their AIDS drugs, and they were so hard to make. Now we know that it's simply not true. The generics make these drugs for pennies, and they make other drugs too. So the secret is finally out. The truth is, the profits in this industry have been just staggering."[49] Once the pricing bottleneck was gone, the prevention-only ideology removed,[50] and funding secured through the Global Fund and PEPFAR, the access battle was on for national governments to make or buy the cheapest generic ARV drugs for a maximum number of citizens. Four of the drugs—efavirenz, tenofovir, lamivudine, and lopinavir/ritonavir—became frontline targets for AIDS activists in Thailand, Brazil, South Africa, India, and China.

Efavirenz (EFV)

In November 2006, the Thai minister of public health, Mongkol Na Songkhla, announced his decision to issue a compulsory license (CL) for efavirenz, which was followed by a similar move for six other ARV and cancer drugs a couple of months later. His bold decision did not go unnoticed; it encouraged his Brazilian and South African counterparts to follow suit shortly after while it also provoked US trade sanctions and virulent attacks by the Pharmaceutical Research and Manufacturers of America (PhRMA). "How did a small and submissive developing country in the global community become the 'Talk of the Globe' as Jack the Giant Killer? Is this an act of 'intellectual property piracy'? Will it destroy innovation in the world?" a Thai activist asks rhetorically.[51]

Listed in the WHO's Model List of Essential Medicines, efavirenz is one of the most important drugs for first-line and second-line ARV therapy, grossing $1.5 billion in annual sales for its originator, Merck. It is recommended in the 2010 WHO guidelines as a preferred first-line treatment in conjunction with two other drugs, one of which should be zidovudine (AZT) or tenofovir (TDF).[52] It is also recommended as the preferred drug for patients starting ARV therapy while on tuberculosis treatment. Merck held its basic patent between 1993 and 2013, and it has held another patent for the crystallized forms since 1998 (due to expire in 2018). Merck's price for a 600 mg tablet for middle-income countries on its Tier II list ($637) is more than ten times the lowest generic price ($61), making it inaccessible in a lot of countries.[53]

Long before AIDS was on the agenda, Thailand had been under relentless US trade pressure. PhRMA claimed to have lost $165 million in export revenue since 1985 because of weak IP protection in Thailand, and it successfully lobbied to extend drug patent protection from fifteen to twenty years through bilateral trade negotiations. Concerned about the impact of patents for pharmaceutical products, the Thai nongovernmental Drug Study Group carried out a study and found that drug imports would have been 72% more expensive with a product patent system.[54] According to Vichai Chokevivat, the president of the Government Pharmaceutical Organization, "The Drug Patent Act (1979) was fair for us because our level of technology was much lower than that of developed countries. It was fair for us to protect only process patents. But since 1985, we were under pressure to amend the Act to further protect product patents. . . . At the end, we were defeated."[55] In response to US pressure, Thailand amended its Patent Act in 1992, introducing patent protections for pharmaceutical products, thirteen years before the 2005 TRIPS deadline.[56] According to a Thai professor, Jiraporn Limpananont, "Thus, Thailand lost a total of 13 years in which it could have significantly developed its domestic drug industry, producing new generics with their own dosage form preparations and expanding their market to the ASEAN countries. This inability to develop a local pharmaceutical industry with R&D capacity continues to be a major barrier to fight the HIV/AIDS epidemic."[57]

By 1999, an explosive spread of HIV among injecting drug users, sex workers, and men who have sex with men meant over a million people were living with HIV in Thailand, out of which 100,000 required treatment. Only 5% were receiving ARV therapy due to the high cost of imported ARVs. After the first attempt to issue a compulsory license for didanosine (ddI) in 1999 failed because of threats of US trade sanctions, two HIV patients and the AIDS Access Foundation sued Bristol-Myers Squibb (BMS) in 2001 (unsuccessfully) for its overly broad patent coverage. The following year, AIDS patients and the Foundation for Consumers brought another lawsuit against BMS for lack of novelty in its ddI patent application of 1991. The case was settled with BMS " 'dedicating' the ddI patent to the Thai people."[58] In 2002, the Government Pharmaceutical Organization (GPO) took advantage of three expired patents to produce its first generic fixed-dose combination of stavudine, lamivudine, and nevirapine (GPO-VIR), reducing the price to one-sixteenth of its previous cost (1,200 baht per month versus 20,000 baht for the brand-name drug). This made it possible for the National Access to Anti-retroviral Program for People Living with HIV/AIDS to provide free ARV initially to 50,000 patients and then to expand it into a universal access program in 2006.

According to Thai AIDS activists, "Thailand's issuance of the indicated compulsory licenses was not a coincidence. Rather, it was the result of years of endless agitation and advocacy by Thai civil society to get these CLs issued."[59] The executive director of the AIDS Access Foundation explains the shift to a treatment focus and the long road to compulsory licensing:

> For eight years from 1991 to 1999, we worked on prevention. We started to work with PLWHA groups to encourage them to do home care visits. We found that many of them got sick and died after one or two years, and we needed to train new leaders of the PWA groups. We realized that we needed to get good treatment for them. Around 2001, ARV drugs were widely available outside Thailand, but in Thailand, we had little experience [with] ARVs. ARVs were too expensive. We thought if we could negotiate with the government, we could get more affordable treatment. We started to work with MSF on home care visits, and we learned from MSF about treatment. We developed [an] OI [opportunistic infections] treatment curriculum. We thought if we could push community hospital[s] to have more capacity to treat people, it would be good for treatment expansion. We started to learn about the capacity and budget of community hospital[s]. We also tried to convince the government to provide free treatment. Between 2001 and 2003, Thai NGOs looked into [a] Thai patent law that has been there for three decades and yet the flexibility to import ARVs had never been used. We found more allies on this issue. That's when we created a network. We worked with MSF and Oxfam. Oxfam was not working on HIV issues, but they had the Make It Fair campaign, and a lot of issues around the WTO, TRIPS, free trade agreements, and compulsory licensing came out. Between 2004 and 2005, we worked together with TNP+ [Thai Network of of People Living with HIV/AIDS], APN+ [Asia Pacific Network of People Living with HIV/AIDS], MSF, Oxfam, ACT UP, Health GAP, and [the] Lawyers Collective to prepare for compulsory licensing.[60]

In late 2005, the president of TNP+, Kamol Uppakaew, submitted a letter to the minister of public health, urging him to use CL to cut the high medicine prices that prevented the poor from accessing drugs. A subcommittee was set up in the ministry by January 2006, and it researched and passed a resolution calling for a CL to domestically produce efavirenz. If approved by the National Health Security Board, the CL would have saved over a trillion baht (roughly $25 billion) of the government's annual budget and provided coverage for six to twelve times more patients.[61] According to Chokevivat, the Thai government only moved as a last resort to issue compulsory licenses:

> Some patients suffered side effects from taking Nevirapine, one of the components of GPO-VIR. We didn't succeed in negotiating the price of Efavirenz. We tried again in 2004. The MSD Company, the patent holder of the drug, agreed to lower the drug price on condition that the Ministry of Public Health must set up a committee, jointly supervised by the FDA and [the] Department of Internal Trade. But the negotiations came to nothing. So we had to look for an opportunity in the intellectual property laws. It was really our last resort.[62]

The Thai Ministry of Public Health and the National Health Security Office explained in February 2007 that "the rationale mainly lies in the mandate to achieve universal access to essential medicine for all Thais, under the National Health Security Act 2002. . . . [The move was] in full compliance with the Thai national and the international legal framework."[63] Merck filed an appeal with the Thai Department of Intellectual Property, arguing that the Ministry of Public Health's compulsory licensing did not follow legal procedures, since no prior negotiations with the patent holder had been held. Abbott apparently offered to reduce the price of Kaletra in exchange for the TNP+'s lobbying of the Ministry of Public Health to cancel the CL. PhRMA denounced the move and threatened to suspend its investment in Thailand.[64] The USTR put Thailand on the "Special 301" Priority Watch List for the following reasons: "While the United States acknowledge[s] a country's ability to issue such licenses in accordance with WTO rules, the lack of transparency and due process exhibited in Thailand represents a serious concern. These concerns have compounded previously expressed concerns such as delay in the granting of patents and weak protection against unfair commercial use for data generated to obtain marketing approval."[65] Ambassadors of the United States, the European Union, France, and Switzerland all signaled their disapproval of Thailand's move.

Seven months later, in May 2007, Brazil followed suit and announced its CL on efavirenz. Touted as one of the greatest AIDS success stories, Brazil adopted a universal access program as early as 1996 and began the local production of ARVs the following year, greatly reducing drug costs. In 1998, the Brazilian minister of public health proposed universal access to AIDS treatment as a human right at the International AIDS Conference in Geneva.[66]

The IP battle in Brazil was little different from the Thai experience. It began with US trade pressure on Brazil to upgrade its patent protection regime. During President Fernando Cardoso's visit to the United States in 1995, PhRMA ran a smear campaign in the *New York Times* and the *Wall Street Journal*, trying to shame Brazil as the "country of pirated patents."[67] The Clinton administration made it clear that Brazil was already on the "Special 301" list. Brazil subsequently adopted the Industry Property Law, which went into effect in 1997, eight years ahead of its 2005 WTO obligation, mandating pharmaceutical product and process patents for drugs introduced after 1997. In 2001, the USTR filed a complaint (labeled as the *Merck* case) in the WTO Dispute Settlement Board concerning Article 68 of Brazil's patent law, which allowed for the compulsory licensing of any drug when its patent holder does not manufacture locally. After considerable negative publicity, the USTR withdrew the complaint, but Brazil agreed to provide the United States with advance notice of any compulsory licenses.[68]

In 2003, Brazil issued a public decree allowing for the local production or import of efavirenz, lopinavir, and nelfinavir without the patent holders' consent after it had failed to obtain a 40% discount on antiretrovirals from pharmaceutical companies (it was offered a maximum reduction of 6.7%).[69] By 2006, efavirenz was used by 38% (75,000) of all patients in treatment. The Merck price for Brazil was $580 pppy, compared to $164 pppy (28%) for the generic drug produced by Indian companies.[70] Even after a proposed discount of 30%, the Merck price was still three times the cost of the Indian generic, which prompted the Brazilian government to issue a CL. According to the former director of the Brazilian HIV/AIDS Program:

> The first battle for efavirenz began in 1999. The then minister of health, Jose Serre, who was an economist, was very committed to public goods. He said, "I need concrete evidence of costs and benefits of this license." He became the strongest supporter of [the] AIDS problem in Brazil. He went to Doha during the WTO discussion and presented the declaration for discussion. He called me and asked, "I want to know what the capacity is for state companies to produce ARVs." The conclusion was that Brazil was able to produce efavirenz. He decided to raise the issue with the company: "If there is not [an] excellent price, we will produce locally." The company promised [a] voluntary license in 2002, but they never did [it]. When I came back in 2004, I took part in the discussion for voluntary licensing. Finally, under Jose Temporao as the minister of health of the Lula administration, the compulsory license was issued. There was a lot of noise afterwards. But in real life, nothing happened. There was no violation of international law. We only used TRIPS flexibilities.[71]

The US Chamber of Commerce condemned the move: "Breaking off discussions with Merck and seizing its intellectual property sends a dangerous signal to the investment community. Merck researchers invested hundreds of millions of dollars to develop this ground-breaking medicine."[72] The *Economist* saw it as a "conflict of goals," helping patients but hurting science.[73] In 2007 alone, using unbranded efavirenz saved Brazil $30 million.[74]

Six months after Brazil issued a CL on efavirenz, the AIDS Law Project, acting on behalf of the Treatment Action Campaign, filed a complaint with the South African Competition Commission in November 2007, alleging that Merck was acting unlawfully and in an anticompetitive way by refusing to license EFV to local producers on reasonable terms. As part of the settlement,[75] Merck licensed four generic drug companies to bring stand-alone, co-packaged or co-formulated EFV products to market. Before these agreements, the EFV patent did not allow any company other than Merck to bring EFV products to market, which had resulted in high prices for co-packaged and co-formulated products involving EFV and other ARV drugs, such as AZT and TDF. AZT was no longer under patent protection, and TDF was never patented in South Africa, so EFV was the only patent barrier that prevented much-needed combination products from being sold in South Africa.[76] The IP victory saved $87.25 pppy: Merck's best international price was $237.25 in contrast to the best international generic price of $150 pppy. The savings for fixed-dose combinations were even more significant. The Clinton Foundation's HIV/AIDS Initiative managed to secure a commitment from an Indian generic company to bring the generic TDF/FTC/EFV to market for $349 pppy, compared to $613.20 for the Merck version.[77]

In India, Merck does not hold a product patent on efavirenz, but a process patent for the preparation of crystalline EFV was granted in 2005, to which representatives of Indian civil society have filed a post-grant opposition. Meanwhile, Gilead applied for a patent for a once-a-day pill combination of EFV, tenofovir, and emtricitabine (TDF/FTC/EFV), which was rejected by the Indian Patent Office in 2009 on the ground that combinations of known medicines are not patentable under its law.[78] But the threat remains since Gilead has filed several divisional applications. BMS has also filed for a patent for its once-a-day pill of TDF/FTC/EFV, to which Cipla filed a pre-grant opposition in 2010.[79] As of 2012, nine generic sources of EFV (600 mg tablet) were quality assured by either the US FDA or WHO prequalification. The impact of global AIDS activism against Merck's monopoly on EFV has been significant: the originator's price went down by 32% and the generic price by more than 90% in the decade between 2002 and 2012.[80]

Tenofovir (TDF)

After Brazil challenged Merck by issuing a compulsory license on efavirenz, its patent office in 2008 rejected Gilead's patent application for tenofovir on the grounds that it lacked inventiveness. TDF is an extremely important ARV drug, which in 2011 brought in $738 million for its originator, Gilead. It has formed the backbone for first-line treatment ever since WHO in its 2009 guidelines recommended that countries phase out stavudine-based regimens because of irreversible side effects. It is also the recommended ARV for second-line treatment in combination with lamivudine (3TC) or emtricitabine (FTC) if patients become resistant to stavudine or zidovudine. Further, TDF is used to treat hepatitis B patients and therefore plays an important role in countries with large hepatitis B and HIV co-infections, such as China. In 2009, the US FDA granted TDF an "orphan drug" designation (meaning that it is used for the prevention, diagnosis, or treatment of a rare disease) for pediatric use. Gilead is entitled to seven years of marketing exclusivity as well as tax credits for clinical research.[81]

In December 2002, Gilead announced an access program that would offer TDF at discounted prices for sixty-eight developing countries, which increased to ninety-seven in 2005; it did not include middle-income countries like Brazil, China, and Thailand. According to MSF, however, the discounts exist in name only, and TDF has remained unavailable in most countries covered in Gilead's access program.[82] The problem is that TDF was registered in only six of the ninety-seven eligible countries as of October 2005. When a drug is not registered in a country, special authorization to use or to import it must be requested by the government, and the rules are complex and only available to institutions, not individual doctors, which further impedes access.[83]

In Brazil, TDF has been incorporated into the country's treatment guidelines since 2003 and is widely used as part of both first- and second-line HIV treatment. The Industrial Property Law, which allows pharmaceutical product patents, went into effect in 1997, and Gilead filed a patent for TDF in Brazil the following year. Though the patent was never granted, the monopolistic market situation enabled Gilead to charge a price ($3,300 pppy) that was unsustainable for Brazil's universal access program.[84] The Brazilian government used the threat of a compulsory license to achieve some price reductions. When the first Indian generic versions of TDF became available on the international market in 2006, Gilead was further pressured to halve the price from $2,766 to $1,380 pppy, but that was still ten times the generic price.[85] An NGO coalition called the Working Group on Intellectual Property of the Brazilian Network for the Integration of Peoples (GTPI/REBRIP) decided to file a pre-grant opposition to prevent the patent from being issued on "not only pharmaceutical arguments but also public health arguments."[86] The GTPI/REBRIP came together around the time that the Pharmaceutical Research and Manufacturers of America and thirty-nine major pharmaceutical companies took the South African government to court because the Medicines and Related Substances Control Amendment Act of 1997 allowed parallel imports (buying the cheapest available patented drug), generic substitutions, and price controls to make medicines more affordable. "Brazilian AIDS NGOs were concerned, and we felt the need to understand IP," explains a GTPI lawyer. "In 2003, we were formally created with the involvement of international NGOs like MSF and Oxfam. The idea was to have a working group on IP issues only."[87] GTPI began pushing in 2005 for compulsory licenses, especially for lopinavir/ritonavir, which at the time accounted for 30% of the budget of the Brazilian Department of Sexually Transmitted Diseases, AIDS and Viral Hepatitis.[88] In 2008, two years after GTPI filed its post-grant opposition against TDF, the Brazilian government declared TDF to be of public interest, and its patent office rejected Gilead's application. Since 2011, TDF has been locally produced through a partnership between a public and a private manufacturer, greatly reducing the price. For GTPI, the price drop for TDF has been one of its biggest successes in AIDS activism, and it also raised public awareness through thousands of educational events.[89] Its former coordinator, Renata Reis, explains:

> The struggle for a compulsory license was a political fight and a dispute [about] concepts. It took a lot of our energy, so we realized the use of oppositions could be a strategy that would put us one step ahead, even before the granting of the patent. . . . The point was that the patent was very questionable, and the government noticed that. . . . We knew also that this patent was very important for Gilead, [which] came to ABIA and were very unhappy. The Gilead representative disagreed with us when we said the patent was being questioned all around the world.[90]

Marcela Vieira, a lawyer working for GTPI, further emphasizes, "The success of the patent opposition also represents the continuity of the thirty-year fight to preserve the principles of equality and universality which underlie the Brazilian response to the AIDS epidemic. . . . We intend to keep using this strategy since it has proven to be effective, replicable, and compatible with our purpose of ensuring improved access to medicines."[91] Several months after the patent rejection, Gilead appealed the decision and also filed for a divisional patent in March 2009, which was also opposed by GTPI and similarly rejected by the patent office on the basis of lack of inventiveness in May 2011.[92]

A year after the Brazilian Patent Office rejected Gilead's TDF application, its Indian counterpart followed suit, rejecting several patent applications relating to TDF in September 2009 on the same grounds that they lacked an inventive step and thereby failed to meet the requirement of enhanced efficacy as stipulated under Section 3(d) of India's patent law.[93] India had inherited from the British its 1911 Patents and Designs Act, which included strong patent protections for both product and process for a sixteen-year period.[94] By the 1960s, the prices of drugs in India were among the highest in the world due to lack of competition.[95] Indian producers got together in 1961 to form the Indian Drug Manufacturers Association for the sole purpose of boosting the national pharmaceutical industry.[96] It fought for years for the amendment of the draconian colonial patent law, and the 1970 Indian Patents Act introduced several significant changes that could have affected the patent regime for the next forty years. The act provided only for process patents, for a limited term of seven years, which allowed different manufacturers to make the same medicines through different processes.[97] The Indian generic industry boomed. In 1971, multinational pharmaceutical companies accounted for 71% of the Indian market. In 2004, the multinationals' share had dropped to below 23%. Seen as the pharmacy of the world by many activists, Indian generic companies have provided ARV drugs for 50% of HIV patients in the developing world. About 85% of MSF's patients have depended on them, and over 90% of all ARVs procured by the Global Fund and PEPFAR have been Indian generic AIDS medicines.[98] India owed its unique position as the supplier of generic drugs to the world to its patent law.[99]

All this changed after 1994, when India signed the TRIPS agreement, which required product and process patent protection for a minimum of twenty years. As a developing country, India had until 2005 to become TRIPS-compliant by modifying its patent law, but it was required to accept patent applications from 1995 onward and to keep such applications pending, in a patent "mailbox." The mailbox was to be opened in 2005, when the applications were to be assessed.[100] By December 1994, however, the Indian Parliament still had not amended the 1970 Indian Patents Act as required by TRIPS, and President Shankar Dayal Sharma responded by issuing a Patents (Amendment) Ordinance, which allowed mailbox filings and the granting of exclusive marketing rights. The Indian Parliament reconvened in 1995 but still failed to pass a law to amend the Patents Act, and both the United States and the European Union took India to the WTO's Dispute Settlement Board in 1997 over the mailbox and data exclusivity issues.

In 2001, the Lawyers Collective's HIV/AIDS Unit conducted a national survey of the impact of the TRIPS-compliant product patent regime on access issues, and then launched the Affordable Medicines and Treatment campaign.[101] In December 2004, when the Indian Parliament still had not amended the Patents Act to provide for product patent protection, the president once again issued a Patents (Amendment) Ordinance to ensure compliance by the January 1, 2005, TRIPS deadline.[102] When the Patents Act was finally amended in 2005, it contained a number of significant public health safeguards from the Affordable Medicines and Treatment campaign against "evergreening" (when an originator that has obtained a patent on a chemical product seeks to enlarge its monopoly by seeking patents on new forms or new uses for the same product) and against frivolous patenting, while it also introduced twenty-year product patents. Sections 2(1)(j) and (j)(a) require a patent applicant to prove "novelty" and "non-obviousness," and they define "invention" as a new product or process involving an inventive step that constitutes a technical advance or economic significance or both, and that is not obvious to a person skilled in the art.[103] In order to prevent evergreening, Section 3(d) was amended to exclude the patentability of new forms of known substances unless there is a significant enhancement of "efficacy."[104] Further, it provides broad grounds for compulsory licensing, including the unavailability and unaffordability of a drug, a national emergency, export, and government use. It also retains the right of pre-grant opposition while introducing post-grant opposition, powerful tools that AIDS activists have taken full advantage of since 2005.

Gilead first filed its TDF product patent in India in 1997 and has filed a number of divisional patents since 2002.[105] In 2006, the Indian Network of People Living with HIV/AIDS and the Delhi Network of Positive People filed a number of pre-grant oppositions against all TDF-related patents filed by Gilead that year.[106] Two years later, in an unprecedented move, a Brazilian AIDS NGO, ABIA, also filed a pre-grant opposition against TDF in India in conjunction with the Indian NGO Sahara, because "a patent in India would not only restrict generic competition in India, but would also directly impact Brazil being able to import and access affordable generic versions of the drug."[107] In 2009, the Indian Patent Office finally rejected Gilead's basic TDF product patent and several divisional applications.[108] Since Indian generic production of TDF began in 2005, the originator's price has remained constant for low-income countries while the generic price has decreased by 84%. As of June 2012, there were six generic sources of TDF (300 mg tablet) that were quality-assured by the US FDA and WHO.[109]

In the same year, 2006, that the Indian Network of People Living with HIV/ AIDS and the Delhi Network of Positive People filed their pre-grant oppositions against all TDF-related patents in India, MSF took the same action in China. Despite a low HIV prevalence rate (under 0.1%) compared to South Africa, India,

Thailand, and Brazil, China received heavy international criticism for its denial of AIDS until the early 2000s. The Chinese AIDS epidemic went through three phases that broadly followed the country's economic transition: it began with poor farmers selling blood and getting the virus through infected plasma in the Henan province in the 1980s and 1990s, which was followed by a rapid spread of HIV among injecting drug users along the country's southern borders, and then in 2007 sexual transmission became the main route among men who have sex with men and among sex workers in five provinces: Yunnan, Xinjiang, Guangdong, Guangxi, and Henan.[110]

According to a prominent AIDS lawyer, the Chinese government's response to AIDS went through three stages: denial—"AIDS is a disease of Western capitalism"—then fear, and, finally, recognition.[111] A UNAIDS publication, *China's Titanic Peril* (2002), put the number of infected patients in 2001 above a million with the potential of reaching 10 million within a decade; this catapulted the AIDS problem of the new economic superpower onto the global map. After the 2003 SARS (severe acute respiratory syndrome) outbreak, China realized the importance of better managing its public health policy, including AIDS.[112] That same year, it passed the Four Free and One Care policy: free antiretroviral drugs to AIDS patients who are rural residents or who are people without insurance living in urban areas; free voluntary counseling and testing; free drugs to HIV-infected pregnant women to prevent mother-to-child transmission, and free HIV testing of newborn babies; free schooling for AIDS orphans; and care and economic assistance for the households of people living with HIV/AIDS.[113] In 2006, the government finally passed the Administrative Regulations for the Prevention and Treatment of AIDS and its first five-year Action Plan to Control HIV/AIDS.[114]

"Nobody knows how many AIDS cases there are in China," says the founder and executive director of the Dongzhen Center for Human Rights Education and Action, who set up the Dongzhen School for AIDS Orphans, which unfortunately was shut down by the government in 2004. "China is too big and the government relies on a lot of sources for its statistics. Perhaps the statistics on sex workers, IDUs, and MSM are reliable. But we are not sure about the number of the blood transfusion patients. Many have died, and so it is hard to know their proportion. Many are still not recognized by the government today."[115] The official statistics put the number of people living with HIV and AIDS at 650,000 in 2006 and 740,000 in 2009. By 2015, an estimated 230,000 more will be in need of treatment.[116]

China is a latecomer in adopting the concept of IP rights. It was not until the promulgation of the national "Open Door" Policy of 1979 that China began to realize that national IP laws are needed to attract foreign investors.[117] It passed its patent law in 1984 and has since amended it four times: in 1992, 2000, 2009, and 2012. Product patents on medicines were introduced in 1992.[118] A number of significant changes were made in 2000, including stronger enforcement mechanisms and infringement penalties, which were designed to narrow the gap between Chinese patent law and TRIPS in preparation for China's accession to the WTO.[119] A compulsory licensing system was also introduced under Articles 48 and 49: "where a national emergency or any extraordinary state of affairs occurs, or where the public interest so requires, the Patent Administration Department under the State Council may grant a compulsory license to exploit the patent for invention or utility model."[120] Around the same time that the Brazilian Working Group on Intellectual Property was lobbying for its government to issue compulsory licenses and the Indian Affordable Medicines and Treatment campaign was fighting for public health safeguards in the amended Indian Patents Law, MSF set up its China team (in 2004), in line with its global Access to Essential Medicines campaign.[121] The co-founder of Access to Medicines Research Group, China, explains how access activism began in China:

> My supervisor was the first campaigner who looked specifically at policy advocacy. She was the one that opened the access debate and created a loose network in China. DFID [the UK Department for International Development] issued a report about pharmaceutical manufacturing. Oxfam–Hong Kong also had a person looking at access. We involved the Third World Network's Beijing office. In addition, the Clinton Foundation was partly looking into the issue because, like MSF, it ran projects in the country. MSF was the one that looked deeper and longer and brought everyone together between 2006 and 2008.[122]

By 2006, MSF campaigners began giving presentations on ARV access issues to local HIV-positive networks, academics, government officials, and generic producers and, with the help of Chinese patent attorneys and pharmacists, completed summaries of the patent statuses of key ARV drugs in China.[123] In July, Chinese AIDS activists used the International AIDS Conference in Toronto as an opportunity to discuss the TDF patent issue with the Ministry of Health and the national CDC. The following month, in the first major collective effort by the Chinese PLWHA community, AIDS activists from a wide range of NGOs, CBOs, and networks, including AIDS Care China, Shanghai Beautiful Life, Ark of Love, Mangrove, Aizhixing, and Yirenping, collected over 7,500 signatures in fifteen Chinese provinces and municipalities on a letter that was submitted to the state Intellectual Property Office, the Ministry of Health, the Chinese CDC, and China's

Food and Drug Administration, requesting that the government block Gilead's TDF patent application. Together with a Chinese patent law firm, Anboyda, MSF filed a pre-grant opposition to TDF the same day.[124] The PLWHA community also demonstrated in solidarity with TDF oppositions filed by their counterparts in India and Brazil. But the state Intellectual Property Office granted a TDF product patent to Gilead in 2007. MSF's effort had failed because of a technical reason: a different standard of inventiveness was applied in China compared to India and Brazil, where the patent was successfully blocked.[125] The campaign process was crucial, however, since it "developed the advocacy capacity of grassroots PLWHA networks and sent a signal to Pharma that our public health message was okay." It also represented "the first attempt by the Chinese AIDS community to participate in an international movement calling for access to medicines at the local level."[126]

MSF-Beijing and the Third World Network did not give up. They took advantage of a narrow political opportunity to submit public-health-friendly commentaries to the Chinese Patent Office through a new communication channel:

The WHO officer was passionate about the access issue and created a sub-working group under the HIV/AIDS theme group for information sharing and technical discussion. It included us, the Clinton Foundation, and [the] Third World Network. It was through this sub-working group that we wrote joint commentaries. Between 2006 and 2008, MSF alone submitted three commentaries on the Chinese patent law to the government, specifically requesting more public-health-friendly clauses, like compulsory licensing and data exclusivity. When the government publicized a draft of the amended patent law and called for commentar[ies], we submitted them indirectly to someone we knew at the patent office by email. Somehow, international NGOs could get access to the patent office, and the government accepted this way of communication, which was quite new, and found our commentary interesting, since very few civil society representatives would go for this angle. . . . In 2007, there was another good opportunity. The Third World Network and MSF co-organized a conference with the Chinese Medical Association, supported by UNAIDS and WHO, and invited experts from Argentina, Thailand, and Europe to discuss access and compulsory licensing in other countries. We invited the bureaucrats from the patent office [and the] Health Ministry and some academics to attend. The patent office requested [that we] coordinate the opinions of the international experts and submit [the opinions] to them. After the conference, a new column on public health was added in the journal of the patent office. The new revised patent law was passed in 2009, and there were some public-health-friendly clauses. Of course, it is hard to prove which clause was from us. We think that it [was] a collective effort.[127]

Among other changes, the 2009 amendments to the Chinese Patent Law specifically address the compulsory licensing issue "where the exercising of the patent right by the patentee is legally determined as an act of monopoly, for the purposes of eliminating or reducing the adverse effects of the act on competition."[128]
The new patent law also allows China to grant compulsory licenses for the purpose of manufacturing and exporting patented pharmaceuticals to other WTO
members that have insufficient or no manufacturing capacities in the pharmaceutical sector, in order to address public health problems. This is in accordance
with the 2005 protocol amending the TRIPS agreement, which was ratified by
China in 2007.[129] Since the amendments, MSF-Beijing's top priority has been to
push for the compulsory licensing of TDF in China because of its high cost and
unsustainability as a treatment option. In 2011, the government paid $396 pppy
for TDF. By 2015, there will be 230,000 Chinese AIDS patients receiving TDF-
based first-line treatment. At the 2011 price level, the government will be paying
roughly $91 million, while local production would cost less than a third of the Gil-
ead price—$124 pppy—for an annual budget of around $29 million with annual
savings of over $62 million.[130] According to the national project director of
MSF-Beijing:

> We've had discussions with the WHO on implementing Treatment 2.0 in China.
> The concept behind [this] is better treatment, better drugs, and [a] highly efficient
> delivery system. The new model is that the . . . ARV clinic will not be operated by
> a hospital but by patient groups. . . . We want TDF for everyone, including for second-
> line treatment, HIV and hepatitis co-infection, and . . . pregnant women for trans-
> mission prevention. So the most important [aspect] is supply security. The Thai gov-
> ernment already issued six compulsory licenses. But Thailand and China are very
> different. The Thai pharmaceutical sector is weak, while the Chinese industry is
> so strong. China has generic capability. The only barrier is [the] patent. . . . It will
> be good to develop the Chinese pharmaceutical industry. It's a game. If China is-
> sues a compulsory license on TDF, Gilead will respond. We don't know how they
> will play the game. . . . We will support the government by writing articles in inter-
> national media to mitigate pressure against the Chinese government.[131]

In June 2012, three months after India issued its first compulsory license for
a cancer drug made by Bayer, China made its fourth revision to its patent law to
allow Chinese manufacturers to produce generic medicines still under patent protection during state emergencies, under unusual circumstances, or in the interests of the public. According to two sources with direct knowledge of the
matter, "China is known to be looking at Gilead Sciences Inc.'s tenofovir, which

is recommended by the World Health Organization as part of a first-line cocktail treatment for AIDS patients."[132] In response, Gilead has offered some concessions, including giving China a substantial donation of TDF if it continues to buy the same amount.

Lamivudine (3TC)

Like TDF, lamivudine is an essential ARV drug recommended by the WHO for first- and second-line treatment for adults. Grossing $110 million in 2011 for its originator, GlaxoSmithKline (GSK), it has been an important component of the fixed-dose combinations that made treatment scale-up possible in many resource-poor settings. Like TDF, 3TC has also been proven to be efficacious against the hepatitis B virus (HBV). The 2010 WHO guidelines recommend using TDF with 3TC or emtricitabine in all HIV/HBV co-infected patients requiring treatment. But unlike TDF, whose clinical trials are still ongoing for pediatric use, 3TC has been recommended for and widely used in children. The WHO List of Prequalified Medicinal Products includes four pediatric fixed-dose triple combinations containing 3TC. Since 2001, the originator's price has decreased by 66% while the generic price has dropped by 70%. As of June 2012, there were nine generic sources of 3TC (150 mg tablet) that were quality-assured by the US FDA or WHO.[133]

In 1997, the same year that Gilead filed its TDF product patent in India, GSK applied for patent protection for its combination of 3TC and AZT simultaneously in India and Thailand. Three years later, Thai activists submitted a pre-grant opposition against this drug, which was followed by the same move six years later by the Indian Network of People Living with HIV/AIDS and the Manipur Network of Positive People. In 2006, a joint civil society action was organized by Thai and Indian AIDS activists with protests in Bangalore outside the office of GSK, in New Delhi, and in Bangkok. A few months later, GSK withdrew its patent application in both Thailand and India.[134]

In China, despite the absence of any product patent on 3TC, the government has been paying a high price to GSK: $1,780 pppy for 3TC compared to $33 for its generic competitor in 2010.[135] The problem is that, in addition to process patents, 3TC is covered by layers of other patent-like protections in China. Before it started granting product patents on medicines in 1992, China was pressured by the United States during the Sino-US bilateral trade negotiations to offer "administrative protection" for US pharmaceutical products.[136] Any new drug that has never been marketed in China gets seven and a half years of protection with the possibility of extension. This exclusive protection functions exactly the same way as a product patent. 3TC has also been under the so-called new drug protection, where exclusive rights are given for a period of five to ten years in order to monitor the safety of a new drug before generic versions are introduced.[137]

This multilayered protection, which creates a strong safety net for 3TC, has caused serious access issues for both HIV and HBV patients in China, where many ARV drugs are not available despite local production capabilities. In 2004, MSF had a pharmacist looking at ARV access for its two treatment projects and found patents everywhere.[138] A former MSF-Beijing campaigner explains:

> There are two formulations [of 3TC] to treat HIV and hepatitis B. When MSF started HIV treatment in China in 2003, we found out that only the hep B formulation was used in China. We have the biggest hep B prevalence in the world with almost 20 million people infected. No HIV formulation was available in China. We also found out that there was no local production of 3TC because of patents. All the 3TC patents in China are process patents, so MSF thought it [would be] okay to import. However, after closer examination, we found out that those process patents functioned as product patents, as nearly every step of the manufacturing process was patented. So it is impossible for Chinese companies to produce [3TC] as they would violate patents. For 3TC alone, MSF had to buy the brand[-name] drug, which was expensive. Internationally, MSF has been promoting the use of fixed-dose combinations, which are 3TC combined with two other drugs into one pill, developed by Cipla. This is easy to use especially in resource-limited settings. But because of 3TC patents in China, importing this cocktail would violate the patents, so MSF made a special application for noncommercial use in pilot MSF projects. It's not sustainable because it only benefited a few thousand patients in the pilot programs. The government didn't bother to do anything; rather, they used stavudine, which was very toxic with high treatment failure. Finally, the government stopped using stavudine and negotiated with GSK, [which] agreed to donate 3TC to China with conditions.[139]

GSK's donation scheme for HIV patients was, of course, bait to keep its dominance in the more important Chinese hepatitis B market. Soon, AIDS activists found numerous problems with the 3TC supply through the donation program:

> Donation was on a monthly basis [and] customs had to be cleared. Whenever there was a delay in customs clearance, the whole countrywide program would be delayed. So there was no guaranteed supply. People didn't realize what the delay meant until international NGOs were involved. MSF brought the case to the government and said, "In order to overcome the problem, you have different solutions, including compulsory licensing." But the government still relied on [the] donation, and believed that as long as GSK donated, it [was] fine. GSK wanted to control the market. From

2007 to 2008, patients in a number of cities, including Shanghai, Henan, and Beijing, experienced 3TC [shortages]. It was after the [shortages] that we found out about the customs clearance bottleneck. We also found out that some of the drugs they donated were very close to [the] expiration date. The activists from Beautiful Life, a peer support group in Shanghai, called the Shanghai CDC and demanded a response and also called the national CDC and called for an investigation. In Henan, they went directly to [the] national CDC. The problem was solved; the stock was replenished. The issue of reliance on GSK [was] serious. But the problem was not solved due to layers of patent protection.[140]

In 2009, some Chinese pharmaceutical companies hired an attorney to challenge the 3TC process patent. The patent reexamination office ruled the process patent to be invalid. "After a long battle, we discovered that we had been fighting against something invalid," said the former MSF campaigner. "The problem with patent law is that unless somebody challenges, the examination [does] not start, and the patent is still valid." Toward the end of 2009, when the administrative protection for 3TC was about to expire, GSK put an announcement on its website about the remaining 3TC-related patents in China, sending a warning signal to Chinese companies. So even though some Chinese companies had already received approval from the state Food and Drug Administration, none produced 3TC until 2010. The 3TC story in China taught the activists many crucial lessons:

> If a country does not have a good patent law, it will trap itself for twenty years per [the] TRIPS requirement. If the government accedes to too many exclusive protections not required by TRIPS, it further traps itself unnecessarily. In the long run, breaking these illogical standards is very important. [The earlier fight was] only about the single-dose drug. There are more patents on 3TC-related cocktails. Hopefully, the Chinese government will learn from this.[141]

Lopinavir/ritonavir (LPV/r)

Lopinavir/ritonavir, commonly known by its brand names, Kaletra and Aluvia, is an important fixed-dose combination recommended by the WHO for second-line treatment, and it has been the subject of global AIDS activism. LPV/r is a blockbuster drug for Abbott, grossing $1.17 billion in 2011. Most patents related to ritonavir also cover LPV/r. Abbott has applied for patents related to LPV/r softgel capsules in many countries. LPV/r is approved for use in children from two weeks old. But the current pediatric formulation, an unpleasant-tasting solution with 42% alcohol that requires refrigeration until dispensing and then storage below 25°C for no more than six weeks, is not adapted to resource-limited settings.[142]

In Brazil, the basic patent for LPV/r was protected under the "pipeline mechanism," which was introduced in the 1996 Industrial Property Act and allows drug companies to apply for patents on medicines that were invented before 1995, when TRIPS came into force. With this measure, many patents on medicines filed in another country well before TRIPS have been given protection in Brazil.[143] As a result, Brazil paid a high price for LPV/r: $1,380 pppy while the lowest-priced generic was a third of that cost.[144] In 2005, after Abbott refused to lower the price, the Brazilian government declared the drug to be of public interest and threatened to issue a compulsory license for LPV/r; it would have been the first country to do so for any ARV drug. However, the CL attempt failed under US pressure, and Brazil signed an agreement with Abbott instead, which fixed the price at $1,380 until 2011 regardless of fluctuations in demand or changes in international price, on the condition that Brazil would not issue a compulsory license.[145] The former director of the Brazilian HIV/AIDS Program explains how their efforts were derailed:

> Around 2004, we prepared everything to issue three compulsory licenses: juridical analyses, meetings with top-level lawyers, academics, ABIA, and the Working Group on IP. The government worked closely with NGOs. I invited James Love [of the Consumer Project on Technology] to come for one week. The CL was almost ready to be issued and announced. Then the US government threatened commercial retaliation. Because of that, Brazil decided to interrupt the process in 2004. In 2005, we had a new minister of health, Dr. Saraiva Felipe, who was committed to the issue, so everything started again. We worked with Renata Reis from the Working Group on IP and some other lawyers and were ready. . . . Suddenly, the authority of coordinating the process was given to the minister of development. Dr. Saraiva Felipe called me on a Monday morning and told me that something bad had happened. The Ministry of Health [was] not coordinating the negotiations any more. The Ministry of Development wanted to have an agreement with Abbott. Dr. Felipe went to the meeting. It was clear that the ministry in charge was not the Ministry of Health. The agreement with Abbott was reached, and that [was] it.[146]

The Working Group on Intellectual Property took the case to court, urging the government to issue a compulsory license. The trial judge first questioned Brazil's technical capacity to produce the drug, and then after proof of Brazil's technical ability was submitted to him, cited Brazil's presence on the "Special 301"

Priority Watch List as an argument against compulsory licensing.[147] Then, in 2007, the National Federation of Pharmacists made a request to the Brazilian prosecutor-general to overturn the entire pipeline mechanism itself on the grounds that it was unconstitutional since many drugs were already in the public domain. While the case is still pending in the Brazilian Supreme Court, in February 2012 the federal Court of Rio de Janeiro ruled in favor of a generic manufacturer's 2009 application and annulled the original Abbott patent on LPV/r, which had been granted in 1997 through the pipeline mechanism.[148] Abbott has made several other patent applications related to LPV/r in Brazil. In November 2011, the Working Group on Intellectual Property filed a pre-grant opposition on the heat-stable formulations of both LPV/r and RTV in "an attempt to avoid monopoly extension over LPV/r and appropriation of ritonavir alone, since this patent, if granted, would allow patent protection for both until 2024."[149]

In India, the patent office rejected the LPV/r application in 2006, and Abbott subsequently withdrew two other LPV/r-related divisional patent applications in 2009.[150] The Thai counterpart took a more drastic step. Two months after the Thai government issued the first compulsory license for efavirenz, the patent office did the same for LPV/r in January 2007, cutting the price by almost two-thirds from $2,200 to $793 pppy by 2011 and stirring a global IP storm. In retaliation, Abbott withdrew all seven registration applications in Thailand for its new products, including the heat-stable LPV/r.[151] The Thai Network of People Living with HIV/AIDS, together with the AIDS Access Foundation, the Thai Foundation for Consumers, the Thai Rural Doctors Society, the Thai Chronic Renal Failure Network, the Thai Alternative Agriculture Network, the Thai Parents Network, the Thai Rural Pharmacist Society, the Thai NGOs Coalition on AIDS, FTA Watch, and AIDS activists in twenty countries immediately called for a global boycott of Abbott products.[152] ITPC-China organized a solidarity boycott against Abbott in China. Angry protestors, including Thai patients, converged in Illinois to protest at Abbott's general shareholders meeting on April 27, 2007, demanding that the company not use drugs as political leverage. The Thai Foundation for Consumers also sued Abbott under the Thai Competition Law, arguing that its retaliation constituted an illegal anti-competitive practice. There was a global outcry. The Delhi Network of Positive People, the Indian Network of People Living with HIV/AIDS, the Affordable Medicines and Treatment campaign, and the Community Health Cell submitted a letter to WHO and UNAIDS over the WHO director-general, Margaret Chan, allegedly saying, "I'd like to underline that we have to find a right balance for compulsory licensing. We cannot be naive about this. There is no perfect solution for accessing drugs in both quality and quantity."[153]

The student-led group Universities Allied for Essential Medicines wrote a letter to the Wisconsin Alumni Research Foundation, which owns one of the patents covering Kaletra, and urged it to take action. ACT UP–Paris organized an online strike in which thousands of activists worldwide repeatedly connected to Abbott's website, shutting it down several times, to which Abbott responded by threatening a lawsuit. The European AIDS Treatment Group and the AIDS Treatment Activists Coalition wrote a letter to the CEO, Miles White, accusing Abbott of betraying its own slogan: "a promise for life."[154]

The Thai Kaletra scandal was reported by all the major news outlets. An editorial in the *Wall Street Journal* called it "Theft in Thailand."[155] USA for Innovation, a pro-Pharma group, ran a smear campaign: it bought advertising in the Thai and foreign print media and created a website that accused the military-backed government of Thailand of turning the country into a dictatorship like Burma by illegally issuing compulsory licenses.[156] The USTR responded to Thailand's compulsory licenses by putting it on its priority watch list. After a discussion with WHO director-general Chan, Abbott announced that it would use "a balanced approach to provide Kaletra/Aluvia (lopinavir/ritonavir) capsules and tablets to more patients in the developing world. Now the new price of Kaletra/Aluvia is $500 per patient per year for Africa and least developed countries and $1,000 for low income and lower middle income countries."[157]

In 2009, Ecuador issued a compulsory license for ritonavir and has considered the same move for LPV/r. In November 2011, the US-based NGO Public Citizen, in conjunction with other public health groups, launched a global campaign in twelve countries to challenge Abbott's patents on LPV/r. According to Peter Maybarduk, the director of the Global Access to Medicines program at Public Citizen:

> Freeing these drugs for competition and co-formulation could save countless lives. . . . These medicines can be manufactured cheaply where patent barriers can be overcome. Licensing and competition could spur the development of new and improved ritonavir-based combination treatments against HIV/AIDS. If patent holders and the pharmaceutical industry will not negotiate, then health advocates will pursue compulsory measures to break their monopolies on lifesaving medicines.[158]

Generic competition has driven the price of LPV/r down from over $10,000 pppy to less than $100. Yet Abbott charges $400 in the world's poorest countries, and from $1,000 to around $4,000 in other developing nations. In December 2012, Indonesia announced compulsory licenses for six HIV and hepatitis drugs, including EFV, TDF, and the combination drug LPV/r. Table 2 summarizes some major events in access to AIDS treatment.

TABLE 2
AIDS Treatment Timeline

Year	Science	Pharma
1987	US FDA approves AZT as first drug against HIV	Burroughs Wellcome sells AZT at $10,000 pppy
1988		
1989	FDA approves use of ganciclovir and aerosolized pentamidine	
1990	FDA approves use of fluconazole	
1992		
1993	Concorde study: no advantage of AZT before symptoms develop	
1994	ACTG 076: AZT effective in PMTCT FDA approves AZT for PMTCT and approves Bactrim and Septra	
1996	Availability of ARV therapy: Lazarus effect	
1997		
1998		39 Pharma companies file lawsuit against South African government on Medicines Amendment Act
1999		
2000		Cipla ARV $350 pppy BMS, Glaxo Wellcome, Merck, Boehringer Ingelheim, Roche reduce ARV prices in least-developed countries
2001		
2002		
2003		

Government	Community	Intergovernmental Organizations
	ACT UP Wall Street demonstration ACT UP takes over FDA ACT UP protest at Burroughs Wellcome office, followed by NYSE action	
Thailand amends Patent Act		
Brazil passes law 9313 on universal ARV access		UNAIDS Accelerating Access Initiative
Brazil begins local ARV production South Africa passes Medicines Amendment Act French president Chirac launches International Therapeutic Solidarity Fund		
	TAC	
Thailand fails to issue CL on ddI	TNP+ camp at Thai Ministry of Public Health demands CL of ddI MSF's Access to Essential Medicines campaign Activists file pre-grant opposition against GSK on combination of 3TC and AZT	
USTR files complaint to WTO against Article 68 of Brazil's patent law	Thai AIDS Access Foundation lawsuit against BMS on ddI IAS Durban: Treatment March Foundation for Consumers and AIDS patients sue BMS against ddI product patent (settled)	Doha Declaration UNGASS UNCHR resolution on access to AIDS treatment Global Fund
PEPFAR Thai GPO produces first fixed-dose combination, GPO-VIR	ITPC	3 by 5 Initiative

(continued)

TABLE 2 (*continued*)

Year	Science	Pharma
2004		
2005		
2006		GSK withdraws patent application for combination of 3TC and AZT in India and Thailand
2007		In retaliation for Thai CL on LPV/r, Abbott withdraws 7 new drug applications in Thailand
2008		
2009		
2010		Cipla files pre-grant opposition against BMS on TDF/FTC/ EFV
2011		
2012		
2013		

Sources: Gorman 2012; UNAIDS 2011c; Terto, Reis, and Pimenta 2009; and http://patentoppositions.org [accessed Mar. 10, 2013].

Government	Community	Intergovernmental Organizations
Brazil public decree for local production of efavirenz, lopinavir, and nelfinavir		
		Global Fund Treatment Round
India amends its patent law Thai universal ARV access Thai CL on EFV USTR puts Thailand on "Special 301" Priority Watch List Indian Patent Office rejects Abbott LPV/r application	DNP+ files pre-grant oppositions against Gilead on all TDF-related patents in India MSF files pre-grant opposition on TDF in China Joint Thai and Indian protests outside GSK in India Global boycott of Abbott products in 20 countries	Political Declaration on HIV/AIDS UNITAID
Thai CL on LPV/r Brazil CL on EFV AIDS Law Project complaint to South African Competition Commission against Merck on EFV Brazilian Patent Office rejects Gilead patent on TDF	GTPI files post-grant opposition against TDF in Brazil ABIA and Sahara file pre-grant opposition to TDF in India	
Indian Patent Office rejects Gilead patent on TDF/FTC/EFV Ecuador CL on ritonavir		
		Medicines Patent Pool
Brazilian patent office rejects TDF divisional patent China amends patent law, allowing local production of generic medicines during state emergencies Indonesia CL on 7 hepatitis B and HIV drugs		Political Declaration on HIV/AIDS
		Global Fund new funding model based on GNP and disease burden

The access struggles, patent by patent, drug by drug, company by company, and country by country, point to the need for a more coordinated and systemic effort to bring Pharma to the negotiating table to develop a mechanism that balances private interests with public health. One such mechanism may be the Medicines Patent Pool, where patent holders voluntarily put their patents in a pool, which then licenses generic manufacturers to produce the drugs in return for a royalty paid to the patent holders. Is the Medicines Patent Pool the solution to the innovation versus access problem?

Medicines Patent Pool: Innovation and Access

We're at a fork in the road: either governments summon the political will and financial resources to treat AIDS in developing countries, or current funding for AIDS treatment stagnates, which means patients will see their treatment delayed, deferred and denied. It's a question of choices: if they don't help us treat AIDS, there will be more graves.
—*Tido von Schoen-Angerer, Director of MSF's Access to Essential Medicines campaign*[159]

For us, it is never purely the market, but a market for public health impact.
—*Executive Director, UNITAID*[160]

We know that the best way to dramatically lower the costs of ARV is through robust generic competition. This is one lesson that has been hammered over the past ten years. We know when generic companies can enter the market, they have an effect on the prices.
—*General Counsel, Medicines Patent Pool*[161]

Civil society played a crucial role in the creation of the Medicines Patent Pool (MPP, sometimes referred to as the pool).[162] The idea was proposed by James Love of the Consumer Project on Technology (now Knowledge Ecology International, KEI) at the Barcelona International AIDS Conference in 1992. His idea of an "essential healthcare patent pool" was modeled on a patent pool that was created by US aircraft manufacturers during the First World War. In 2006, together with MSF, KEI proposed a patent pool for medicines to UNITAID, which had been created to look into innovative market solutions to increase access to essential medicines. Patent pools were discussed by the World Health Assembly in 2008 and considered a feasible mechanism to accelerate access to essential medicines in developing countries. UNITAID's constitution explicitly acknowledges intellectual property barriers; it was the first international organization to recognize the importance of the issue.[163] A subcommittee, set up in UNITAID with the push of Ellen 't Hoen of MSF, concluded that there was a sufficient basis to move forward. UNITAID voted for the creation of the MPP as a separate entity in 2009, and the MPP was established the following year. The idea is to negotiate with patent holders and create a pool of relevant patents for licensing to generic manufacturers while paying a royalty based on sales to the patent holders. The goal is to increase access to high-quality, safe, effective, appropriate, and affordable treatment for HIV in low- and middle-income countries by bringing down the prices of HIV medicines and by facilitating the development of better-adapted HIV medicines, such as simplified fixed-dose combinations and special formulations for children.

As the acting executive director of the MPP explains, the global treatment crisis is acute, and the treatment landscape and financial situation are different from those of twenty years ago:

> We have to recognize that despite enormous progress over the last two decades in treatment scale-up, a lot [of] people continue to need treatment. Close to 8 million are in urgent need of treatment in the developing world. On top of that, ambitious political commitments . . . at the UN High-Level Meeting on HIV/AIDS set the goal to treat 15 million people by 2015. The challenge has to be viewed in the current economic crisis, [which] impacts on funding for treatment. Funding has either declined or remained flat. There is a need to find innovative ways to do more with less. . . . In 2000, a triple combination therapy cost upward of $10,000. Now it costs less than $70 per person per year. But the problem is that it is outdated treatment. The standard of care has improved with less toxic drugs. An increasing number of people need to be migrated from these first-line [drugs] to newer drugs.[164]

In the post-TRIPS context, where most ARV drugs are or will be protected by patents, the MPP can play an important role in increasing access globally by bringing costs down, accelerating generic manufacturers' access to technology, and developing fixed-dose combinations that currently depend on multiple patent holders. He continues:

> The problem is that the global IP landscape has changed dramatically in the past ten years. Post-2005, there are TRIPS and TRIPS-plus obligations in the world. Pre-TRIPS, drug compounds were sparsely covered in the developing world, but now, the new drugs are vastly covered under patents until 2025, 2030 for many of them.

Unless some corrective actions are taken, we will not be able to meet the huge treatment needs because of TRIPS. One mechanism is voluntary licensing. What the patent pool tries to do is negotiat[e] on a voluntary basis with pharmaceutical industries from public health perspectives to include the IP within the pool for sublicensing or outlicensing . . . with three aims: (1) to enable robust generic competition; (2) [to] promote development of fixed-dose combinations (when the IP of each component is owned by a different entity), for example, by creating a one-stop shop where a generic sublicensee can come to MPP and manufacture a fixed-dose combination; and (3) [to] facilitate the development of specific formulations that are necessary and adapted to developing world needs, such as pediatric ARVs, which are still largely neglected.[165]

MPP-Gilead Agreement

In September 2010, without much fanfare, the MPP signed its first licenses with the US National Institutes of Health for patents related to the HIV medicine darunavir. Ten months later, however, its first licensing agreement with a pharmaceutical company patent holder, Gilead Sciences, created much division among AIDS activists. In return for a 3%–5% royalty based on generic sales (waived for new pediatric formulations), Gilead agreed to put into the MPP the patents of its blockbuster TDF, emtricitabine (FTC), and three other new drugs in the pipeline: cobicistat (COBI), elvitegravir (EVG), and the much talked-about, single-tablet, once-daily, supposedly more tolerable so-called Quad, which is a combination of TDF, FTC, COBI, and EVG. As already mentioned, TDF is an important ARV drug for first- and second-line HIV treatment and for hepatitis (co-)infections. Cobicistat is known to improve the efficacy of other ARV drugs by boosting their availability in the blood, making the ARVs more effective, and decreasing their negative side effects. Elvitegravir is an integrase inhibitor that helps to prevent virus replication. Emtricitabine blocks an enzyme needed for viral replication and is used in both first- and second-line treatment for adults.

Gilead agreed to allow the supplying of tenofovir and emtricitabine in 111 countries, cobicistat in 102 countries, and elvitegravir and the Quad in 99 countries. The aim of the MPP-Gilead licenses is to make access to these medicines easier and less expensive. By 2012, five Indian generic companies—Aurobindo Pharma, Emcure Pharmaceuticals, Hetero Drugs, Laurus Labs, and MedChem—were signed up as sublicensees. On the same day that the MPP-Gilead licenses were publicized, Gilead also announced that it had signed separate voluntary licenses for the same drugs with four major ARV producers in India.

Prior to the MPP-Gilead licenses, Gilead in 2006 had entered into voluntary licensing agreements with a number of Indian drug manufacturers covering ninety-five countries. The MPP argues that its licensing improves on the prior agreements in several important ways. The MPP itself is a critical step toward changing the norms of voluntary licensing by making global access initiatives more transparent and improving their focus on public health. Voluntary licenses outside the MPP are always privately negotiated, and the terms and conditions are confidential. In contrast, the MPP publishes the entire text of its licenses on its website, allowing generic companies to understand their rights and obligations and encouraging public health stakeholders to provide feedback. Importantly, the MPP negotiates licenses that are favorable to public health objectives by including a number of critical IP flexibilities, for example licensees can supply to countries outside the territory where a compulsory license has been issued. Data exclusivity rights are also waived, removing a key non-patent barrier to access to medicines. Further, the MPP-Gilead agreement covers a far greater number of developing countries and 93,200 more people living with HIV than any previous Gilead license or any other company's voluntary license. In particular, previous Gilead voluntary licenses only allowed the use of TDF in HIV treatment and prevention while the current licenses allow for its use also in the treatment of hepatitis B, which kills 600,000 people a year worldwide. This is also the first time that COBI, EVG, and the Quad have been licensed. The licensing of products still in clinical development is rare and is considered to be an important success of the MPP. These licenses should spur competition and drive prices down by facilitating early generic competition for these new products, and since the MPP licenses are nonexclusive (within India), any company that meets the eligibility criteria may receive a license from the MPP. The agreement also contains special provisions for pediatric formulations to be made available outside the licensed territory; a "one-time technology transfer of know-how" to the licensees; and "unbundling" whereby licensees are allowed to terminate for any reason the license of one medicine while retaining those of other drugs, a novel provision compared to previous Gilead TDF licenses.[166]

With such a long list of benefits that go beyond the industry norms, the MPP-Gilead license looks almost too good to be true. The MPP acknowledges four main limits of the groundbreaking deal, however. It recognizes that "the Pool is a voluntary mechanism that negotiates with the aim to create the largest possible benefits for the largest number of people. But it is not in a position to dictate terms and conditions to licensors."[167] Despite some improvements in the expansion of geographical scope, now covering between 83% and 88% of people living with HIV in low- and middle-income countries, there are still developing countries with high HIV burdens, including Argentina, China, Egypt, Peru, Thailand, and Ukraine, that the MPP was unable to negotiate into the licenses. For instance, nine countries included in the TDF geographic area are excluded from both the COBI and the EVG areas—Botswana, Ecuador, El Salvador, Indonesia, Kazakhstan, Namibia, Sri Lanka, Thailand, and Turkmenistan, some of which have high HIV burdens—due to Gilead's "semi-exclusive" voluntary licenses with these countries as "preferred partners."[168] But the MPP is mandated by UNITAID to seek the inclusion of *all* developing countries and considers geographical scope to be a key area to be improved in future licenses. Another limit of the current agreement is that licensees must purchase all active pharmaceutical ingredients (API) only from other licensees or directly from Gilead or Gilead distributors. Further, it restricts API manufacturers to Indian producers. The MPP recognizes that these restrictions are not ideal and need to be improved but notes that India already manufactures 90% of the world's ARVs. A third limit of the MPP-Gilead agreement is that while the MPP is mandated under its statutes to support countries' use of TRIPS flexibilities, "on its own, the Pool will not be able to remove all barriers to access. . . . It must be viewed in the context of the range of different policy options available to governments and other actors to promote access to HIV medicines."[169] Finally, the hands of the MPP are tied when it comes to access to fixed-dose combinations, since there are patent barriers. Fixed-dose combinations that include products from more than one patent holder usually require additional licenses. For instance, for Atripla, which contains TDF, FTC, and EFV, a licensing agreement with Merck, the patent owner of efavirenz that has not yet entered into negotiations with the MPP, will be necessary. Similarly, for a combination of TDF, FTC, and rilpivirine (RVP), which is currently under development, a license for RVP from Johnson and Johnson, which is also not yet in negotiations with the MPP, is necessary.

The MPP hails the Gilead agreement as "a milestone in managing patents for public health." According to its former executive director, Ellen 't Hoen:

> The licence agreement with Gilead Sciences will help make medicines available at a lower-cost and in easier to use formulations without delays. . . . In particular, the licensing of elvitegravir, cobicistat and the Quad while they are still in clinical development should significantly accelerate availability. People in developing countries often have to wait for years before they can access new health technologies. Today's agreement changed that.[170]

The MPP views the agreement as "a first step—a floor, not a ceiling—and will continue to work with Gilead and others to improve this and future licences. . . . These licences are a proof of [the] concept that the Pool can negotiate constructive, public-health oriented licences with pharmaceutical companies that represent an improvement on the status quo."[171] UNITAID naturally endorses its own baby as the best possible generic licensing agreement that could be negotiated currently, even though it recognizes the limits of the MPP's geographical scope in excluding important middle-income countries such as Brazil and Chile. While "wanting to see things go faster," it also adopts a realistic approach by acknowledging that the nature of the MPP is "a permanent negotiation; if you want more and more, the company won't sign."[172]

Gilead views its agreement with the MPP as a step forward in its continuous commitment to access:

> The success of global HIV is that we are now seeing treatment being more available. Seven million people being on treatment [was] unheard of ten years ago. It is a huge victory. Having the products is a big part of that, but also making it available. We have gone through a lot of versions of our access program. We needed to get the product out by registration and [by] developing a local distribution model with local companies. That was the first thing we did. Then came the issue of costs. What we found out is that costs became a huge issue even for nonprofits. We looked at the generics market. Instead of copying them, we partnered with them. We went to India and broadly licensed tenofovir with fourteen Indian companies in 2006. It is a very successful model. The ramp[-up was] incredible, with access going up quickly. That was when we became interested in the patent pool to work with Indian manufacturers to bring [the] price down to drive the access. It has worked phenomenally well for us. We do need a robust pipeline in HIV, and we will continue this path with the goal of making medicines available in the developing world as in the developed world. No one has the perfect model yet. We continue to [tweak] this. The Medicines Patent Pool has been pushing us for more changes, and we continue to adapt. We hope to make medicines more broadly available [at] high volumes and low margins.[173]

Gilead's public health rhetoric has its limits, however. The company does not hide its bottom-line thinking when it comes to treatment coverage: "When we negotiated on the scope of the territory, we asked ourselves which countries needed this license. There are countries where price is not a barrier. Why are China and Brazil not included in the agreement? Because they have the capacity to pay. They are not paying for innovation. For us, the criteria is: What is reasonable? Our current China market is $10 million."[174] Concerning the controversial provision on restricting API production to only licensees and Indian manufacturers, Greg Alton, the executive vice president of Gilead, responds, "Our goal is to drive the costs down. We could accomplish that in India. Our concern is that once we open the door to others, the other manufacturers can drive the prices up."[175]

The US government hails the agreement as "breaking new ground in using voluntary licensing agreements as a tool to improve access to medicines for people in developing countries,"[176] even though there is still concern about pricing competition and transparent negotiations. "Aren't you concerned that the low-priced drug will come back to your commercial market?" asks a US representative in Geneva, to which the executive vice president of Gilead replies, "In the field of HIV, it didn't happen due to strict regulations. The bigger challenge is price diversion, where Americans want the Canadian price, the Canadians want the Mexican price, the Mexicans want the Brazilian price, and the Brazilians want the Chinese price."[177] The general counsel of the MPP confirms, "We don't see diversion as a key risk, unlike erectile dysfunction drugs available on the internet."[178] There was also concern that the negotiations were *too* transparent, which could discourage other pharmaceutical companies from following suit. The *Pharma Times* welcomed the licenses as "a major step forward for MPP given that pharmaceutical companies have not been rushing to sign up [for] the initiative."[179]

Civil Society Division over the MPP-Gilead Agreement

Among AIDS activists, however, the MPP-Gilead agreement has provoked bitter disputes, claims and counterclaims, and polarizing responses that pit northern NGO "pool enthusiasts" against southern NGO "pool skeptics." The division lies between KEI and MSF (two early MPP advocates), the Treatment Action Group, Health GAP, Health Action International, Oxfam, Coalition PLUS, the UK Stop AIDS campaign, the Cameroon Coalition against Malaria, the National Empowerment Network of People Living with HIV/AIDS in Kenya, and the African Services Committee (most of which are community or NGO delegates on the UNITAID board), on one side, and the ITPC and a majority of AIDS NGOs worldwide, on the other.

KEI, the originator of the MPP idea, is unsurprisingly supportive of the MPP-Gilead agreement overall: "the pool has rapidly positioned itself as a dynamic and ambitious international actor, focused on the public health aspects of controversial and complex intellectual property issues. [The agreement] demonstrates the benefits of the collective licensing approach, and sets the stage for the next round of negotiations with other companies controlling key HIV treatment patents."[180]

It particularly lauds MPP's efforts in publishing all the information on its website as a precedent for transparency in intellectual property policy. It does note, however, that the MPP license agreement follows in many ways the approach used by Gilead in its earlier voluntary licenses for TDF and FTC, which is the subject of an antitrust complaint by KEI to the US Federal Trade Commission. In particular, KEI is concerned about the exclusion of important developing countries and about the restriction of API sourcing to Indian manufacturers only, which are "reflection[s] of the relative bargaining power of the parties at this stage in the negotiations. It is an important step forward, but there is much more to do."[181] Like UNITAID, KEI recognizes "realpolitik. . . . Given [the agreement's] voluntary nature, it is the best we have got. We have to live with it."[182]

Likewise, MSF, the NGO most active in advocating for the MPP for years, endorses the agreement in general. In a comprehensive review in December 2011, it reiterates an observation based on a decade of MSF treatment field experience that only market competition will drive drug costs down: "In the absence of intellectual property rights, or where these have been opposed or expired, the price of first-generation ARVs has fallen from over $10,000 in 2000 to under $70 today."[183] In the post-TRIPS world, however, patents have become a major barrier for newer medicines. For example, because of patent barriers there are no generic sources, including in India, for etravirine (ETV) or raltegravir (RAL), two important drugs to treat people who have failed on first- and second-line treatments. Company price discounts are often insufficient to make these drugs affordable for developing countries. Without generic competition, a potential third-line regimen of RAL, DRV, and ETV could be available for the poorest countries only at the prohibitive price of $2,766 pppy, at best.[184] In this sub-ideal world then, MSF considers well-negotiated and properly implemented voluntary licenses as "one tool in the fight for access" by ushering in some restricted competition. It especially endorses the licenses managed by the MPP, "an independent organisation free from commercial interests, focusing on public health objectives and with a clear mandate to address intellectual property barriers in developing countries to increase access to ARVs."[185]

However, MSF does raise seven major concerns about the agreement and broader IP trends. First, voluntary licenses (VLs), including the MPP-Gilead agreement, can but do not necessarily lead to competition and improved access:

> The Gilead-MPP voluntary licences should be seen as part of a growing trend in relation to voluntary licences: Driven partly by commercial considerations of seeking to increase ties with and leverage over their main competitors, pharmaceutical

companies started to actively pursue voluntary licences with generic companies based in India—who had started to pursue patent oppositions—from 2005. Coupled with increased pressure on patent-holding companies to do something about the lack of affordable medicines, this has led to a growing trend towards voluntary licences. . . . Many VLs have allowed patent-holding companies to segment the market by determining in which countries the licensee can sell its product. All VLs have differing geographic scopes, reflecting differing "red lines" for patent-holding companies. There is no company VL that covers all developing countries. By excluding certain countries, companies can protect their own market access in what they see as key emerging markets. VLs do not address the problem of affordability of medicines in excluded countries. Gilead's 2011 licences show a deliberate attempt to side-step the Pool by directly signing separate VLs with four of the major ARV producers in India, three of which also supply API to other generic manufacturers of TDF and therefore have a large role in determining prices.[186]

Second, like the MPP, UNITAID, and KEI, MSF took issue with the limited geographical scope of the MPP-Gilead agreement: "Several of the countries that are excluded are among the first in which MSF provided HIV treatment ten years ago. We do not take their exclusion lightly. . . . For TDF, where the 2006 licences included 95 territories, the MPP licence includes 112. It is unlikely TDF is patented in any of the additional territories, so the significance of this licence extension is minimal."[187] For the other drugs, "the four licensees that have signed an agreement with Gilead outside the MPP benefit from a wider geographical scope."[188] Since not all countries have parallel provisions in their laws, which allow the importation of a lower-cost medicine without the patent owner's consent if that product has been put on the market in another country, excluded countries are unlikely to be able to access these drugs through parallel importation.[189]

Third, MSF objects to the restriction of API sources to Indian manufacturers since that fails to help build the generic production capacity of countries such as the Philippines, Argentina, Pakistan, and China. Fourth, the provisions concerning pediatric formulations are too complex and require Gilead's prior written consent for some of the drugs. Instead, MSF proposes a "non-assert" declaration—where the patent holder agrees to not assert its intellectual property rights—covering all formulations in all developing countries.

Fifth, a provision that "a licensee will still have to pay royalties to Gilead, and will still be forbidden from selling the drug in excluded countries, until all patents and patent applications have been held invalid and no further appeals can happen in India" discourages generic manufacturers from exporting drugs to excluded countries.[190] Sixth, some civil society organizations have argued that another provision requiring generic licensees to receive WHO prequalification or US FDA conditional approval within one year of signing the agreement may prove onerous to some manufacturers. The issue was apparently discussed at length by the UNITAID board before the MPP was established, and language has since been inserted into the memorandum of understanding between the MPP and UNITAID that requires the provision of alternative temporary arrangements through a WHO expert panel in cases of prequalification difficulties. Finally, the current dispute settlement mechanism stipulates that the "MPP will not be able to enforce the licences or participate in any dispute between Gilead and a generic licensee and that the MPP will not be able to undertake legal proceedings against Gilead unless Gilead breaches payment obligations to the MPP."[191] MSF believes that it is important that the MPP be able to interfere in disputes in order to ensure the integrity of its mission.

On the other end of the spectrum, civil society organizations (CSOs) from Asia, Russia, Central and Western Europe, North and South America, the Middle East, and Africa led by ITPC ask, why did MPP accept this flawed agreement despite its recognition of several shortcomings? In early October 2011, ITPC and a group of AIDS activists met with UNITAID and the MPP. A letter entitled "Concerns about the Process, Principles of Medicines Patent Pool and the Licence" was co-signed by seventy-three leading AIDS activists representing a wide range of HIV-positive networks, NGOs, CBOs, regional networks, and global coalitions, such as the Thai Network of People Living with HIV/AIDS, the Argentinean Network of Positive People, Grupo Pela Vidda, the Lawyers Collective, the AIDS Rights Alliance of Southern Africa, the Central Africa Treatment Action Group, the Asia Pacific Network of Sex Workers, the Latin American and Caribbean Council of AIDS Service Organizations, the Egyptian Initiative for Personal Rights, AIDS Care China, and the AIDS Access Foundation. They objected to the Gilead deal and believed that MPP had failed to uphold its mandate and had ignored concerns that CSOs have consistently shared with UNITAID about the Medicines Patent Pool since 2009 and about the Gilead agreement more recently.[192]

According to ITPC's executive director, people came together, and ITPC took the lead:

> The movement was divided. I didn't realize I was stepping into boiling water. I was sold by MPP. When I started looking into it and asked the lawyers to do an analysis, I realized the limitations of the license. Lots of people from the Global South have criticisms about the patent pool, and they had written to UNITAID about them

around 2008–2009. NGOs like MSF and Oxfam, etc., think that somehow we criticized the idea of [a] patent pool, which we [didn't]. We just had issues about the terms
and the process.[193]

Based on an October 2011 legal analysis by a US-based NGO, Initiative for Medicines, Access, and Knowledge (I-MAK), ITPC has raised eight objections about
the terms of the agreement, half of which duplicate MSF's concerns: (1) the reliance on the original 2006 Gilead voluntary license as the template; (2) the restricted geographical scope of the TDF license, which excludes over half a million patients in more than forty-three countries, with an even greater number
excluded for the pipeline drugs; (3) the circumvention of TRIPS flexibilities by
requiring the prior consent of Gilead when sublicensees export drugs to excluded
countries that have issued compulsory licenses, by allowing Gilead to cancel agreements if sublicensees are found to be providing drugs to excluded countries
through parallel importing, by requiring royalties to be paid until all related patents, including undecided applications, go through the entire legal appeals process and are finally rejected, and by allowing MPP's licensing of Gilead patents
to legitimize and endorse weak patentability standards for medicines; (4) requiring royalties on the sale of drugs even in countries where patents are nonexistent
or are not granted; (5) restrictions to Indian-only sublicensees and API production, limiting local generic production worldwide, which is essential to enhancing competitiveness and self-sufficiency and is one of the few options for countries excluded from the licensing agreement; (6) that MPP did not negotiate a
separate license for each drug and instead championed the "unbundling" provision of the license; (7) the failure of MPP to explain to the public that if a generic
company severs the license for TDF, it also loses the ability to produce and supply emtricitabine; and (8) the "incomprehensible waiver of its legal standing and
right to enforce the provisions of the license in any dispute between Gilead and
a sub-licensee at a secret arbitration . . . [which] neuters the MPPF's [Medicines
Patent Pool Foundation] ability to affect much of what occurs after a sub-licensee
agreement is signed, including ensuring that the license is implemented in a
manner that increases access to medicines."[194]

Further, the ITPC-led group raises questions about process and denounces "an
absolute lack of transparency on the terms of reference, roles and responsibilities,
selection criteria and selection process of the ad hoc expert advisory group (EAG),
which was consulted during MPPF's negotiations with Gilead, and the permanent
EAG currently being assembled" as well as the refusal by the foundation's staff
to disclose the contents of the review by the ad hoc EAG on the Gilead licensing

agreement prior to its approval.[195] It also objects to the provision whereby the MPP will receive 5% of all royalties paid by sublicensees to Gilead up to the amount of $1 million per year. Finally, the ITPC-led group finds the celebratory tone taken by UNITAID and the MPP in the media to be "misleading and damaging as they allow originators and decision-makers to be complacent and satisfied with the notion that MPPF solves most issues regarding access to medicines."[196] The activists have demanded a substantial revision or termination of the MPP-Gilead agreement, an immediate moratorium on the negotiation of any new license agreements, and a reevaluation of the current structure of the MPP.

Should civil society welcome the licensing agreement despite the fact that half a million HIV-positive people have been left behind by it? Should northern NGOs show solidarity by refusing to endorse it because the ones who are going to suffer are people in the Global South? Is the division in civil society a strategic or ideological one? Does accepting the MPP-Gilead agreement mean legitimating the Pharma-led and -dominated global IP landscape? Is it better to have a flawed agreement than no agreement at all? Have the severe attacks on UNITAID and the MPP been misplaced? Should the energy of civil society focus on Pharma, which largely sets the terms for such negotiations? The co-founder of the US-based Treatment Action Group, which is on the KEI-MSF end of the spectrum, thinks all this opposition to the Gilead deal is a lot of sound and fury:

> There were a lot of activists in Bangkok. . . . They issued a manifesto. Some of us thought that it was over the top. MPP was new; it hadn't achieved anything yet. It's a kind of international experiment in global IP pooling, which in theory could lead to an expansion of access. Why direct all this fire [at] them? Some of us thought the fire should be directed [at] Gilead. They have the licenses and have control over twelve generics and API. Some of us thought it is not MPP, but only Gilead that can change the situation. What is the point in attacking an institution with no power? . . . We stand back on the IP issues. We let the experts do their job. This whole thing has been more than divisive. It reveals differences in strategy.[197]

The MPP's position is that the civil society groups led by ITPC represent a vocal but minority view.[198] But it acknowledges their legitimate concerns about licensing territories and API restrictions. Those were among the most contentious areas of negotiation:

> One of the most difficult areas was definitely the fact that licensees have to be based in India and that API can only be bought from other Indian licensees. We felt that should be changed. Another key negotiation area was licensing territory. We were

glad that [Gilead was] willing to expand from 95 to 112 countries. We tried to get more but failed. A third key area of negotiation was that Gilead was initially [unwilling] to give the license[s] separately. It was a package. If a licensee wants emtricitabine, it has to take tenofovir as well. We didn't find bundling acceptable, particularly because of the tenofovir patent structures. . . . There was a real risk that MPP would walk away on the unbundling issue. It was the expert advisory [group] that evaluated and submitted their opinion to our board, and then the board made the final call . . . to go ahead. There was a possibility that Gilead would not make a concession on unbundling and that the EAG would advise us not to sign the agreement. We successfully opposed that. It was a significant concession that Gilead made in the eleventh hour of the negotiations. That is a major victory. We have signed three sublicenses so far. Two of them have decided to terminate the tenofovir license and continue with the other ones.[199]

At the same time, the MPP confirms that Gilead was motivated by profit rather than public health in excluding important middle-income countries:

We made it clear in all our communications that the licenses should cover all lower- and middle-income countries. Gilead's starting position was 95 countries. We wished we had leverage. Gilead had the option of walking away. I do think there are people in low- and middle-income countries that need access. Our mandate is to seek to cover as many low- and middle-income countries as much as possible. There are probably more poor people in middle-income countries than [in] low-income countries. We did make the case from [the] moral perspective, [from the] business perspective, and from [the] access perspective on why Gilead or others ought to include countries like Ukraine, [which] has huge treatment needs. But Brazil is not the same as Burundi. It certainly has lower prevalence and [a] higher ability to pay. There is this recognition and what we tried to do was to introduce a mechanism to take account of the difference. We proposed tiered royalt[ies] based on a country's GDP and disease burden. There are several different ways to do the analysis about reasonable revenue stream. None of the licenses that MPP has signed has tiered royalt[ies]. We put tiered royalt[ies] as an incentive for Gilead, but it was not a big enough financial incentive.[200]

There seems to be less concern about API restriction to Indian manufacturers, however. "From a political perspective, it is quite significant as many other countries focus on local production initiatives," the general counsel of the MPP explains. "From an access perspective, it is not as significant because of the dominance of Indian generic [manufacturers] in supplying drugs and API to the world."[201] In response to criticism, the MPP amended the Gilead licenses twice, first by making it clear that Gilead would not have to agree before a sublicensee could provide drugs to an excluded country that had issued a compulsory license, and then by removing any appearance of a conflict of interest by waiving the royalty to the MPP, as stipulated in the original agreement. Further, MPP has committed to greater transparency, adding more people nominated by HIV-positive communities to its expert advisory group and publishing all evaluations and board decisions on its website. It is clear, however, that the MPP does not see itself as the solution: "I think the patent pool can only succeed if other mechanisms are in place. There is a laundry list of TRIPS flexibilities. Some of the alternative models under discussion right now are promising solutions, such as models that seek to delink the costs of research and development."[202] The biggest challenge lies in getting more pharmaceutical companies, such as Abbott, Merck, Johnson and Johnson, Bristol-Myers Squibb, and Roche, to the negotiation table. Despite all of the Gilead agreement's shortcomings, its biggest impact, according to MPP, lies in expanding TDF access and speeding access to future medicines by reducing the time lag in the availability of a drug from developed countries to developing countries from ten years to two.

For ITPC, however, the issues that the agreement raises are much deeper than the specific contents:

> The thing is that the idea of MPP was based on a little group . . . running ahead with something even when they met initial resistance from the Indians, South Asians, and Brazilians. It's like they were saying: "You don't know what you are doing. We have bigger fish to fry. This is a more important issue than your regional concerns." They made political miscalculations. The IPR [intellectual property rights] regime remains very much firmly in place. It has not gone anywhere. With second- and third-line drugs patented, Big Pharma hasn't conceded much at all. They make one voluntary license with MPP and four with generic companies. MPP is irrelevant. It is not a better deal; it is irrelevant. . . . there are much more serious issues like about the generic companies getting into the market. It is not about IPR; it is about market share. So how are going to meet treatment needs? This is another disaster coming. I don't think it is an IPR issue. The point is that we have to keep banging on Pharma, just trying to ensure that they keep the pressure on pricing, to protect India's ability to produce and see if China can produce. . . . MPP is a little bit driven by its own institutional survival and perpetuation rather than having its own critical discourse about IPR. . . . [It] is setting the terms for the debate on access to medicines for the rest of the movement, and getting the consent of groups like

Health GAP, MSF, and TAG. . . . [This] has created a big fight between northern and southern NGOs. From southern NGO perspectives, the deal between Gilead and MPP is against the intent of the patent pool. It discriminates. Only some countries can make use of the patent pool.[203]

AIDS activists from the excluded countries and regions are dismayed that they could be left behind in such a major so-called global access initiative. An ITPC–Eastern Europe and Central Asia campaigner expresses his shock and disappointment: "UNITAID thinks this is an initiative for Africa because it's not as bad in other regions. I understand the focus is on Africa. We have a black joke here. You know Treatment 2.0? Eastern Europe and Central Asia will be 'Africa 2.0.' Donors are moving away, governments are not stepping in, and community activism is not well developed. Sometimes when you listen to Pharma, it looks like a catastrophe [needs to] happen everywhere [before] they will pay attention."[204] The ITPC–Latin America coordinator explains how the MPP-Gilead agreement divided Brazilian civil society from the international AIDS civil society:

Civil society in Brazil was concerned about this because for the countries involved, the deal was good. At the same time, we have to be in solidarity with those countries excluded. Our Ministry of Health [has] constraints in the budget. We feel betrayed. After a close look at the deal, we realized [that] even for the countries included, it was not such a good deal. The deal undermines local production and is bad for everyone in the long term. In the long term, we need to foster local production. The Brazilian civil society was divided, with some organizations preferring to abstain and wait for the reactions of other poor countries and others saying the deal was good for poor countries, that we could not afford to cancel the deal. . . . In the international arena, the split was even clearer. Some big NGOs are on the UNITAID board: Oxfam, Health GAP. They were there when the vote was taken. They hoped the pool would bring benefits. . . . MSF was part of the creation of the pool but started rethinking . . . it. MSF's position is not as hard as ITPC and I-MAK but not like Oxfam and Health GAP. Some southern NGOs believed that northern NGOs were supportive of the pool and had access to information before the license was announced.[205]

Other AIDS groups and coalitions have adopted a wait-and-see attitude. For example, the AIDS and Rights Alliance for Southern Africa was wary of the influence of the Gates Foundation, which supports several of the northern NGO pool enthusiasts, such as the Treatment Action Group, and decided not to take a formal position by signing the ITPC letter but to monitor the work of the MPP.[206]

Meanwhile, the Indian Pharmaceutical Alliance is concerned about the detrimental impact of the MPP-Gilead agreement on potential compulsory licenses issued by the Indian government:

> The brand-name industry is very crafty, very resourceful. They are not convinced that they need to share the[ir] intellectual property with anyone. The model that can work is [the] non-assert declaration whereby the patent holder agrees not to assert [or] enforce patent rights. Then you are free to manufacture and supply the drugs. It will be a free interplay of market forces. UNITAID is not a free interplay of market forces; it decides to whom it licenses. Civil society and UNAIDS should continue to keep pressure on the industry [for the] non-assert declaration. The patent pool has become a buffer against that pressure. In India, we are working on the compulsory licensing of a few ARVs and cancer drugs. If brand-name companies say they already give patents to the patent pool, compulsory licensing may not work.[207]

Cipla, the Indian generic manufacturer that slashed ARV prices and made the treatment revolution possible back in 2000, chose not to be a sublicensee of the MPP-Gilead agreement:

> The problem is that the freedom to operate is very restrictive. They tell me I can only sell [to] the list of ninety-five countries. How can I recover my costs? These countries don't have patent laws. I want the freedom to manufacture and freedom to market, and pay a royalty. You can't tell me not to sell in Latin America because you are strong there. They won't let me sell in the US and Europe, where the money is. In the Third World countries, you only sell on tender, which is at cost price. The patent pool concept should be based on the Canadian bill S91 [which was revoked after Canada joined NAFTA in 1994], where generic manufacturers can copy any drug and pay the patent holder a 4% royalty. I want an automatic license of rights. I don't [want to] have to ask Pharma. The patent pool does not work. I don't see [that] it's financially beneficial to Cipla. I don't earn in Third World countries.[208]

In February 2013, MPP announced a new license with ViiV Healthcare—a joint venture of GlaxoSmithKline, Pfizer, and Shionogi—to increase the market access of pediatric ARVs. The license includes major improvements over the Gilead agreement. It has broader geographical coverage, allowing generic abacavir to be supplied in the 118 countries where 98.7% of children living with HIV reside; does not require royalty payments; does not designate specific countries where the drug can be manufactured; and allows the product to be used in new fixed-dose combinations or formulations.[209]

Lessons Learned from AIDS Treatment Advocacy

It is clear that access to essential medicines continues to be impeded by the global IP regime that was negotiated by "twelve incredibly efficacious individuals" back in 1988 and that culminated in TRIPS in 1995. TRIPS was completely off the radar screen of early AIDS activists, who were busy burying their friends and fighting against government inaction.[210] Yet, when you look at all the issues surrounding HIV, perhaps the "biggest impact is the TRIPS agreement that was negotiated with no community input into the WTO."[211] By the time AIDS activists realized the IP bottleneck and got public health legitimated in international law through the 2001 Doha Declaration, it was already too late. Most countries never took full advantage of the transition period afforded by TRIPS. Thailand amended its patent act in 1992, thirteen years before the 2005 TRIPS deadline. Brazil amended its Industrial Property Law and South Africa amended its Medicines Act in 1997, eight years before their TRIPS obligations. In each of these countries and many others, Pharma started applying for patent protection for their blockbuster drugs long before countries' TRIPS deadlines, all the while pursuing TRIPS-plus provisions through bilateral and regional trade agreements, national administrative protections, patent linkages, evergreening, data exclusivity, voluntary licenses, and anti-counterfeiting regulations.

The success of any mobilization against the de facto market monopolies imposed by Pharma depends on a number of factors, one of which is the strength of the national patent legal framework in terms of TRIPS flexibilities and grant oppositions. India is a prime example: AIDS civil society managed to lobby for public-health-friendly clauses in its amended national patent law in 2005, including the possibilities for both pre- and post-grant oppositions, which activists have been fully exploiting with great successes and far-reaching consequences since 2006. In countries like South Africa, where the domestic patent legislation does not allow for pre-grant or post-grant oppositions, activists have to go for other legal angles, such as anti-competition, to bring down access barriers. An MSF–South Africa campaigner explains, "If you compare the number of patents in Brazil and South Africa, you will see that 2,000 patents are granted in South Africa each year compared to 300 in three years in Brazil. Here, any patent you file for will be granted. We do not have a strong patent office. When [a] patent dispute comes up and generic companies say they will go ahead, patent holders will take them to court."[212]

Another factor is the ability of civil society to form a mass-based movement and/or a broad-based coalition. Thailand offers a great case study on the efficacy and limits of coalition work involving over a thousand local HIV-positive networks, national and international access advocacy groups, lawyers, academics, and public health and consumer groups. Since 1991, over 200 AIDS groups have come together as the Thai Nongovernmental Coalition on AIDS, a community mobilization model that has spread to other areas, such as drug-user networks. In India, it is the cooperation of the trinity of HIV-positive networks, MSF, and the Lawyers Collective that accounts for its remarkable fight against Pharma. The president of the Delhi Network of Positive People, which filed and won many of the grant oppositions, reflects:

> In Delhi, we are very lucky to have good working relationships with the Lawyers Collective and MSF. The lawyers, we need them for all the patent and IP work. MSF has good evidence and communication. And we are the people on the street. The three of us have an unwritten agreement almost. It's amazing. We understand what we need to do, and they understand what they need to do. We mobilize the people, the lawyers file the cases, and MSF does all the communication[s] and media thing[s]. This combination is very good. We can't do without them. . . . One of our most important roles has been our resistance against Pharma. This is our biggest fight, and we are not losing that fight. We are able to resist so far. It's a big victory for us and an eye opener for our politicians as well.[213]

In China, the access movement is led by MSF and the Third World Network, in conjunction with local, regional, and national HIV-positive networks and legal groups, such as the Access to Medicines Research Group, China. This confirms the importance of broad coalition work involving state actors (the Ministry of Health and the patent office) as well as international organizations and foundations (WHO, UNAIDS, and the Clinton Foundation).

None of the fights for access in the twenty-first century would have been possible without treatment literacy, a rights-based approach pioneered by ACT UP that has spread to Latin America, Russia, Africa, China, and the Middle East. Since the 1980s, ABIA has been talking about AIDS treatment access not just from a narrow health perspective, but also from the point of view of discrimination and citizenship rights.[214] In Thailand, treatment literacy at both the grassroots and policy levels paid off in the radical transformation of treatment policy and access around the mid-2000s. As the former executive director of the AIDS Access Foundation emphasizes, "At the time, the NGOs working on AIDS that had previously been engaged in campaigning and training had to learn all about ART [antiretroviral therapy], patenting, TRIPS, and the WTO. . . . We had to travel far and wide, giving information to nearly 100 forums about patents, drugs and various movements at regional and provincial levels."[215] The current executive director continues:

> Every change that we see happened because we worked on it, because we protested and had dialogue with the government. If we had not worked on it, it would not have happened. We cannot stop. At the policy level, we educate and convince policymakers about ARVs. Even when we are able to procure ARVs, we have to educate doctors and policymakers about them. At the field level, we mobilize people around ARV knowledge to make them understand why they need ARVs and why ARVs are so expensive.[216]

Brazilian AIDS activists started their patent oppositions and other civil and legal actions after they met with and learned from the Lawyers Collective. In order to build the case for opposing the TDF patent, GTPI looked at similar grant oppositions in India:

> I was in Toronto for the 16th International AIDS Conference in 2006, on behalf of the ABIA, when my colleagues and I met the Lawyers Collective. . . . We talked a lot and began to understand how oppositions work. We were very inspired by their experiences with oppositions in India. . . . The close contact with Indian activists after the AIDS conference led to the sharing of documents, especially the patent application they were opposing. We compared it to the Brazilian one in order to identify corresponding claims, and then decided which arguments used by the Indians could be replicated in Brazil.[217]

Despite the huge gains in the twenty-first century, many barriers to universal access remain: it is a lucrative $13 billion market, and the margin for some products is over 95%, so there is little incentive for pharmaceutical companies to lower their prices.[218] In addition, the demand for second- and third-line treatment will dramatically increase between 2015 and 2025. In Khayelitsha, South Africa, 14% of the patients on first-line treatment for five years needed to switch to second-line treatment, and 25% of those who switched developed resistance within two years, necessitating third-line treatment. As of 2010, the most affordable WHO-recommended second-line treatment cost $465 pppy, three times that of first-line regimens.[219] "The crisis is not going away," stresses the advocacy officer of MSF–New Delhi. "What we have is a very compromised situation, solving patent issues for a few ARVs. We haven't resolved the more fundamental patent regime issue. [Despite] setting up a patent pool on ARV, the issue of Pharma is still there."[220] In India alone, there are over 10,000 patent applications for medicines pend-

ing. Patient groups have opposed only a dozen so far. Opposing patents is difficult and time-consuming, and requires tremendous human and financial
resources:

> [Even for lawyers,] the patent system is very hard to understand. We never know
> how many patents cover a medicine because nothing is disclosed. . . . AIDS is sup-
> posed to be regulated by UN bodies, but there are side systems advocating for TRIPS-
> plus with pressure coming from all sides. It is impossible for NGOs like ABIA, [which]
> can't even pay the rent of our office, to face this [on] every front. Even by issuing
> compulsory licensing, we are legitimating a system we don't agree with. We need
> to find another possible system. Every time, we are just throwing [drops of] water
> [on a] fire.[221]

Pharma has increasingly taken bolder actions to preempt civil society's patent
oppositions. After Novartis lost its appeal of the Indian Patent Office's rejection
of a patent application for a cancer drug, Gleevec, in 2005, because it failed to show
an increase in therapeutic efficacy in what is essentially a new form of a known
substance, the pharmaceutical giant decided to challenge the national patent law
itself by launching a lawsuit on Section 3(d). This section of the amended Indian
Patents Act, which requires the patent holder to demonstrate inventiveness and
non-obviousness in its application, was specifically lobbied for by the Affordable
Medicines and Treatment campaign as a safeguard against patent evergreening.
It is the legal basis for many of the patent oppositions filed by AIDS and other patient groups. If Novartis won the case, the consequences would have been far-
reaching, affecting not only AIDS drugs, but also those for TB, malaria, heart disease, and asthma. MSF, Oxfam, and Care spearheaded a global Drop the Case
campaign against Novartis.[222] On April 1, 2013, the Supreme Court of India rejected Novartis's appeal for Gleevec. Anand Grover, the senior counsel and director of the Lawyers Collective's HIV/AIDS Unit, who represented the Cancer Patients Aid Association, said, "The Supreme Court's interpretation of section 3(d)
keeps it intact. It is alive and kicking. It gives life to Parliament's intent of facilitating access to medicines and of incentivizing only genuine research. By refusing patent monopolies on minor changes to known molecules, this judgment will
facilitate early entry of generic medicines into the market for other medicines and
diseases too. The impact will be felt not only in India, but also across the developing world."[223]

Adding to this hostile pharmaceutical landscape is donor AIDS fatigue, which
has a fatal impact on treatment. After years of considerable funding increases,

AIDS funding fell in 2010 (to $7.6 billion from $8.7 in 2009).[224] MSF immediately felt the effects on the ground:

> Disruptions of supply have been more frequently noted in 2009 and 2010 in almost all countries studied. Whereas previously, MSF-supported health facilities would receive the majority of the ARV needs through government channels, financed by the Global Fund, UNITAID/CHAI [Clinton Health Access Initiative] and PEPFAR, with a relatively limited need for MSF to complement ARV supply, in 2009 and 2010, MSF had to increase its buffer stocks significantly and provide more regular emergency supplies to MSF-supported clinics in Mozambique, Malawi, Uganda, and DRC. In Uganda's rural northwest, after a period of more effective decentralization of care to clinics closer to patients, these decentralized sites received no government-supplied ARVs and had to be fully supported by the MSF ARV[s].[225]

In October 2009, the US CDC sent out a letter asking its partners in Uganda to "only enroll new ARV patients if they are sure that these new patients can continue to be supported without a future increase in funding."[226] In Zimbabwe, Uganda, and South Africa, PEPFAR-funded clinics were asked to reserve treatment slots for pregnant women and children. Treatment scale-back also has an impact on patients developing resistance. Margie Hardman, who works in a PEPFAR-funded treatment program in South Africa, explains:

> I think the consequences of someone that has been tested HIV-positive and that can't get on treatment very quickly are really terrible. Those patients have plucked up the courage to have the test, they know that people who get ARVs got better. So, they are very disappointed. And because their CD4 counts [are] quite low, they will pick up TB, they will get sick with pneumonia, meningitis, many things. If we could have . . . them on ARVs quickly, this would [be] prevented.[227]

Finally, little has been done to ensure treatment research sustainability. There are a couple of global public health proposals that have been suggested by the Nobel-winning economist Jeffrey Sachs, including some form of foreign aid to be granted to pharmaceutical companies that develop new medicines to treat neglected tropical diseases. In April 2012, the Consultative Expert Working Group on Research and Development (CEWG), established by the WHO in 2010, published a groundbreaking report recommending concrete mechanisms to deal with market failures. These include the creation of a new binding agreement to provide billions of dollars annually for R&D to address the special healthcare needs of people in developing countries, open innovation models, technology transfer, and the delinkage of R&D costs from product prices.[228] At the annual World

Health Assembly in 2012, governments had the opportunity to vote on the issue. Health Action International delivered an open letter to WHO member states that was endorsed by over sixty NGOs, reiterating the severity of the problem: "More than ten years of debate and discussion and the publication of three expert reports all have arrived at one conclusion: medical technologies, such as medicines, diagnostics and vaccines, too often remain unaffordable, unavailable and unsuitable for the people who need them."[229] Despite the passionate call to member states to adopt the measures proposed in the CEWG report, however, governments chose to shelve the initiative and opted instead for a global R&D "observatory."[230] According to KEI, "A number of negotiators from developing countries pressed for a much more ambitious outcome, building upon the bold report of the WHO Consultative Expert Working Group on R&D Financing, but the United States and the European Union, both dealing with large financial crises, were dead set against any action [on] the R&D Treaty proposal until 2016."[231]

This was yet another major setback for treatment activists. It is clear that unless immediate action is taken to restore funding, to address fundamental IP issues, and to invest in research and development for the majority around the world, the grandiose commitments—universal access, Treatment 2.0, 15×15, the Millennium Development Goals, Countdown to Zero, Born HIV-Free, and AIDS-Free Generation—will remain slogans only.

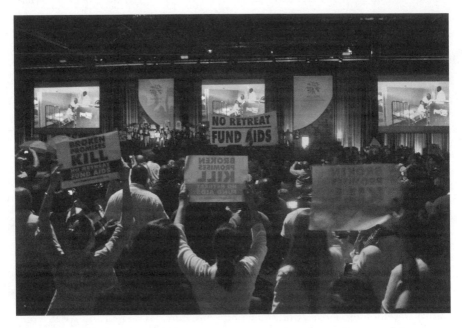

No Retreat, Fund AIDS, 2012 International AIDS Conference, Washington, DC
Photo by author

CHAPTER FOUR

Against Governance and the
Oligopolization of Power

AIDS is the biggest success in UN history.
—*External Relations Officer, UNAIDS*

AIDS is a kind of window through which we see global governance.
—*Executive Director, ABIA*

While science regulates the at-risk body and while the market controls who lives or dies, an enormous global governance apparatus has arisen over the past three decades that sets the AIDS agenda, determines the scientific and technical guidelines and the normative contours of how the world talks about AIDS, slots funding, and decides the strategic future of the epidemic by investing or divesting political energy. This AIDS bureaucracy employs an impressive elite corps of professionals in epidemiology, procurement, finance, grant and project management, monitoring and evaluation, auditing, risk management, innovation, resource mobilization, MARPs, and donor relations—a global AIDS industry. Above all, AIDS has brought forth a new public health perspective that is marked by the global cooperation of a wide range of actors, including people living with HIV and AIDS.[1] If AIDS is the biggest success in UN history, is it an exception in global governance because of the confluence of specific political factors, or has AIDS transformed global governance in some fundamental ways from which other social movements can draw lessons? What role has AIDS activism played in this transformation?

Using a nexus of power-knowledge-subject-resistance, this chapter looks at the emergence of a global AIDS governance structure and the intrusion of AIDS activism into this structure since the late 1980s in the context of an ongoing legitimation crisis of democratic deficits, inefficiency, and the ineffectiveness of the United Nations. I first lay out the political and organizational contours of this regime of power by discussing the division of labor among UN agencies and funding organizations. Then I analyze AIDS activists' battles for inclusion and involvement in governance. I end by examining activists' reform proposals in five areas of the global AIDS architecture: donor coordination; governance harmonization; health system integration and national leadership; intellectual property and the private sector; and civil society engagement and capacity building. At the center of these discussions are broad questions of legitimacy: Who holds the power to set the global AIDS agenda? On whose and on what terms is inclusion being negotiated? To what extent has AIDS activism changed the traditional rules of global governance based on state sovereignty and economic power?

Who's in Charge: Division of Labor or Turf War?

Despite what must be counted as a formal consensus, international cooperation in response to AIDS aroused public controversy and resistance, doubts and divergent responses from some governmental authorities and social groups. This contention extends from broad social issues to more technical and legal questions. These include voluntary versus compulsory testing, issues of confidentiality, antidiscrimination, AIDS and HIV infection in the workplace, the control of "high-risk" behavior, access to clean needles and syringes and the contention of novel education programs. Other related issues include whether AIDS should be classified as being a sexually transmitted disease, how the infected should have access to experimental drugs and how these should be tested. Moreover, strife among organizations over the scope of their work, the control of resources and a wide variety of other "normal" interorganizational frictions have frustrated and complicated cooperation.

—*Gordenker et al.*, International Cooperation
in Response to AIDS[2]

The history of the international response to AIDS—which has been marked by "bargaining, compromises, uncertainties, unintended consequences, [and] differences in perceiving 'reality' and in approaches to both policies and programs of international cooperation"[3]—can be grouped roughly into four phases: 1981–1986, 1987–1990, 1991–1999, and 2000–2010.

1981–1986: Inaction

The first years of the epidemic were defined by little multilateral cooperation. In June 1983, the Committee of Ministers in the Council of Europe passed a recommendation on the prevention of AIDS transmission from blood donors. A few months later, the Parliamentary Assembly of the Council of Europe adopted a resolution "to denounce the use of this disease as a pretext for campaigns against homosexuals."[4] The resolution reaffirmed the 1981 commitment of the Council of Europe that upheld the right to sexual self-determination and called upon the WHO to remove homosexuality from its International Classification of Diseases. Still stuck in its colonialist thinking about tropical medicine, the WHO did not respond to AIDS until after the first International AIDS Conference in Atlanta in 1985. The director-general of the WHO, Halfdan Mahler, confessed that he had to be convinced that AIDS, which had up until that point primarily caught the attention of North American and European governments, was a problem that would affect the developing world.[5]

1987–1990: Fragmented Multilateral Response

The second phase was marked by an initially uncoordinated response under individual leadership. In the United Nations, there were two parallel structures on AIDS: the Department of International Economic and Social Affairs (DIESA, but now more commonly DESA), designated by the secretary-general through a 1987 UN General Assembly resolution to coordinate various agencies in the UN's response to AIDS, and the Global Programme on AIDS (GPA), which was set up within the WHO that same year. While the Steering Committee on AIDS organized by DIESA, which included the UN Children's Fund (UNICEF), the UN Population Fund (UNFPA), the UN Development Programme (UNDP), and later WHO, achieved little and became practically dormant by 1992, GPA's strategy of donor relations and putting in place national AIDS programs was highly successful. Under the leadership of Jonathan Mann, the program expanded rapidly, and its budget increased from $30 million in 1987 to $214 million in 1991, half of which flowed directly to or through the WHO. By 1990, almost every country in the world had a national AIDS program, and 159 out of 167 WHO member governments had received some support from GPA.[6]

But the rapid expansion of GPA and the meteoric rise of Mann as an AIDS star, eclipsing his boss, the newly appointed WHO director-general, Hiroshi Nakajima, soon spelled the end of this initial phase of multilateralism. According to a former staff member, the GPA was not a typical WHO program. The new operational and communication procedures demanded by the urgency of a global AIDS response bypassed the traditional lines of regional authority in the WHO and angered many.[7] GPA also inserted itself as the gatekeeper for all external support for national AIDS programs, which created much jealousy and animosity among other UN agencies. GPA was concerned about each UN agency pursuing an independent AIDS agenda. For instance, UNICEF wanted to focus its AIDS program uniquely on children, ignoring other vulnerable populations.[8] More important, GPA was created with its own supervisory structure called the Global Management Committee (GMC), which was funded mostly through extrabudgetary, that is, voluntary, contributions from a few key donor governments, notably the United States with an initial endowment of $100 million. While the World Health Assembly (WHA), consisting of all WHO members, retained final authority over GPA, "the emphasis on oversight of programs and financing leaves little doubt as to where the final decisions [were] prepared."[9] A 1989 GMC-mandated review of the GPA found that the WHO/GPA leadership role vis-à-vis other UN agencies was not clarified and that there were duplicated duties and undefined responsibilities in the United Nations.[10] Rumor had it too that donors, led by the United States, would divest from GPA in opposition to the reappointment of Hiroshi Nakajima as the WHO director-general, because he had caused the abrupt resignation of Jonathan Mann.[11] In 1991, contributions to GPA declined, marking the end of this initial, short-lived, multilateral response.

1991–1999: UN Division of Labor in AIDS

The third phase, the 1990s, was characterized by the search for a new coordinating mechanism that would be acceptable to all the major stakeholders. An ad hoc working group headed by Ulf Rundin, a Swedish diplomat who had just directed the Nordic UN Reform Project, proposed the creation of a new organization outside the WHO, with representation from bilateral donors, UN agencies, and NGOs, to coordinate AIDS policies and programs in the United Nations.[12] This is what scholars in international relations call "forum shifting": moving an agenda from one organization to another in order to achieve certain specific objectives.[13] The idea of a joint and co-sponsored UN program on AIDS, proposed by a Canadian representative, was adopted by the 1993 World Health Assembly. At the heart of the subsequent negotiations was the role of the WHO in this new structure. While a 1994 WHO press release continued to argue for its central role in housing the new UN program on AIDS, rekindling lingering suspicion among other UN agencies about WHO's control, the final July 1994 resolution by the UN Economic and Social Council (ECOSOC), which gave birth to UNAIDS, got rid of the traditional hierarchical ordering of the United Nations: "Explicitly seeking to avoid 'verticalization' of AIDS issues, it promotes a multisectoral approach. By 'integrated programming' officials of all participating organizations will need to consult each other in each step of assistance projects. The new secretariat for the UN program would reflect the 'co-ownership' of the program."[14]

Touted as UN reform in action, UNAIDS, established in 1996, represents a new form of partnership where each co-sponsoring UN agency—initially, WHO, UNDP, UNFPA, UNICEF, UNESCO, and the World Bank, and then expanded to include the International Labour Organization (ILO), the World Food Programme (WFP), the UN High Commissioner for Refugees (UNHCR), UNODC, and UN Women—contributes to the global AIDS response according to its "comparative advantage."[15] The collaborative model is "premised on the technical competency, leadership and facilitating roles of the Secretariat and the Cosponsors at the various levels and how they deliver results."[16] UNAIDS is charged with the mission of uniting UN efforts in conjunction with civil society, people living with AIDS, national governments, the private sector, and other global institutions; taking up a human rights agenda; mobilizing resources; empowering agents of change with information; and supporting inclusive country leadership.[17] Its main governance structure is the twenty-two-seat Programme Coordinating Board, which has representatives from governments from all geographic regions, representatives from UNAIDS co-sponsors, and five representatives from NGOs, including associations of people living with HIV. Its biggest success has been in mobilizing leadership, which has translated into advocacy in each subfield of the global response, including funding and treatment.[18]

WHO's GPA funding was diverted to the newly established UNAIDS secretariat, and WHO was forced to scale down and mainstream its HIV work through some thirty different departments focusing on nutrition, medicines, technology, human rights, children, youth, and so on.[19] Although an HIV/AIDS Department was reestablished in 2001 after the UN General Assembly Special Session on HIV/AIDS (UNGASS), WHO never regained its GPA-era stature or funding for its AIDS work. In the division of labor, WHO takes the lead on HIV and TB treatment and care, and co-leads on preventing mother-to-child transmission (PMTCT). As a result of significant funding cuts, it has been reduced to providing technical guidelines and assistance. The expectation is that it will do all the standard setting, for example, on PMTCT or harm reduction despite a lack of resources, all the while continuing to provide support to member states.[20] The major achievements of the WHO are its AIDS treatment and prevention guidelines, its PMTCT guidelines, and the 3 by 5 Initiative (to treat 3 million people in the South by 2005) under the leadership of Jim Kim. Although the 3 million target was not achieved until 2007, the political momentum of the initiative encouraged the adoption of

the universal-access agenda reflected in the 2006 Political Declaration on HIV/
AIDS at the UN General Assembly's High-Level Meeting on HIV/AIDS.

UNDP played a very significant early role through the 1987 WHO/UNDP Alliance to Combat AIDS, even though "the formal act did not quickly achieve much of the sought-after result."[21] The early partnership arose out of a mutual recognition of the complementary structures of the two organizations with the WHO leading in the scientific and health dimensions of AIDS and the UNDP providing the much-needed field response from the wider perspectives of development and poverty. As the director of the HIV/AIDS Group of the UNDP recalls:

> From 1987 to 1991, Elizabeth Reid and . . . other colleagues within the UNDP developed the notion that the AIDS epidemic did not just come from [a] virus, but from patterns of development, poverty, and gender. Poverty shaped the way HIV spread and in turn HIV had [an] impact on gender and development. Jonathan Mann at the WHO had a very similar analysis, but focused more on human rights terms. The shorthand was that UNDP were the AIDS and development people, and the WHO were the AIDS and human rights people. There was a bureaucratic element as well when the Special Programme on AIDS became GPA. WHO wanted to facilitate the transfer of money to countries to set up the NAP [national AIDS program]. But the WHO had always had operational limitations, and so WHO and UNDP together set up a WHO/UNDP trust fund in which traditional donors would then help get national AIDS committees off the ground.[22]

According to this director, the mandate of UNDP has changed little since the early days. The conceptual distinction in the work of UNDP vis-à-vis the WHO is crucial. The WHO has always been central to the health sector response, using biomedical public health interventions, whereas UNDP focuses on the socioeconomic dynamics of the epidemic.[23] When UNAIDS was created, UNDP was tasked with planning, governance, gender issues, and human rights. According to the HIV/AIDS Group director, this is UNDP's most significant contribution to the AIDS response:

> UNDP is the premier and central UN organization that draws attention to the role of poverty and gender as social factors that drive vulnerability. UNDP did not pioneer multidimensional community response to address those things; ActionAid did on how to address gender and inequality. UNDP was central, however, in showing that you can implement at scale and that you can incorporate [those perspectives] into policies. . . . UNDP has [had some] huge success on law and rights. I give Jonathan Mann credit [for] put[ting] law and rights on the AIDS agenda initially, and

then more recently Michel Sidibé has been doing the same thing. But UNDP does deserve credit for [working] country by country, initiative by initiative, working on advising parliamentarians on legislation, building political consensus, and repealing bad laws . . . translating leadership into actions. In the area of IP laws, UNDP has done a huge amount to let countries know how to use compulsory licensing, procurement for small states, looking at different ways such as competition laws. . . . Again, we weren't the first to talk about TRIPS, but UNDP has been out there helping countries to put these ideas into laws.[24]

UNFPA is the convenor on sex work and the co-convenor with UNDP on men who have sex with men and transgender populations. Its four main activities are engaging with sex worker community organizations; providing sexual reproductive health services for key populations; condom programs for sex workers, MSM, and transgender people; and working with key affected young people.[25] UNFPA has been successful in providing global guidance for specific key populations but struggles to mainstream HIV across all UNFPA agendas from the headquarters to the country level. One of the main challenges for UNFPA is its controversial mandate—involving issues such as abortion and sex work—that makes it hard to work with some governments.[26]

Within UNAIDS, the mandate of the World Bank is planning, accountability, and governance of the HIV response. Most of the bank's work on AIDS, however, has been channeled through its own Multi-Country HIV/AIDS Program (MAP) for Africa, which has a bigger annual budget than UNAIDS. Its independence from the rest of the UN system means that the bank often does not even appear in the UNAIDS work plan at the national level even though it receives money to supposedly fulfill its mandate.[27] A more fundamental problem relates to the bank's ideology of neoliberal market reforms.[28] How can it strengthen health systems through MAP while capping public spending on health and other social services in other bank operations? For example, in some African countries, new healthcare workers cannot be hired in areas with chronic shortages even if donors are willing to finance the human resources because the bank has put wage ceilings on the public sector and quotas on healthcare posts.[29] This fundamental contradiction between the bank's financing ideology and its role in the global HIV response remains unresolved.

The ILO is the lead agency for workplace policies, programs, and the private sector. It addresses HIV from the point of view of labor rights, and its major contribution has been the 2001 ILO Code of Practice on HIV/AIDS, which positions HIV as a workplace issue. The ILO affirms principles of nondiscrimination and gender equality, and provides guidelines for the development of national policies and employer programs in prevention education, training, testing, care, and support.[30] While it has been successful in advocating for better workplace HIV policies, scaling up national responses and the mobilization of the private sector remains a challenge. As of 2012, only thirty-two countries had developed national policies on HIV in the workplace. According to the senior technical advisor of the ILO Programme on HIV/AIDS and the World of Work, global recognition of the criticality of workplace responses is still largely missing. In high-burden countries, governments or private companies might put in place some kind of programming in specific sectors, such as mining, but do not look at the economy as a whole, assuming that other workers are not at risk. The ILO might work with a country on a project for two years, but its impact is limited if the program is not then continued by the Ministry of Health or a national AIDS program. How to position HIV in the private sector is also an issue. The majority of private sector responses to AIDS are framed as corporate social responsibility activities: the company supports a small one-time intervention and then checks the box "funded and delivered."[31]

On paper, the demarcation of responsibilities among various UNAIDS co-sponsors looks rather straightforward. In reality, however, continuous competition among UN agencies "is painful" to acknowledge.[32] A veteran bureaucrat confesses that UNAIDS has at least partially failed in coordination when one member of the UNAIDS family goes against another in competition for Global Fund money.[33] Overlapping governance and organizational structures, funding shortages, and ideological conflicts are to blame for failures in UN agencies' cooperation in AIDS.

One of the greatest challenges of UNAIDS is the different governance structures of its co-sponsors. WHO, for instance, is a specialized agency accountable to the WHA, which is composed of 194 member states, while UNDP answers directly to ECOSOC instead of member states. The confusion comes because "decisions made at the Programme Coordinating Board (PCB) of UNAIDS often may not take into consideration . . . the governing bodies of the co-sponsoring organizations."[34] Hence, while the formal mandate of the WHO comes from WHA, as a UNAIDS co-sponsor WHO is also supposed to abide by PCB decisions, which are made by a much smaller subset of states and nonstate actors. Decision-making processes concerning AIDS thus vary, depending on the actual country and delegation, from the Ministry of Health reporting to the WHA to the national AIDS program reporting to the PCB to the Ministry of Development working with UNDP. A concrete example of governance conflicts is the Unified Budget and

Work Plan of UNAIDS, which is supposed to be binding on all co-sponsors, creating the expectation that they will all report to PCB. Yet each co-sponsoring UN partner also has its own budget mechanism based on its mandate.[35] This structural governance problem remains unresolved. Some member states maintain that they cannot be held accountable for adherence to PCB decisions that they have never been part of, while others challenge UNAIDS strategy as a whole.

The WHO is explicit in arguing that it should focus on health sector responses, given that 75% of HIV work is undertaken by the health sector and that the predominant vertical strategy of HIV work compromises many other aspects of public health. Ultimately, the question of AIDS governance requires an assessment of the value of having a dedicated HIV response compared to integrating HIV into wider health system changes.[36] The governance structure has also enabled some states to use the smaller PCB as a forum to voice their ideological objections, bypassing the more cumbersome 194-state WHA. For example, at the 2012 PCB meeting, two Middle Eastern governments—Iran and Egypt—opposed the inclusion of MSM in the discussion concerning the enabling legal environment.[37]

The structural impediments to UN cooperation in AIDS include different organizational structures, funding competition, and ideological opposition among UN agencies. Some co-sponsors, such as UNDP, UNFPA, WFP, and UNHCR, are well established in the field while others, like ILO and UNESCO, have only regional or subregional offices. So while UNESCO may be enthusiastic about leading the global AIDS response on stigma and discrimination as they relate to cultural and social barriers, it has a limited field structure to support such a response. Meanwhile, on issues where there has been substantive funding, such as gender and HIV, turf wars inevitably arise. UNDP became the convenor on gender based on the recognition that gender has many dimensions in addition to AIDS, including poverty, migration, and human rights; UNDP has deep roots working in these areas and hosts UNIFEM.[38] Feminist health activists, led by Adrienne Germain of the International Women's Health Coalition, however, have been vocal against UNDP's lead on gender and HIV, and are concerned that too much AIDS funding will take away from family planning and sexual reproductive health within UNFPA.[39] When the feminists' push to take gender away from UNDP failed, the solution was to "divide the pie" by having UNFPA co-convene with UNDP on gender.[40]

Even when the division of labor is more or less clear on paper—with UNFPA focusing on reproductive health and UNDP on key populations—"it takes a lot of time to clarify" the roles in UNAIDS.[41] With the coming on board of UN Women in 2012 as the newest UNAIDS co-sponsor, a whole set of new negotiations among the three agencies has been opened. How about MSM? If UNDP is the lead convenor on gender, should it not also perform the same role for MSM? Some think that UNDP's work on MSM has been "disastrous" since it simply does not have a tradition of dealing with such issues. Critics charge that the only reason for UNDP to cling to its ill-adapted responsibility is to "have a share of the budget."[42] Further, UNDP's role as the principal recipient of last resort of Global Fund grants in post-conflict societies and corruption-ridden countries, delivering $300 million worth of AIDS services per year, has attracted considerable jealousy as well as criticism from both within and without the UN system. International NGOs consider grants in these contexts to be their line of business and would rather see themselves instead of the well-endowed UNDP as the principal recipient.[43]

Finally, ideological opposition also stands in the way of a coordinated UN AIDS response. Both harm reduction and sex work are examples par excellence. According to the former communications manager of the Asian Harm Reduction Network, assigning UNODC to be the convenor for HIV among injecting drug users has been disastrous:

> This organization does not have a legitimate reason for existence. Giving them the mandate of HIV prevention among IDUs and harm reduction is one of the worst mistakes in the past ten years. UNODC is a very unique UN agency. It's the only one that works with a law enforcement paradigm. The others have a humanitarian paradigm. Do you think the cops are going to tell us how to save lives? I don't think so. It's a fundamentally flawed design. That said, they have improved in the past ten years, though not by much. They have improved in that they are open to consultation [with] civil society. I would not say "genuinely," but more open. They are somewhat supportive of harm reduction now. In front of [representatives from] civil society, they . . . speak out with brio about harm reduction. When they are with law enforcement, they won't say a peep about IDUs.[44]

In regard to sex work, no UN agency was willing or ready to convene until 2006. WHO was doing some programmatic work, but the doctors did not want to take the lead. ILO could have done it from a labor perspective, but never got to the point of leading the response. UNDP does not have technical expertise in this field.[45] So UNFPA became the convening agency by elimination. A UNFPA senior technical advisor admits:

> To say that it has been an easy journey within the UNFPA would not be telling the truth. I still think . . . at the headquarters level, there is a 10% buy-in [on sex work]. I would say that is being honest. . . . Since 2006, we have gone from five-country

office programming on sex work to seventy-nine-country programming, which is a gigantic leap. . . . I mean, it has really been incredible. So I think the [lack of] political buy-in [at] headquarters is really shocking. . . . And I say openly to them . . . from the executive director down, that they really should accept strongly that UN-FPA leads in this area of work, and it is a legitimate area of work.[46]

"The real question to be asked in terms of division of labor and the uptake of mandate," continues this activist turned UN bureaucrat, "is the extent to which a co-sponsor organization has a strong, medium, lukewarm, weak, or barely existent commitment to HIV."[47] While enthusiasm and commitment were strong around 1996, when UNAIDS was created, it may no longer be the case today, as donors push UN agencies to go back to their core mandates. For instance, HIV was completely dropped from the UNFPA mission statement in 2012. As for other co-sponsors, one should ask: Which have retained a focus on HIV as a really critical part of their functioning?

2000–2010: High-Level Political Commitment and the Oligopolization of AIDS Funding

The global response to AIDS in the first decade of the twenty-first century was marked by high political commitment matched with unprecedented levels of funding and a proliferation of actors and partnerships beyond the traditional intergovernmental structures. A number of high-level UN meetings, declarations, and resolutions catapulted AIDS from a narrow health concern to an issue of global security, human rights, and development.

In July 2000, the UN Security Council passed a resolution on a health issue (resolution 1308), the first in its history, to address the severity of the crisis, especially in Africa, and to urge international cooperation on access to treatment, care, and prevention.[48] Two months later, the UN General Assembly adopted the Millennium Declaration in which time-bound goals were set in eight major areas of human rights and development: end poverty and hunger; achieve universal education; eliminate gender inequality; promote child health; improve maternal health; halt HIV/AIDS, malaria, and other diseases; ensure environmental sustainability; and develop global partnerships. In particular, goal 6 establishes the ambitious targets of halting the spread of HIV/AIDS, reaching universal access to treatment, and reversing malaria and tuberculosis by 2015.[49] In April 2001, recognizing that the "access to medication in the context of pandemics such as HIV/AIDS is one fundamental element for achieving progressively the full realization of the right of everyone to the enjoyment of the highest attainable standard of physical and mental health," the UN Commission on Human Rights passed the Access to Medication in the Context of Pandemics Such as HIV/AIDS Resolution to urge nation-states "to facilitate, wherever possible, access in other countries to essential preventive, curative or palliative pharmaceuticals or medical technologies used to treat pandemics such as HIV/AIDS or the most common opportunistic infections that accompany them."[50] The commission also passed other resolutions on intellectual property rights.[51]

Two months later, in June 2001, the UN adopted the historic Declaration of Commitment on HIV/AIDS at UNGASS, which for the first time named AIDS a global emergency that requires the urgent, coordinated, and sustained response of all nation-states. The 2001 declaration acknowledges all of the key issues of the epidemic: poverty, underdevelopment, and illiteracy as the principal contributing factors to the spread of HIV/AIDS; stigma, silence, and discrimination; gender inequality and the need to empower women; the availability and affordability of drugs and related technologies; the lack of high-quality health systems; the debt problem; and the particular role and significant contribution of people living with HIV/AIDS. It sets time-bound goals in leadership, prevention, treatment, human rights, vulnerability, the care of children made vulnerable by AIDS, social and economic impact, research and development, and conflict situations. Above all, UNGASS calls on nation-states to "reach an overall target of annual expenditure[s] on the epidemic of between US$7 billion and US$10 billion in low- and middle-income countries" by 2015.[52]

UNGASS was followed by two more high-level meetings and declarations of commitment to AIDS. In 2006, states met to review the progress toward the targets set out in the 2001 declaration on HIV/AIDS and adopted a new Political Declaration on HIV/AIDS that reaffirmed both the 2001 declaration and the Millennium Development Goals, highlighting in particular the goal of universal access by 2010. Clearly, the latter goal was not met. The 2011 Political Declaration on HIV/AIDS refined the goals, targets, and indicators to ten specific areas: reducing sexual transmission; preventing HIV among drug users; eliminating new HIV infections among children; reaching 15 million people with treatment; reducing TB deaths; closing the resource gap; eliminating gender inequalities and gender-based violence; eliminating stigma and discrimination; eliminating travel restrictions; and strengthening integration in health systems.[53] AIDS activists continue to use these various declarations of commitments as an accountability mechanism to monitor intergovernmental and state activities through regular progress reports.[54]

One of the most significant outcomes of the high-level visibility of AIDS on the global agenda was the unprecedented financial mobilization for a single disease. Some would go so far as to argue that this was the biggest advocacy success of the UN in recent years.[55] In April 2001, the UN secretary-general, Kofi Annan, who had made the battle against AIDS his personal priority, called for a "war chest" at the Abuja Special Summit on AIDS.[56] The establishment of the Global Fund to Fight AIDS, Tuberculosis, and Malaria in 2002 brought sea changes in the AIDS funding scene. As of 2012, the Global Fund had approved $23 billion of funding for more than a thousand programs, which have provided AIDS treatment for 4.2 million people, anti-tuberculosis treatment for 9.7 million people, and 310 million insecticide-treated nets for the prevention of malaria in 151 countries.[57]

Wary of its lack of control in a multilateral fund, the US government chose to set up its own organization, PEPFAR, and committed a total of $67 billion between 2003 and 2013, almost three times the money raised by the Global Fund. Meanwhile, the World Bank launched its first HIV/AIDS strategy, *Intensifying Action against HIV/AIDS in Africa: Responding to a Development Crisis*, in 2000, committing a more modest $2 billion for its Multi-Country HIV/AIDS Program for Africa over a fifteen-year time frame.[58] Above all, the Bill and Melinda Gates Foundation, with a handsome $60 billion endowment, has created what Okie calls the "Gates-Buffett effect."[59] By increasing the foundation's annual giving from US$1.36 billion in 2005 to about US$3 billion in 2006, or nearly $1 per year for every person in the poorer half of the world's population, the Gates Foundation became by far the largest charitable organization with great potential impact in global public health. A major difference that sets the Gates Foundation apart is its conspicuous absence from the treatment scene. The Gates strategy rests primarily on medical and preventive technologies in vaccine research and development, antiretroviral prevention methods, service delivery, voluntary medical male circumcision, diagnostic tools, and scaling up HIV prevention programs.[60]

Adding to these major investments in AIDS was the emphasis on innovative financing beyond traditional bilateral and multilateral aid mechanisms. Supported by France in partnership with Brazil, Chile, Norway, and the United Kingdom, UNITAID was created in 2006 to strategically channel innovative funding to underserved health product markets, such as pediatric HIV treatments or cutting-edge diagnostic tools. Its business model is "commodity-driven" with the goal of developing sustainable and affordable health products. Over half of its funding comes from an airline levy, which ranges from $1 for economy-class tickets to approximately $40 for business- and first-class travel, that has been implemented so far by nine countries: Cameroon, Chile, Congo, France, Madagascar, Mali, Mauritius, Niger, and the Republic of Korea.[61] Since 2006, UNITAID has raised $2 billion and funded projects in ninety-four countries. According to its executive director, the impact of UNITAID is not so much on financing per se, since the airline levy does not bring in a huge amount of money. Rather, "the impact is much more [from] using the small [amount of] money to reduce the price of second-line drugs, especially in pediatric ARV, . . . and financing the WHO Prequalification Program, which [has] made forty-three drugs available since we started funding."[62] UNITAID's market initiative has resulted in price reductions of 10%–40% for medicines and diagnostics.[63] Beyond the airline levy and initiatives such as Product Red—where 50% of the profits go directly from the manufacturers to the Global Fund[64]—a promising new avenue is a financial transaction tax (FTT), already adopted in various forms in over forty countries, which is expected to bring in an additional $15 billion per year.[65] The question, however, is whether the new funding will be used for development or for neglected health markets.

What has been observed in the twenty-first century in AIDS funding is oligopolization—the market becoming dominated by a small number of players—with PEPFAR, the Gates Foundation, and the Global Fund bypassing the traditional UN structure. PEPFAR is a bilateral aid agency under the sway of US national interests. The Gates Foundation is a private entity accountable only to the Gates family. The Global Fund mixes traditional multilateralism with private sector and NGO participation, but is accountable only to its own board.

With $67 billion committed by the US Congress between 2003 and 2013, PEPFAR became the most important funder in AIDS. From the anti-prostitution pledge to its abstinence-only prevention policy, the prohibition of needle exchange, and earlier purchases of expensive brand-name ARV drugs, its impact on setting the global AIDS agenda according to US interests is undeniable. The effect of PEPFAR "conditionalities" on African recipient countries has been profound. According to a Ugandan activist, "Organisations taking PEPFAR money have to stop doing all this other work for fear of losing their funding. It becomes a nightmare for people, juggling their work and how they present it to different people—and there is a deep fear of legal action. This is paralysing people and organisations."[66] In 2005, Human Rights Watch published a scathing report, *The Less They Know, the Better*, detailing the devastating impact of the PEPFAR ideology of abstinence on Uganda.[67] "This whole abstinence-only agenda is based on falsehoods," Beatrice Were, a Ugandan AIDS activist, says. "They target girls but they never talk about gender and power relations. Girls are told to abstain but boys in our culture are still encouraged to explore—and to experience different sexual relations. Male promiscuity is socially accepted or even expected. . . . This whole abstinence agenda is profoundly out of touch with cultural and social norms in Uganda and makes no attempt to address them."[68]

PEPFAR is omnipresent and yet invisible in the African AIDS scene. According to a veteran Health GAP activist:

> The Global Health Initiative we helped create is opaque, dysfunctional, and entirely secret. . . . PEPFAR is massive in the African health sector and yet hidden behind multiple layers of things. People don't even think of PEPFAR, but it is so much bigger than everything else. Every single INGO that is out there is PEPFAR. Every single USAID and CDC truck is PEPFAR. Every single Department of Defense truck, every single government truck is PEPFAR. About half of the staff in most of the public clinics is PEPFAR. They are everywhere. They are almost everything. Nobody knows. We know how to go and fight with the government for the tiny sliver, but hardly anybody realizes the huge actor.[69]

PEPFAR's invisibility makes it difficult for AIDS activists to monitor how funds are being used on the ground. For example, only after extensive consultation with local Kenyan grassroots groups in preparation for a PEPFAR extension did US AIDS activists find out that PEPFAR had a policy against buying drugs for opportunistic infections that were killing people despite the fact that those drugs were really cheap compared to ARVs.[70] More recently, according to a report on Uganda leaked to Health GAP, as part of its pledge to treat 6 million people by 2013, PEPFAR started claiming a number of people under Global Fund programs as its own. A Health GAP activist calls this PEPFAR "lying and cheating to get their road to 6 million."[71] The organization has also been criticized for its high internal overhead and central administration charges, reliance on high-priced expatriate consultants and technical assistants, excessive training costs, and high overhead paid to the INGOs that are implementing PEPFAR projects.[72]

The role of the Gates Foundation in global AIDS governance is even more difficult to ascertain due to its nontransparency.[73] Its flagship AIDS initiative, Avahan, was established in 2003 to build an HIV-prevention model at scale in India, to encourage others to take over and replicate the model, and to disseminate lessons learned from India.[74] In its first five years, it spent $338 million providing prevention services to more than 220,000 female sex workers; 80,000 men who have sex with men and transgender people; 18,000 injecting drug users; and 5 million other men at risk along India's major trucking routes in six states: Tamil

Nadu, Karnataka, Andhra Pradesh, Maharashtra, Nagaland, and Manipur.[75] It works with 20 international NGOs, 150 grantees, and hundreds of thousands of clients on the ground in six key intervention areas: peer-to-peer outreach; testing and treatment of sexually transmitted diseases; condom distribution; community mobilization and program ownership; stigma reduction; and access to HIV testing, care, and treatment.[76] In the context of the large Indian epidemic, however, it is hard to gauge Avahan's role relative to other actors. "The scale-up work of Avahan [that] has led to the containment of high-risk groups, which then has led to a decrease in the spread of HIV in the general population" should be considered as a contribution rather than being attributed solely to Avahan, admits its executive director.[77] In the absence of national STI (sexually transmitted infection) prevalence data, Avahan had to make a number of adjustments as the prevention programs developed:

> We decided that our primary objective was to scale up rapidly. We didn't go for the approach whereby we had the time to fine-tune our program and then scale up. We took the view that rapid scale-up was urgent, and scaling up was a technology that was not well understood. We work with 82 districts in 650 towns in 6 states and the national highway system. We managed to work at scale between year two and three of the Avahan program. We made a number of mistakes: the design was off, and we changed the design. For example, in the truckers' program, we did not have data on the movements of truckers along the national highway system, and we had too many stations. We learned that there are certain nodes within that network, and we reduced the number of stations. Another example is our STI franchising. Again, we had no data on STI prevalence in India (the existing studies covered only small areas), and we had over 6,000 franchises. Once we found out that there are hot spots, we reduced the number of franchises to 800. I think our success is our ability to learn from the doing and simultaneously change the program.[78]

Several other critiques have been made about Avahan. Its executive director acknowledges that the business model causes "considerable tension, to put it mildly," in its partnerships with various implementers.[79] Others have argued that the Avahan program is too expensive: it has a high cost per intervention (US$18 per beneficiary compared to US$5 per beneficiary spent by the Indian National AIDS Control Organisation), it has high managerial costs, and it is difficult to convert it to a national program because of the expense and the lack of community involvement.[80] According to Prasada Rao, the director of the UNAIDS Regional Support Team for Asia and the Pacific, "[i]t is an established fact [that] community programmes are better managed by communities themselves. Avahan itself has started with this philosophy but the transition model does not sufficiently articulate . . . how to ensure it in a publicly funded programme."[81]

The impact of the Gates Foundation, however, goes way beyond the modest Avahan initiative, which began its transition into the Indian national AIDS program around 2013. Unlike PEPFAR and the Global Fund, the Gates Foundation decided early on to focus on the niche areas of preventive research and technologies, such as AIDS vaccines, diagnostics, and microbicides. The People's Health Movement criticizes the Gates Foundation for its skewed funding decisions divorced from local needs, its nontransparency, and its conflict of interests.[82] In 2009, the UK physician and PHM activist David McCoy led a team of researchers that analyzed 1,094 Gates Foundation global health grants between 1998 and 2007 and found that, out of a total of $8.95 billion, 65% ($5.8 billion) was granted to only twenty organizations, most of which are premier research institutions in the United States. McCoy and his team challenged the foundation's primary focus on new technology and questioned who it is supposed to be serving.[83] The *Lancet* editors add, "The grants made by the Foundation do not reflect the burden of disease endured by those in deepest poverty. . . . The concern expressed to us by many scientists who have long worked in low-income settings is that important health programmes are being distorted by large grants from the Gates Foundation."[84] For example, a focus on malaria in countries where other diseases require more urgent attention creates damaging incentives for governments and health workers. The editors urge the Gates Foundation to improve its governance by visibly involving diverse leaders, making its decision making more transparent and accountable, explaining its strategy openly, devising a grant mechanism that more accurately reflects the global burden of disease, aligning itself more with the needs of those in greatest suffering, and investing in health systems and research capacity in low-income countries.[85] Another example of controversial funding by the Gates Foundation pertains to stavudine trials. WHO has phased out stavudine since 2010 due to irreversible toxic side effects, but the Gates Foundation continues to fund trials in South Africa and Uganda despite opposition.[86]

Further, the Gates Foundation's partnership with Coca-Cola (an $11.5 million venture to enable mango and passion fruit farmers to use the company's supply chain) has raised issues about conflicts of interest. Over 10% of the Gates Foundation endowment is invested in two companies: McDonald's and Coca-Cola. Over half of the endowment is invested in Berkshire Hathaway, which owns an additional 8.7% of Coca-Cola and shares in GlaxoSmithKline, Sanofi-Aventis, and Johnson and Johnson.[87] PHM activists ask whether "community partnerships" with Coca-Cola are self-serving and self-contradicting (the foundation funds global public health programs but invests in companies that cause obesity and diabetes). Above all, "philanthrocapitalism" may hide the corporate lobbying of public and civil society organizations. In addition to AIDS NGOs and CBOs, the Gates Foundation contributes to the WHO prequalification program and to the Global Fund ($19 million in 2009 and 2010). Michael Edwards, a former director of civil society programming at the Ford Foundation, comments: "The concentration of wealth and power among philanthrocapitalists may be having a negative influence on the non-profit sector both in the United States and internationally, with civil society groups reporting increasing constraints on their flexibility and independence as a result of an obsession with performance reviews."[88]

Of the three most important financiers in the AIDS funding oligopoly, the Global Fund is the only multilateral organization that is supposed to answer to the broad spectrum of constituents on its board, which includes donor and recipient countries, the private sector, and representatives of civil society, including people living with HIV, TB, and malaria. Is the Global Fund only a funding organization, or does it play a role in shaping global AIDS governance through its innovative principles of transparency, country ownership (the greater involvement of each nation), and civil society partnership (which set it apart from PEPFAR, the Gates Foundation, and almost all other international organizations)?[89] The manager of Civil Society and Private Sector Partnerships at the Global Fund explains:

> Originally, the idea was that it would be a funding mechanism but a different one. It recognized that business as usual would not work. There was understanding at the time that you couldn't just put money into a country. You had to understand the environment [that] the money was going into. Because of the structural adjustment programs of the World Bank, [which] had destroyed the health systems of the countries, there was recognition that the fund would have to help put in place structures in the country to ensure that the money would have impact. It was supposed to be based on partnerships. So it was designed to be more than a funding institution.[90]

In some countries, the Global Fund has helped create new ways of thinking and working in AIDS. In China, for example, in contrast to other international funding bodies, such as the Clinton Foundation, the Global Fund has forced the government to think about what it wants and needs and to draft a proposal that is part of the national strategy. In preparation for Round 6 applications, where the objective was civil society participation, different participants in the Country Coordinating Mechanism (CCM) realized that they had different definitions of participation (*chan yu*), and those differences were exposed and discussed for the first time. "Only the Global Fund could have made such discussions happen," says a Chinese AIDS activist. "So the Global Fund brought conceptual change, management structure, but also the opportunity to raise questions. And the government promised 'I will change.'"[91]

But others point to the lack of sustainability of programs financed by the Global Fund. A Global Fund Grants Program manager at UNDP-Kyrgyzstan says:

> Take the countries where Global Fund money has implemented programs. Pull out the money, nothing will be left tomorrow. It is also a problem for other donor-funded programs, but the fact that the Global Fund is linked to ARV treatments, harm reduction, and other high-risk programs means if the money stops, 100,000 people on treatment risk having no medications because no system is in place by the governments to continue the Global Fund programs. While Global Fund money has been a huge asset for the country, it's time to reconsider the model of funding. It should be linked to structural changes. The amount of money is huge, but structural changes have not been happening anywhere.[92]

GIPA: The Challenge of Inclusion

> There was a table set out under a tree in front of the house. . . . The table was a large one, but the three were all crowded together at one corner of it: "No room! No room!" they cried out when they saw Alice coming. "There's *plenty* of room!" said Alice indignantly, and she sat down in a large arm-chair at one end of the table.
>
> "Have some wine," the March Hare said in an encouraging tone.
>
> Alice looked all around the table, but there was nothing on it but tea. "I don't see any wine," she remarked.
>
> "There isn't any," said the March Hare.
>
> "Then it wasn't very civil of you to offer it," said Alice angrily.
>
> "It wasn't very civil of you to sit down without being invited," said the March Hare.
>
> "I didn't know it was your table," said Alice; "it's laid for a great many more than three."
>
> —*Lewis Carroll*, Alice in Wonderland[93]

> Civil society is now so vital to the United Nations that engaging with it well is a necessity, not an option.
>
> —*Panel of Eminent Persons on United Nations–*
> *Civil Society Relations*[94]

Where have AIDS activists been at the AIDS "tea party"? Is the GIPA princi-ple rhetoric or reality in global AIDS governance? We need to remember that non-governmental participation in the United Nations historically was limited by its member-state governance structure. The first time that NGOs took part in for-mal UN deliberations happened in ECOSOC in 1946 through the provision of Ar-ticle 71 of the UN Charter on NGO consultation.[95] In the WHO, only a few pro-fessional and biomedical NGOs have been given access to attend meetings, to submit documents, or, on specific occasions, to make statements to the annual WHA.[96]

The initial opening, at least rhetorically, for more NGO participation came with the 1981 Global Strategy for Health for All by the Year 2000, which was based on the principles of the 1978 Declaration of Alma-Ata on primary health care, where the WHO talked of partnerships with nongovernmental bodies.[97] In other areas of UN operations, NGO representation was regulated largely through ECOSOC's formal accreditation system. By the Rio Conference on Environment and Development in 1992, the ECOSOC list of NGOs had grown beyond 1,000, with over 2,400 NGO representatives attending the official conference and 17,000 participating at the parallel NGO global forum. A certain "NGOization" of the UN occurred throughout the 1990s and 2000s with a series of conferences on human rights (1993), women (1995), housing (1996), the commercial sexual exploitation of children (1996), trade (1999, 2001, 2003, 2005, 2009), racism (2001), the environment (2002), indigenous issues (2002), and climate change (2002), which led to different kinds of mechanisms for NGO participation in the global governance system broadly speaking. Despite increased recognition, however, the majority of the more than 3,700 ECOSOC-accredited NGOs con-tinue to keep their traditional role as service providers and sometimes occupy a watchdog role. For instance, the World Bank now has 120 civil society focal points in its headquarters and over 100 country offices where NGOs are supposedly being consulted, but it is unclear how their participation has had an impact on the bank's governance structure or policymaking.[98]

As soon as the Global Programme on AIDS was established within the WHO in 1987, the search was on for the most appropriate mechanism for NGO inclu-sion in order to ensure an effective global response to AIDS. An early GPA strat-egy paper specifically named NGOs as indispensable actors: "Legitimacy, author-ity, resources, and a credible community base can only be obtained through the tri-partite cooperation of governments, WHO and other intergovernmental orga-nizations, and NGOs. Each provides some of the components missing from the others."[99] The GPA, however, was internally divided. One group, which "saw [itself] as possessing a comprehensive appreciation of the pandemic and as standing above allegations of being linked to specific interests," wanted to maintain the traditional role of NGOs in program execution and information exchange.[100] The other, led by Mann and his like-minded colleagues, wanted to ensure that NGO "experiences contribute to planning, implementation and review of national and international programs" and proposed the creation of an informal working group to implement a comprehensive strategy of NGO inclusion in the global response to AIDS.[101]

AIDS service organizations and NGOs themselves started lobbying in Geneva as early as 1988 for "official acknowledgement of the legitimacy and competence of ASOs," "representation on AIDS-related bodies," and the removal of "structural impediments such as attitudes, laws, and regulations that hinder the prevention of HIV."[102] Mann tried to provide funding support from GPA, administered through GPA-funded national AIDS programs, but this turned out to be cumbersome and unworkable. Some WHO staff members continued to question "what exactly NGOs or ASOs had to offer the global strategy in return for WHO support" and saw "ASO requests as excessive and impermissible under WHO regulations; these provided that consultative bodies could not make specific requests of the Director-General for use of staff, services, or funds but only could offer advice."[103] The final compromise, in the form of a partnership program that provided limited funds to NGOs for about a hundred projects between 1989 and 1993, did not last long. It and GPA disappeared when donors divested money from the WHO. A more conventional mechanism in the form of a GPA recommendation in 1991 to urge national AIDS programs to set a target of 15% of their resources for AIDS NGOs also failed to bring much inclusion.[104]

Organizational Interfaces

The most significant achievement of AIDS activism in the early days of multilateral cooperation was the formation of an umbrella group for more systematic engagement with GPA. The idea came from the Canadian AIDS Society, which wrote to the WHO in early 1988 seeking assistance in setting up an international forum to house all ASOs under one roof. The International Council of AIDS Service Organizations (ICASO) was formed in 1990 after a series of consultations with the GPA's NGO liaison officer and the first international ASO conference in June 1989 in Montreal.[105] The long process of mobilization and the subsequent recognition by GPA meant that by the time a new joint UN AIDS program was proposed in 1992 and adopted by ECOSOC in 1994, there was no question that civil society would play a role in AIDS governance:

> When ECOSOC created UNAIDS, it was [the] first time that NGOs had a seat at the table. . . . It was in HIV, and HIV started it. . . . It was the only [area] that had human rights at its core and that had civil society engagement at its core. And the whole response has been built around those two things, built around communities, built around human rights. It is not about morals. It is about fundamental human rights, the fundamental human right of everybody to have access to health, to the services, to the support, to community engagement. Now, for people who come from conservative agendas, that is a bit shocking. For the people who have been nurses, who have been running health clinics, who have been telling people all their life what it is that they have to take, what it is they have to do, what it is that they have to think, it is a radical departure. . . . The HIV response has been unapologetic about that.[106]

Setting aside five seats out of twenty-two for NGOs, including associations of people living with HIV and AIDS on its PCB, UNAIDS has often been credited as the first intergovernmental organization that included civil society in its governance structure. The fact that the NGO representatives have no voting rights makes little practical difference, since PCB operates by consensus.[107] NGOs, including the GNP+, ICW, and ICASO, were asked to sit as board members while efforts were made to ensure that people living with AIDS were also present in the secretariat. Although not a funding organization, UNAIDS does provide direct funding support to nascent HIV-positive networks and to sex worker, drug user, and MSM networks to enhance their capacity at both the country and global policy levels. For instance, after the Global Fund changed its funding criteria in 2009, excluding lots of ASOs and NGOs in middle-income countries, UNAIDS convened a meeting between donors and NGOs at the 2010 International AIDS Conference in Vienna and in 2012 launched the Robert Carr Civil Society Networks Fund, which gives $5–$6 million per year to sustain the work of civil society organizations in the new tightened AIDS-funding environment.[108] Without doubt, the UNAIDS partnership with civil society is considered to be a model for other UN bodies and multilateral organizations.[109]

Other organizations that include civil society representation in their governance structures are the Global Fund, the Roll Back Malaria Partnership, the Stop TB Partnership, and UNITAID. The Global Fund reserves three voting seats—for communities, developed country NGOs, and developing country NGOs—out of twenty on its board.[110] The Roll Back Malaria Partnership dedicates two out of twenty-one voting seats to NGOs, and the Stop TB Partnership has five (three for NGOs and technical agencies and two for TB-affected communities) out of thirty-four members on its coordinating board.[111] UNITAID gives two out of twelve seats to civil society, one for NGOs and the other for people living with HIV, TB, or malaria. Other mechanisms for civil society participation include representation on funding organizations, advisory groups, and focal points. In 2008, the Global Fund introduced dual-track financing: civil society NGOs, for the first time, can apply to be principal recipients along with governments, another innovative idea that some would like to see become a required feature of all proposals, thereby forcing CCMs to bring civil society to the center.[112] Like UNAIDS, the Global Fund also has advisory structures on various populations, including sex workers, men who have sex with men, injecting drug users, and youth.

Another area where the GIPA principle has made a clear difference is the governance of and representation at international AIDS conferences. Throughout the 1980s, the "white coats" and the "T-shirts" represented completely different epistemologies and embodied completely different AIDS politics. In 1991, for example, the scientists attended the main conference, "Science Challenging AIDS," while the much smaller NGO conference, "Communities Challenging AIDS," was an afterthought that met for only two hours during the lunch hour of the main scientific conference.[113] The prevailing attitude among leading scientists was that "NGOs and PWAs simply did not have the capacities or skills needed to understand the complexities of the scientific data and research findings," and they found the activists' protests to be counterproductive.[114] Finally, at the 1992 International AIDS Conference in Amsterdam the NGOs were involved in the planning process and were well represented in the opening and plenary sessions; some scientists complained that the conference was not scientific enough.

Discursive Interventions and Resource-Transfer Interfaces

Few of these gains in various organizational interfaces in global AIDS governance would have been possible without discursive interventions by activists. It was people living with AIDS who put the GIPA principle front and center in 1983 in order to frame AIDS as a human rights issue. The combination of GIPA (for the first time, patients themselves took charge) and a right-to-health framework rather than a narrow biomedical definition of AIDS (which made funding the AIDS response no longer a question of charity) paved the way for unprecedented changes in organizational, funding, policy, and legal interfaces at the global level.

Some interviewees go so far as to claim that the entire global AIDS response would not have happened without civil society's reframing of AIDS beyond traditional epidemiology.[115] Donors did not warm up to the idea of an AIDS war chest on their own. Activists from ACT UP, the Treatment Action Group, Health GAP, MSF, Oxfam, ActionAid, ICASO, GNP+, and ICW had been lobbying for it for a decade. Similarly, NGOs sitting on the Global AIDS Roundtable ensured that the United States increased overall funding with new money for global AIDS programs through PEPFAR. Before the first five-year funding expired in 2008, they lobbied heavily for a substantively improved PEPFAR with increased funding to $48 billion, including $9 billion for TB and malaria, and a bigger contribution to the Global Fund, with the goals of increasing the number of people on treatment (6 million by 2013), increasing the emphasis on nutrition, funding 140,000 new health professionals, repealing the abstinence-only policy and the funding ban on sex worker organizations and programs, and a new partnership framework.[116] AIDS activists also pushed for innovative financing, including the establishment of UNITAID and a financial transaction tax.

Policy and Legal Interfaces

In global AIDS governance, activists have made imprints in treatment, harm reduction, and gender mainstreaming. The hard-won 2001 Doha Declaration on the TRIPS agreement and public health continues to provide a much-needed counterbalancing force against TRIPS in the ongoing battle for universal access to treatment. As discussed in chapter 3, several governments have chosen to amend their domestic patent laws to take advantage of TRIPS flexibilities explicitly permitted in the Doha Declaration. Intergovernmental bodies such as UNDP, the Global Commission on HIV and the Law, and the Global Fund have repeatedly urged states to do so in spite of Pharma pressure.

In regard to harm reduction, AIDS activists have managed to radically reframe drug use away from the traditional criminal control perspective within the United Nations. Harm reduction has now been accepted as the norm in prevention with methadone, for example, included as part of WHO's essential medicines list. Although the battle is not over (belligerent states such as the United States, Russia, China, and Thailand continue to deny clean needles and/or substitution therapy to drug users), discursive and policy gains in the WHO mean that UNODC is now on the defensive if it goes against the new scientific norm on harm reduction.

Finally, AIDS activists have brought new knowledges on human rights and gender mainstreaming to global AIDS governance. While central to the AIDS response, human rights and gender are such political minefields that most inter-governmental organizations prefer not to adopt any formal framework, or when they do, the framework remains on paper only. For instance, UNAIDS has never passed any human rights framework to formally guide its work even though its executive director has personally championed the cause. The adoption of the Sexual Orientation and Gender Identity strategy (SOGI) by the Global Fund in 2009 is another good example of the vacuousness of a so-called rights-based approach that lacks clarification and substance. Several years into its operation, the Global Fund learned that its grant recipients, which were often marginalized populations, were unable to deliver the intended results due to punitive laws and a lack of power, representation, capacity, and access. SOGI was designed without the recognition that without specifically addressing political and social realities on the ground, the Global Fund could only go so far to address the epidemic:

> The Board should ensure that the Global Fund shows leadership in recognizing the importance of decriminalization as an essential element in responding to the three diseases. The Board is requested to create more scope for human rights based proposals that seek to influence the enabling legal and policy environment for successful outcomes for the three diseases in relation to criminalized and vulnerable groups. Proposals should require an analysis of legal and policy barriers to implementation of effective programs for sexual minorities and a plan to address those barriers. Indicators should be developed to track the impact of these interventions.[117]

While a civil society imperative is amply clear both from within the United Nations to increase effectiveness (reform in action) and from without to enhance democracy (notably through GIPA), the problem with sustaining civil society's inclusion in global AIDS governance has less to do with a chronic funding shortage for capacity building and meaningful participation, which has been repeatedly pointed out in numerous reviews, and more to do with a fundamental problem of "misrecognition" by a Westphalian international system of states that impedes parity of participation.[118] The much-celebrated proliferation of global health partnerships, such as the African Comprehensive HIV/AIDS Partnerships, the Alliance for Microbicide Development, and the Global AIDS Vaccine Initiative, has done little to change the marginality of civil society. A study in 2005, based on a sample of twenty-three global health partnerships, found that NGOs were the least represented.[119] This is a problem that confronts not only the AIDS movement, but also practically all other human rights and development social movements. Having five seats on PCB will mean little if donors decide to retreat from AIDS and close UNAIDS, as they once did to GPA. Similarly, having a war chest only raises the hopes of 10 million more people waiting for treatment if the G8 countries, faced with their own economic crises, decide to end vertical funding for AIDS. We need to ask the difficult questions: With the political and funding retreat from HIV that began in 2010, which of the significant gains that AIDS activists have fought for are going to stay? Is the "shell of national state sovereignty" impenetrable,[120] or can it be made amenable to GIPA and human rights?

Global AIDS Governance Reforms

Money makes the dance.
                    —*Executive Director, CARAM*[121]

"NATO": No Action, Talk Only.
        —*National Program Director, MSF-Beijing*[122]

Global AIDS governance reforms? I will give everyone a lie detector [test]. . . . Don't write another commitment. Implement the stuff you promised in 1979.
            —*Senior Researcher, AIDS Accountability*
                        International[123]

More than thirty years of activism has taught us many lessons about global AIDS governance. Activists have proposed five areas where reforms are needed: donor coordination; governance harmonization; health system integration and national leadership; IP and the role of the private sector; and civil society engagement and capacity building.

Donor Coordination, Accountability, and Transparency

Donor fatigue sets in. AIDS seems like a never-ending story. International AIDS funding has been flat-lining since 2010. The Global Fund canceled Round 11 in 2011 and struggled to fulfill its next replenishment round for the funding period of 2014–2016. At the replenishment meeting in Washington, DC, in December 2013, donors had pledged US$12 billion, falling far short of the estimated $87 billion needed to finance urgently needed programs for HIV/AIDS, TB, and malaria.[124] PEPFAR funding has decreased rather than increased AIDS money since 2009. UNAIDS operates with a miniscule biennial budget of $485 million.

Funding is, of course, always political. In the entire history of international cooperation, no group has ever admitted to having too much money to solve an urgent global problem. Just when an AIDS war chest was finally built up to face the challenge, critics charged AIDS of stealing the show in global public health. Conservative politicians talk of a "treatment mortgage," with the developed world financing the bulk of AIDS treatment in the developing world.[125] A senior research scientist at the Harvard School of Public Health, Daniel Halperin, argues in 2008 that the "rigid focus on AIDS" has led to a deadly waste of resources:

> This year [Botswana] will receive about $300 million to fight AIDS—in addition to the hundreds of millions already granted by drug companies, private foundations and other donors. While in that sparsely populated country last month, I learned that much of its AIDS money remains unspent, as even its state-of-the-art H.I.V. clinics cannot absorb such a large influx of cash. As the United States Agency for International Development's H.I.V. prevention adviser in southern Africa in 2005 and 2006, I visited villages in poor countries like Lesotho, where clinics could not afford to stock basic medicines but often maintained an inventory of expensive AIDS drugs and sophisticated monitoring equipment for their H.I.V. patients. H.I.V.-infected children are offered exemplary treatment, while children suffering from much simpler-to-treat diseases are left untreated, sometimes to die.[126]

In July 2012, the question was once again put to global public health experts at a World Bank debate: What makes AIDS, which kills 720,000 people every year, more urgent than diarrhea, which kills 760,000?[127] Some scientists and feminist activists ask: How about maternal and child health? Each year hundreds of thousands of women die during pregnancy or childbirth, and close to 7 million children die before reaching the age of five; many of these deaths are entirely preventable with cost-effective interventions. Two researchers from the Netherlands Interdisciplinary Demographic Institute, Hendrik van Dalen and Mieke Reuser, find that AIDS funding increased from 10% to 90% of all global health funding, including basic research, family planning, reproductive health, and AIDS, between 1995 and 2007, greatly distorting the health priorities in many countries.[128] Why not invest more in nutrition, which is fundamental to all health issues, including AIDS? And if we do, what about other social determinants of health, such as housing, the socioeconomic status of the poorest people (including those living with HIV), and political participation, without which marginalized populations continue to die because of stigma and discrimination rather than directly from the virus itself? These have all been specifically pinpointed by the WHO as indispensable factors in the attainment of the right of health for all, and yet they have never received the same kind of political attention as AIDS.[129] More fundamentally, some development economists, including the Nobel laureate Jeffrey Sachs, argue that the heavy vertical funding for AIDS in the first decade of the twenty-first century has not translated into overall improvement for the health system; rather, it has created dysfunctional, parallel health systems.[130] As a Kenyan nurse puts it, "The patients who receive AIDS treatment leave with a smile. Those here for other problems do not. As I've told my ministry, we now have two systems of health care in Kenya."[131]

It is a fact that AIDS programs now receive more money per patient than those for any other disease. But it is also a fact that the current level of funding will fail to meet the goal of universal access by 2015. In 2011, a group of experts from UN-AIDS, the Global Fund, PEPFAR, the Gates Foundation, the World Bank, WHO, and academic institutions proposed a new investment framework for AIDS based on a more rational resource allocation model in order to maximize the benefits of the HIV response by prioritizing three areas: basic program activities, critical enablers, and synergies with development sectors. The investment framework "takes as its starting point a human rights approach to the HIV response, to ensure that it is universal, equitable, inclusive, and fosters participation, informed consent and accountability."[132] At the core are six evidence-based programmatic activities: focused programs for key populations at higher risk, elimination of new HIV infections in children, behavior-change programs, condom distribution, treatment, and voluntary medical male circumcision. Two kinds of critical enablers are identified in the new framework as crucial to the success of HIV programming: social enablers, such as testing outreach, stigma reduction, human rights advocacy, and community mobilization; and program enablers, such as strategic planning, management, and capacity building for community-based organizations. The last component emphasizes synergies between HIV-specific efforts and development, including the strengthening of social, legal, and health systems; social protection; access to education; legal reform; poverty reduction; and reducing gender-based violence. The total bill for this vast framework stands at US$22–$24 billion per year until 2015, after which it should decline because 7.4 million deaths and 12 million new infections would have been averted between 2011 and 2020.[133]

Yet, as of 2010, only $15 billion was available every year, split almost equally between international assistance and domestic sources. If we count international aid only, $7.6 billion was available, out of which roughly $5.3 billion (70%) was bilateral aid and the rest multilateral funding through the Global Fund and UNI-TAID.[134] The mathematics seems straightforward: the world is $7–$9 billion short of AIDS funding per year. Bilateral aid will need to be increased from the current $5 billion level. Multilateral aid also needs to jump from its current meager $2 billion mark. The Global Fund requires $5 billion per year to achieve its impact. Domestic funding, as committed at the Abuja Special Summit in 2001, which set a target of allocating at least 15% of each nation's annual national health budget for HIV/AIDS, needs to match if not surpass international aid. Yet the economic crisis in the G8 countries makes it unrealistic to expect any immediate funding scale-up. A veteran public health activist puts it bluntly:

> There is a financial crisis out there. The multilaterals are not responding; they just didn't see it. In this current financial environment, it is very hard for politicians— [David] Cameron in the UK, [Barack] Obama in the US, and [Angela] Merkel in Germany—to get their electorates to agree to give more funding to AIDS. People have been asking: Why are we giving to Africa? Imagine the G22 governments. At the very time of the worst financial crisis, [we are] ask[ing] them to sign a check to commit $25 billion per year until 2015. Would you sign a check? I am not sure I would if it were my money. It is a critical question now.[135]

By emphasizing "core" programs and critical enablers, is the investment framework an indirect admission that "some of the things that we have been doing and paying for in the last decade have been wrong"? Or is it part of a survival strategy for intergovernmental organizations and NGOs—the writers of the investment framework—"whose jobs depend on the AIDS budget"?[136] How about innovative funding? Will the financial transaction tax be the missing link in the future of AIDS funding if it brings a few extra billion dollars per year? France adopted a 0.2% transaction tax on share purchases in August 2012, and expected an increase of €530 million in 2012 and €1.6 billion in 2013 in its national coffers. The European Parliament has also approved the FTT to be introduced in eleven countries, which is expected to bring in about €37 billion per year. There is no commitment yet on how this new money will be spent, but activists have been lobbying for some of it to be earmarked for poverty reduction and climate change.[137] Meanwhile, smart investors have already found a way to escape the tax through a new instrument called "contracts for difference"; offered by prime brokers, it allows investors to bet on a stock's gain or loss without owning the shares.[138]

A certainty is that there will be less money for AIDS, and whatever money is available will have to be spent more efficiently, in what the Global Fund calls the "value for money" framework, which emphasizes the strategic allocation of resources to achieve maximum sustainable health outcomes and impact. It means more efficient secretariat operation, smarter grant investments, and improved evidence of value received for money spent.[139] In May 2011, the Global Fund Board adopted a new eligibility, counterpart financing, and prioritization policy that focuses its funding on poor countries with high disease burdens. All low-income countries are eligible to apply regardless of disease burden. Lower middle-income countries can apply but must focus on special groups and/or interventions. Upper middle-income countries are eligible only if their disease burden is measured as high, severe, or extreme. All high-income countries are ineligible.[140] Using these new eligibility criteria, the Global Fund announced a new funding model in December 2012. Beginning in 2013, eligible countries must submit a concept note with a "full expression of demand," including a national strategy that incorporates funding in the budget. According to the Global Fund, the new funding model is different from the old one because it has more active portfolio management; timelines largely defined by each country; ongoing engagement by the secretariat; higher predictability in terms of timing, success rates, and funding range; and disbursement-ready grants.[141] While it might be too early to judge the impact of the new model, many on the ground know already that a "value for money" model will leave many countries and even entire regions out of the Global Fund, putting existing programs at risk. In Latin America, for example, 95% of the response to AIDS is paid for by governments. In China, 80% of the response is funded by the government. But how do governments spend the money? As Javier Hourcade Bellocq, a veteran AIDS activist and former member of the Global Fund's Communities Delegation Board, points out:

> And this is the crux of the matter, even where regions like LAC [Latin America and the Caribbean], Asia and Eastern Europe have already invested substantial domestic resources in the response. These are regions where the epidemic is concentrated in most-at-risk populations. Governments refuse to work with these populations and, in some cases, refuse to even acknowledge their existence. Will domestic funding be obtained for the human rights work that needs to be done in our countries?[142]

The funding crisis is not just one of level, but also one of coordination. Several interviewees are concerned about the possible impact of a donor-driven agenda and a lack of coordination. According to the Global Fund Grants Program manager at UNDP-Kyrgyzstan: "Each bilateral donor wants to be in the driver's seat. No one wants to coordinate the AIDS response. Everyone wants to be visible. With such a high level [of] funding to Central Asia, if there were coordination among donors and proper leadership among donors and governments, a lot of things could be changed. But for this to happen, donors need to sit down and forget their own agenda. They have to be prepared to give away [control]."[143] An MSF–South Africa Access Campaign worker agrees:

> The global response to AIDS is still very fragmented. UNITAID pays for pediatric drugs. The Global Fund pays for others. PEPFAR funds something else. Governments wait for funder 1 to pay X and funder 2 to pay Y. Different donors have different agendas with different funding cycles. Coordination would be key. It is good to have both bilateral and multilateral funding, but we have to make sure no two donors overlap. It makes it so difficult for NGOs to work. NGOs spend half of their time . . . writ[ing] proposals to fit different donor agendas. Governments don't know what to expect in terms of what money [is] coming in for which area. It is so difficult to have a coordinating mechanism like a UN body or someone with a strong fist. Basically, whoever has the . . . pull will set whatever priorities.[144]

More fundamentally, some activists challenge northern donors' vision of development and "project rationality." The executive director of ABIA emphasizes a different globalization, not one from the North with values from the North: "When a donor gives $5,000 to ABIA, it is not just $5,000 to ABIA. It fosters more democratic accountability. If we reinforce democracy in the South, it will help the crisis in the North in the sense that we could create a more pro-democratic environment in the whole world. I believe in a globalization from the South to the North. The Gates Foundation doesn't see this. It sees only the market."[145] Development oriented activists also urge the broadening and linking of AIDS governance to wider debates about aid effectiveness:

> I would try to align AIDS governance with the progressive discussions that are happening elsewhere in aid effectiveness discourses. The AIDS world has been reigning for so long, not watching what is happening elsewhere. There was this Busan aid effectiveness conference in December 2011 that brought aid into the twenty-first century. It is not based on money. It is much more about South-South collaborations, triangular relationships between countries. Emerging economies are going to be much more important in providing assistance than G8. There is a very contemporary group of activists talking about development assistance and the future of that. Some of the countries in this region, like China, Korea, [and] Indonesia, are going to be really important emerging donors. It's changing now; they are writing the future of aid now. I think the AIDS governance structure should look much more into that.[146]

Governance Harmonization, Inclusion, and Alignment
with Human Rights

Having lived intimately with the international AIDS bureaucracy for over two decades, activists are vocal about a UN governance system that is outdated, costly, bureaucratic, cumbersome, and preoccupied more with its own survival than with local needs:

> I don't overestimate the importance of the UN in a global context. But when it comes to HIV, I think they have placed equal emphasis [on] turf battle[s]. If you look at the co-sponsors, e.g., UNICEF, there is evidence of failure in rolling out mother-to-children prevention and pediatric ARVs. . . . UNFPA was pretty good with their priorities on adolescents, sexual reproductive health, and condom promotion. But they were hamstrung because they unfortunately had this issue of abortion that nobody wants to talk to them about. UNDP has helped us think about the relationship between HIV and development. They have forced [the] inclusion of a lot of issues, but they are not there to deliver anything. Others, like UNESCO, forget it. Go to UNESCO, you have to blow the dust off the desk just to have a meeting. UNODC wouldn't even mention harm reduction for years and still [doesn't]. They would never talk about legalization. It is the UN Office of Drugs and Crime; it is not the UN Office of Drugs and HIV. They were given the mandate to work on drug use and harm reduction, but they didn't believe it. It is against their principles and mandate. They didn't want to talk about it. . . . The WHO doesn't deliver. Have you been to any country office of the WHO? They don't have a mechanism to deliver. . . . We trust these UN agencies. They are very capable individuals but, as organizations, they are working on a sixty-year[-old] model. It is very easy for everybody to ignore them. . . . UN agencies reacted to HIV as something exceptional, but it wasn't. It shouldn't be. It is all vested interests. Every time there [was] an issue, they spen[t] an awful lot of energy and ask[ed] what is the comparative advantage of each UN agency. They never talked about what is the comparative advantage of this UN agency against the rest of the world. They didn't realize they were slipping behind all the time. I don't think they were ever in the position to deliver.[147]

The executive director of CARAM says, "We are fed up with the hierarchical structure of the UN. We raised our voices, but it seems like the UN agencies have their own agenda. Their agenda does not respond to our needs. It's a waste of time."[148] For the executive director of Chi Heng Foundation, the problem of the United Nations is weak leadership: "There are times when people expect the UN to take a position. Yet it remains silent so as not to jeopardize its relationships with national governments. . . . For example, Chinese CBOs wanted Peter Piot, the then director of UNAIDS, to speak out on the compensation issue of AIDS patients infected through contaminated blood. He didn't do so until the day before he stepped down. A lot of NGOs and CBOs felt that we lost advocacy opportunities because of weak UN leadership."[149] The former program director of the Eurasian Harm Reduction Network points out the duplication due to the lack of coordination: "One of the things I saw in my early years was how much we wasted when we had the same guidelines developed six different times in six different countries, sometimes paid [for] by the same UN agencies."[150] The president of the Delhi Network of Positive People concurs: "Most of the resources are lost in the system. It comes in billions of dollars but then [is distributed] in trickle[s] of cents because the system consumes everything. My friend who worked at UNAIDS for eleven months told me, 'They paid me a heavy salary and hired this consultant to do my work plan.' But when it comes to community work, they expect it to be voluntary. They hire a lot of experts, but I think we are the experts."[151]

Thai activists from the AIDS Access Foundation charge that the UN system is state-centric, opaque in its decision making, and evasive when it comes to certain sensitive political issues: "Our experience is that the UN agencies provide more support to governments rather than [to] civil society. Another issue is [the] decision-making process by UN agencies, for example, Getting to Zero. Where does that come from? On political issues like free trade agreements, compulsory licensing, or counterfeiting, we had to fight against Pharma. No one came to support us until we won the game. These are structural issues that UN agencies failed to pick up."[152]

Some activists have chosen to focus on the reform of specific organizations.

UNAIDS

The vice president of the Global Business Coalition for Health thinks that UNAIDS, unlike the World Bank, simply does not have political weight, legitimacy, or authority: "If [Michel] Sidibé had real power to influence policymaking, he would have come to meet the president and prime minister of Russia and said, 'I heard that in your country the principles adopted by the WHO and UNODC are not adopted by you. Please tell me your reasons. As the head of UNAIDS, I will tell you why these principles matter.' He never did it."[153] The national project director of MSF-Beijing also questions the role of UNAIDS in the Chinese government's AIDS decision-making process and its extremely limited mandate in enforcing human rights by changing the legal, social, or political environment.[154] "UNAIDS is constrained by governments," says the director of the International

Harm Reduction Development Program of Open Society Foundations. "It is hanging by a thread. It can't do anything to jeopardize its relationships with governments. . . . It talks about civil society and strategic involvement, but since [it] serve[s] at the pleasure of rogue governments, it is reluctant to criticize them."[155]

A country coordinator with UNAIDS admits, "We are not a UN agency, and we don't have the human resource[s] and finance[s], which limits our ability. We are considered as a second-rank organization and have to rely on many UN organizations to work, which delay[s] things. We are a secretariat. Being a broker of all those relationships, we have to get consensus. When co-sponsors fail to deliver, UNAIDS does not have the mandate to enforce."[156] The social mobilization advisor of UNAIDS-China also acknowledges the constraints on pursuing a broad human rights and civil society agenda:

> I don't think any international organization has the kind of political weight to change Chinese government policy. That takes a long time. If you step back and look at the kind of issues that have been promoted and the access of UNAIDS to political leadership here since 2003, UNAIDS has fairly good political weight compared to its actual size and its standing in the UN system. We are not even a UN agency; we are a joint program. . . . Human rights issues are beyond the mandate of the Ministry of Health and [the] CDC. They say they can't handle these issues, which have to be taken up by other government departments. We have limited partnerships with these other departments, like civil affairs, justice, and public security, which have been more reluctant to engage with us. For example, [on] crackdowns on sex work, gay venues, and [the] arrest of activists, we have very little influence whether these happen. . . . A major obstacle in our work is that we can create the space and [we can] support capacity building, but we cannot . . . talk for civil society ourselves. We cannot be the voice. In China, civil society['s] voice is very diverse and not effective.[157]

Sometimes, UNAIDS has to find a "back door" or rely on diplomatic channels to carry out its human rights work. The IP issue also has proven to be difficult since realpolitik means that there is little room for UNAIDS to intervene. A longtime UNAIDS bureaucrat puts it frankly: "If you realize that the US is a major donor to UNAIDS and that PCB say[s] trade agreements are not part of our mandate, when it comes to decision making, our scope is limited even if our ED [executive director] loudly says the US is not right."[158] Suggestions for reforms of UNAIDS are polarized, with one end believing that while it served its purpose really well, "UNAIDS' time is finished; it should go back to all co-sponsors,"[159] and the other suggesting that it should become a "stand-alone agency, endowed with a more significant budget, and with a role reconfigured from the ground."[160] What is clear is that a decision will have to be made on the future of UNAIDS.

WHO

Proposals for WHO reforms are equally divided between staunch WHO believers and harsh WHO critics. On one end are activists from the People's Health Movement who are vigilant about private sector intrusion in AIDS governance; they recommend a WHO reclaiming of global health stewardship through proper financing.[161] On the other are those who think that the WHO is too constrained by governments and has rendered itself irrelevant in the rapidly evolving global public health landscape. A former Civil Society Team officer of the Global Fund says, "The WHO got complacent. They don't do any fundraising and don't deliver enough results. People start[ed] asking: What are you doing?"[162] His colleague adds:

> WHO should have taken a much stronger political lead on the efficacy of human rights. Yet they don't. They don't challenge governments. WHO carries . . . weight in the country, but compromises too much. I think they should protect the rights of people. They need to make that shift. They need to speed up their processes. Can the WHO be reformed? Probably not. Close it down. It is a natural process for something as big and as long [lasting] as the WHO. It is a different world now than when the WHO was conceived. It hasn't moved quickly enough. It is unfortunate, but [that] is reality.[163]

A European AIDS activist concurs: "We cannot expect the WHO to fix the shape of the nations. It cannot be effective against the country's will. What the WHO should do more is expos[e] bad practices. It could be a little bit more harsh."[164]

Short of scrapping it, other activists argue that the WHO should occupy only a normative and technical role in standard setting.[165] According to the executive director of the Roll Back Malaria Partnership, the governing board of the WHO itself came to the perhaps inevitable conclusion that it should focus on what it does best: developing norms rather than implementing programs or hosting partnerships:

> Traditionally in the past, WHO was a primary provider of technical assistance. Today, within its financial envelope, it is less equipped to do so. Technical assistance is where people with the money come in. WHO complains about why it doesn't get the money to do its job. There are certain aspects when money [should be] channeled to the WHO, for example, for strategic planning. But when it is about procurement and supply chain[s], donors don't want to give money to the WHO. . . . At the end, [this] is helping the WHO to adapt its mandate to a new world.[166]

One controversial issue pertains to the future of the WHO governance structure. Should it be broadened to include nonstate actors? Advocates see this as an opportunity to increase WHO responsiveness while opponents are concerned about private sector influence, which already permeates the WHO through funding.

GLOBAL FUND

The Global Fund is viewed by many as one of the most significant achievements in the AIDS response, saving countless lives, encouraging each country's ownership of its AIDS agenda, and ushering in a new norm of partnership at the country level by forcing nongovernmental representation to be accepted at the same decision-making table as the national ministry of health and AIDS program. Critics, however, point to a number of problematic issues, including the fund's governance, bureaucracy, lack of capacity building for civil society engagement, fostering of NGO competition, absence of a clear human rights strategy, and failure to generate local change.

At the governance level, the Global Fund embodies many contradictions in its design. The executive director of Aidspan, an independent watchdog of the Global Fund, explains that traditional aid in the 1950s and 1960s was very much top-down, for example donors would fill up planes of doctors and nurses when there was a crisis. The model in the 1960s and 1970s evolved but was still supply-led. UN agencies would send managers to run projects. Then the Global Fund model came along and asked the countries: What do you need the money for? How would you spend it? The problem is, though, "when it does not work, should the Global Fund from Geneva say to the country 'this is what you must do'? This is the thing that the Global Fund has not clearly resolved, and there is no easy answer. It has probably funded things that didn't deserve funding."[167] So the very principle that makes the Global Fund unique in international aid—country ownership—also renders it susceptible to steering failures in terms of interventions. As an Aidspan consultant asks, "If Nigeria didn't put enough money into maternal and child health, whose fault is that?"[168]

Meanwhile, the board spends too much time on micro-management instead of strategy.[169] There are also power imbalances between donor countries and implementing countries. Western governments have more resources and are well prepared for board meetings, but the Global Fund failed to bolster the capacity of implementing countries. The representation of implementing countries—eight seats, allocated by region (e.g., ten to twelve governments rotate for the seat representing Africa)—changed frequently.[170] Similarly, civil society representation on the Global Fund, while mandated, is not funded. Participation remains a volunteer activity. The expectation is that civil society will continue to deliver out of goodwill. The president of the Delhi Network of Positive People shares his experience: "For a year, I served on the Community Delegation. They asked me [for] 20% of my time, but one document was thick like this! It's madness. I told the Global Fund people, we could say the same thing in one page. Instead, they hired a consultant and produced a fifty-page document to say the same thing. They make simple things difficult, and those who do that are called consultants and they are paid a lot of money."[171]

At the country level, the Global Fund is plagued by a tricky triangle: the Global Fund receives grant proposals from the CCM (which serves as the oversight structure) but disburses money directly to principal recipients (PRs), who alone are legally and contractually bound to the fund. The Global Fund then contracts with local fund agents (LFAs, which are mostly big accounting firms) to keep any eye on the PRs and catch any fraud. The problem is that while the Global Fund vets the PRs seriously to assess their capabilities before any grant is disbursed, assessment at the subrecipient level has often been lacking. In addition, the respective roles of LFAs, CCM, and the portfolio managers in the Global Fund secretariat have not been clearly defined. Who really should be the one uncovering fraud? In Mauritania, for example, fraud went on for over five years. The Global Fund secretariat did not think it was its job. The fund portfolio managers failed to monitor properly. The CCM has no contractual obligations vis-à-vis the Global Fund. The LFA did not catch the problem. Who should be held accountable?[172]

Besides oversight issues, there is also tremendous confusion about the function of the CCM. It was never meant to be an alternative structure in parallel to national AIDS programs, but often it turned out to be so. The founding document of the Global Fund mandates the CCM to be chaired by a government representative, which reinforces state dominance. Having PRs and sub-PRs sit on the CCM also raises serious issues of conflict of interest. An ITPC, Eastern Europe and Central Asia, advocacy officer observes: "I haven't seen a single example of an effective CCM in this region. Many governments have created a body inside the Ministry of Health to be the major coordinative thing, and only government representatives sit on this decision-making body. CCM is there only to deal with Global Fund money. So there are two bodies instead of one, which violates the Three Ones principle [one action framework, one coordinating authority, and one evaluation framework]."[173] Further, the Global Fund Grants Program manager at UNDP-Kyrgyzstan thinks that CCM representation comes at the cost of professionalism:

> CCM has a life of its own. . . . It does not have an effect on the grant programs. They . . . discuss . . . memberships, salary, or some other trivial issues. But when it comes to substantive issues, there are very few discussions. For me, the initial idea of making Global Fund programs nationally owned through the CCM [has] fail[ed]. NGOs are only there to defend their own pot. Some don't know why they are there. Some ministries are not obviously linked to HIV. Representation is fine, but . . . the people are so far away in their daily life from HIV. You have to do advocacy again and again.[174]

Activists have also charged the Global Fund with strengthening state coffers rather than civil society and for failing to take a strong stand on human rights. In China, which is the largest international donor to the AIDS response, the Global Fund has been recognized by the government for bringing international experience and performance-based funding into the national AIDS system. But AIDS activists criticize the Global Fund as the Chinese government's cashier, benefiting mostly the government-organized nongovernmental organizations (GONGOs), and they have organized a "Global Fund, Get Out!" movement.[175] By granting money to many small, nascent NGOs and CBOs, the fund has created dependence and bitter infighting. According to the executive director of the Dongzhen Center for Human Rights Education and Action, "The money is very small: as far as I know, [a] maximum [of] 80,000 yuan [under US$13,000] per organization. It is very hard to run an organization with just this amount of money. Many individuals just wanted the money rather than building an organization. The role of the Global Fund has been to let NGOs appear but not really sustain their development."[176] The executive director of the Shanghai AIDS Prevention Center, which focuses on young MSM, explains the unintended effects of the Global Fund on the ground:

> At the time, the Global Fund Round 6 was calling for proposals. Until then, no Shanghai NGOs [had] ever received any Global Fund money. The government was looking for thirteen CBOs and found twelve. So I gathered five people and created this "NGO." We had no name, no office. We didn't even know how to write a proposal. In April 2008, the NGO was registered. In 2009, because the funds increased, we needed full-time staff. Our salary is very low, about 3,000 yuan, plus social insurance, which makes about 4,000 yuan [US$650] per month. The problem is that donors do not fund salaries. This is why there is a development in China: fraud. You can't do [your work] without fraud. If there is no salary in a project, how

can you do it? . . . In China, a lot of MSM groups were born because of Global Fund grants of about 20,000–30,000 yuan each [US$3,200–$4,800]. The biggest problem with the Round 6 and 7 Global Fund grants is that you can receive the funds regardless of ability if you are [an organization dedicated to] MSM or sex worker[s] or HIV-positive [people]. So a few friends would get together, buy some water and fruit and do some visits and distribute condoms. Global Fund money was spent this way. There was simply no service. There are too many groups. Next year, these two grants will end. . . . It is going to be very difficult. In 1978, when China open[ed] its economy, many state companies collapsed. Chinese NGOs are in this situation now. I am not sure my colleagues are prepared for this revolution.[177]

Elsewhere, NGOs have become so preoccupied with applying for money and reporting to the Global Fund that they have forgotten about their mission. An advocacy officer of ITPC, Eastern Europe and Central Asia, says:

I have heard the point quite often in this region that the Global Fund is an NGO killer because once NGOs have applied to the Global Fund, people start to do everything to fulfill the indicators and do not focus on other things. You need a huge amount of people to cope with reporting. . . . Because of the need to show effectiveness in order to reapply in the next round, there is no more time to push the government to provide the money or time to stop to think whether what we are doing is effective. The Global Fund considers our Round 3, 4, 5 grants [to be] one of the best. But how come the Global Fund didn't affect the Russian government? After these rounds, all programs are now closed. How come we didn't manage to prove to the government the money saved? Normally, if you show the government savings, they will go for it. This is very strange. So the Global Fund might have been "effective" in disbursing the grants, but we don't see any change with the government.[178]

The former communications manager of the Asian Harm Reduction Network thinks that the Global Fund uses "a very ivory tower, bureaucratic interpretation of how services should be rolled out. Members of the Technical Review Panel are so removed from the particularities of [the] lives of MARPs."[179] A Global Fund manager acknowledges that the fund should have been much more vocal in terms of human rights:

There is overwhelming evidence that the Global Fund refused to have a human rights strategy. It refused to take a stand. Michel Kazatchkine [the Global Fund's executive director] did on a personal level. But he didn't make the case with the partners, and he didn't put it at an institutional level. If you are not prepared to do that, how would you influence the AIDS agenda? When you don't insist on, for example, providing multidrug-resistant TB drugs in prison in order for a country to get Global Fund money, it makes it too easy for governments to just go around an issue. Whether the Global Fund admits it or not, it is already part of the agenda. SOGI [the Sexual Orientation and Gender Identity strategy] was pushed by civil society. PMTCT as well. We should have pushed for it. Activists have pushed human rights to the point that it is now one of the five pillars in the . . . Global Fund 2012–2016 strategy. But the problem is senior management. Human rights are not important to them. The fund was not going to have a dedicated employee on human rights issues until it realized [there was] pressure and the need to have a dedicated person. We need a human rights activist, not a human rights academic, who will push human rights across the secretariat, who is not afraid to speak up, who doesn't mind being ostracized. We are not yet there.[180]

The Global Fund is not unaware of its own various shortcomings. A number of governance issues were already identified in the first five-year evaluation, covering the fund's operations from 2002 to 2007.[181] In 2011, the High-Level Independent Review Panel issued a scathing report with recommendations for wholesale changes in governance, management, funding mechanisms, and risk control. For a body founded on the principle of transparency, the High-Level Independent Review Panel was controversial and shrouded in mystery. Concerns began when the Associated Press ran a story in January 2011 on fraud that the Global Fund's Office of the Inspector General had reported four months prior.[182] The amount of money misspent, fraudulently misappropriated, or unaccounted for was no more than 3% of all grants, but donors panicked. Germany said it would suspend its contribution until the issue was cleared up. Sweden, Ireland, and Denmark followed suit. According to a Global Fund observer, the reaction did not seem to be justified: "First mystery: the Global Fund did have a number of problems, but nothing that suggested that it had to throw everything out and start all over again."[183] The Global Fund decided to appoint a panel, which was filled with 90% Americans and Canadians, including Michael Leavitt, who served as the secretary of the US Department of Health and Human Services under President George W. Bush and is the founder of Leavitt Partners—a healthcare intelligence consulting firm—as the co-chair of the panel; Charles Johnson, a partner and senior advisor at Leavitt Partners, as co-leader of the support team; William Steiger, a godson of George W. Bush, also a senior advisor at Leavitt Partners, and also a former employee of the US Department of Health and Human Services; and Matthew Robinson, an advisor for multilateral diplomacy in the Office of the US Global AIDS Coordinator. The Global Fund observer continues: "Second mystery:

No one knows how the panel was composed. It was never talked about except when it was announced. Third mystery: The panel was given a specific mandate to review the fiduciary and oversight mechanisms, but it went way beyond its terms of reference. The final panel report covered all aspects of the fund's operations."[184]

The impact of the panel should not be underestimated. According to the report, the Global Fund will "change or wither": it must transition from an emergency to a sustainable response; develop new risk management approaches; strengthen internal governance; reform the onerous grant approval process; strengthen secretariat management and decision making; and "get serious about results."[185] Two months later, the Global Fund Board hurriedly adopted the Consolidated Transformation Plan to implement "transformations," including a new investment approach to resource allocation; corporate and operational risk management frameworks; streamlined grant management procedures; a refocused executive management team; a new board committee structure; and new financing options.[186] In early 2012, an investment banker, Gabriel Jaramillo, was brought in as the new general manager, and the executive director, Michel Kazatchkine, then chose to "resign." Throughout the rest of that year, the Global Fund was shaken by seismic change: "They brought in the GM. He was brutal. Some senior managers were told to leave the[ir] desk by 5 pm. . . . Then he restructured the secretariat. The fund portfolios became the emphasis of the world. He changed the country team structure. . . . The civil society team is completely gone. The CCM team is also completely gone. The Partnership Unit is gone."[187]

A subsequent series of high-level appointments and events at the Global Fund hint at increasing control by the United States and the pharmaceutical companies. Without any transparency, several of the members of the High-Level Independent Review Panel went on to occupy top positions at the Global Fund. Bill Steiger stayed on as the special advisor to the general manager. According to a KEI researcher, Steiger, the "scion of a political dynasty," is publicly known for his pro-Pharma stand.[188] Steiger was the representative of the US secretary of Health and Human Services to the 2001 World Health Assembly of the WHO, and a Health GAP report writes: "The US will not allow its contributions to go toward any purchase, bulk or otherwise, of generic versions of HIV medications that [are] under patent protection in the US, regardless of price difference. There is also talk that the Administration is threatening to try to kill the fund unless generic manufacturers are excluded from participation altogether."[189] Further, in June 2012, three Global Fund insiders indicated that Steiger was taking over the Global Fund's voluntary pooled procurement,[190] which is responsible for the procurement and management of pharmaceuticals and other health products that represent 40% ($8 billion) of the Global Fund's total funding commitment of $20 billion.

Meanwhile, on April 13, 2011, US senator Orrin Hatch, who received over $800,000 from Pharma in campaign funds between 2007 and 2012, wrote a letter to the secretary of state, Hillary Clinton, complaining about the Global Fund's policy on generic procurement and compulsory licensing.[191] He asserted that Global Fund money was being used to procure generic drugs rather than branded drugs (all Abbott products) and alleged that "officials of the Global Fund are promoting compulsory licenses and verbally conditioning these licenses for the Global Fund grants."[192] In September 2012, Abbott, one of the private sector members on the Global Fund Board, approached senior staff of the Global Fund to assert that the fund had encouraged PRs to purchase generic lopinavir/ritonavir and thus "violate" patents on Kaletra. That same month, on September 28, 2012, Hatch requested a meeting with the Office of the US Global AIDS Coordinator to discuss Abbott's concerns.[193]

Charles Johnson of Leavitt Partners stayed on first as the acting chief risk officer and then as the chief financial officer until Daniel Camus, formerly of Aventis (now Sanofi-Aventis), was appointed in August 2012. More important, the search was on for a new executive director who would steer the Global Fund through this turbulent phase. Compared with the last search, the "selection process [was] conducted in the utmost secrecy," with scant information made available to the public and the names of short-listed candidates withheld until the final appointment.[194] Despite the fund being a health financing institution focused on the Global South, emphasizing diversity and GIPA, all four finalists—two women, two men—were White and from the North: Canada, France, the United Kingdom, and the United States.[195] The appointment of Mark Dybul, who had led PEPFAR under George W. Bush and had been criticized for his abstinence-only ideology, only added to the concerns of some critics about the increasing influence of northern countries.[196] In the same month, the Global Fund appointed a new chief procurement officer, Christopher Game, formerly of Abbott and of Novartis.

Close observers are puzzled by and critical of these changes, which suggest donor (US) control of the Global Fund. According to one, the review exercise was all smoke and mirrors: "It was only political; we had to do this in order to regain the confidence of donors."[197] Another argues, "The US is pushing its way. It decided that it didn't like [the] Global Fund and seized the AP story to push its way."[198] A former Global Fund staff member sees an ongoing power struggle:

I think the US wanted more control. It is clear from the High-Level Panel Report. At the Global Fund Board, the US used to lose pretty much every decision. When PEPFAR had $1.5 billion underspent, the US government needed to put money into something. The Global Fund was an option, but the US wanted more control over it. . . . The US was the main pusher for the review. But then the French had an issue too after Michel Kazatchkine was asked to leave. France had their concern as the second biggest donor. We have always felt the power struggle between the US and Europe for the fund.[199]

Others believe that the "putsch" reveals a fundamental discomfort among some northern donors about their inability to control the agenda of a specialized, multilateral AIDS funding body:

Donors themselves do not publish evidence of fraud of their grants. The OIG [Office of the Inspector General] ran slightly amok, acting so independently as to jeopardize the confidence of the overall structure. The Global Fund didn't know how to handle this stuff. At the secretariat level, it had not had a risk management approach. Most importantly, it revealed profound ambivalence [among] donors about the degree [to] which they control the fund's priorities and the wisdom and value of yet another funding structure independent of their own. . . . DFID [the UK Department for International Development], the Australians, [the] godson of Bush, etc., all have perpetual discomfort with the idea that the fund is so open-ended, country-driven. Then there is debate among development people [about] why specialized money is put aside for AIDS instead of health strengthening. All these pressures converged to produce the coup. To understand what happened, you have to go back to US history of the 1960s with the distrust of multilaterals [and] the UN. The Bill Steigers of the world have always regarded the UN as weakness. . . . The truth is that the US government will not pay for harm reduction, needle exchange, sex work, and sexual health.[200]

Further, critical observers are concerned that the Global Fund will now swing to the other side and become data-driven:

Now I worry. Let me give you an example. I am trained as an economist and am comfortable with data. When the implementer said, "I have done it," the evidence should not be [the number of] mosquito nets delivered but rather the decrease in child mortality. So the idea is to get better data to prove the impact and outcomes, not just the number of meetings held. The danger now is the Global Fund will swing too wildly under a technocratic leader, someone from the corporate sector, . . . to worship number[s]. He might say, "We can't prove grant A saves lives." If grant A is buying ARV pills and distribut[ing] condoms, you can prove with evidence that it's saving lives. But if grant B is for health system strengthening, building a clinic, or training a doctor or nurse, that in itself does not save lives. He might say it's fussy stuff. Let's do concrete stuff. But that's dangerous. If you have people coming into [a] clinic with a leaky roof, you can send a thousand pills [to that country] but still have the same clinic and one nurse, who cannot deliver a thousand pills. In fact, health system strengthening is an important part, but the impact is delayed. If you give pills on Monday, you save lives on Tuesday, there is immediate impact. But building a clinic, providing a bike, etc., all this takes time. We can't say we spent $20,000 on clinics and that saves x number of lives. But if you don't do it, you can't disburse the pills to save lives. I won't say, change the model. Get data, yes, but [do] not worship data.[201]

Many ponder whether global AIDS leadership should be taken outside the UN system altogether. The executive director of UNITAID says: "A whole set of new actors are coming. These new organizations are very quick. The UN is an old and heavy machine. One would want something more responsive with a capacity to think in a less traditional way and have a dialogue not just with the country but also with civil society without being stuck with a whole set of constraints."[202] The executive director of the Stop TB Partnership echoes, "We should detach from the way we were thinking before into operating in partnerships . . . with the flexibility to bring to the table key players without being constrained. [This is] the way forward."[203]

Health System Integration and National Leadership

After three decades of building a global AIDS response, international bureaucrats and activists finally realize the importance of returning to national drawing boards. AIDS mobilization has transformed many aspects of health governance, few of which have yet translated into changes in national health systems. People have increasingly questioned the AIDS exceptionality assumption, upon which the global AIDS response has been built. According to the co-founder of the Health and Development Network:

The island created by HIV has been indifferent to the rest of the world. I just use health system[s] as an example. HIV has been so well funded while health systems have . . . atrophied. Since the World Bank structural adjustment programs came into the country, the health system has . . . decayed while HIV has been completely over-funded. It has been completely distorted. It can't continue like that. It is actually morally wrong to do that. You can't keep people alive because there are not enough immunizations, because they die of pneumonia or they don't have a bed net, but then you pump billions of dollars into HIV programs. . . .

What didn't we do in activism around HIV? We had minimal civil society mobilization around health; we still do. What about universal health care? This is the corner the WHO has been stuck in; they could be much broader. I think there will be a lot more pragmatism now. There is this whole argument about the transition of HIV and its non-exceptionality. People one by one are doing U-turns. AIDS is not that exceptional any more. Other global issues are catching up. There is no way that emphasis on AIDS is going to be able to be sustained no matter how much energy, how loud the voices are because there will be always other people who say, how about the other issues? You are not being equitable. You are actually contradicting your equity and human rights framework that you claimed at the beginning. The moral high ground that the AIDS world took on its own twenty years ago is now available to everybody.[204]

A Russian ITPC advocacy officer agrees: "Donors are very tired because HIV is a never-ending story. It's more effective to work on system changing. We have separated AIDS [from other diseases] for thirty years. It's enough. It's a normal disease. . . . People think they are specialists in HIV. But we cannot separate HIV work from the health system. I don't see any good example in this region where HIV interventions have changed the system."[205] According to her, the absence of the integration of community system strengthening and health system strengthening shows that the work supported by the Global Fund is not sustainable. The senior program officer of the Global Campaign for Microbicides also notes: "There needs to be more integration of HIV prevention programs. These programs operate in [isolation] with a big impact on costs. With the recession and [the] reduction of global funding, we really need to see more integration of these programs. We have all these programs in Africa; they need to come together to be more effective with a better output through more collaboration."[206]

The chronic shortage of healthcare workers in national health systems continues to undermine a robust AIDS response. A Global Health Workforce Alliance advisor explains:

The thing we would like to see among the key actors is what the Global Fund and GAVI [Global Alliance for Vaccines and Immunisation] have done in revising their mandate to focus more on horizontal support [for the] health system [rather] than [a] vertical focus, maximizing synergies between the vertical and horizontal approach[es]. But the funding is still very vertical. . . . The Global Fund has actually backtracked. We had close policy discussions with them, but we have not been successful so far. On the other hand, some other bilateral donors are paying greater attention than before. Everyone agrees it is a priority. The issue is whether donors [will] fund recurrent salaries. We don't see a coherent approach. Typically, it is an issue not reflected in explicit ways in policy [and] strategy document[s]. Different positions are adopted in different countries. We tried to put it on the agenda, e.g., in the 2011 G8 Accountability Report. We are not even arguing for one size fits all, that all countries should fund all. Right now, donors may supply salaries for five years but then pull out. In the long term, the answer is domestic financing. But we are not there yet.[207]

Similarly, an Indian member of the People's Health Movement argues that the biggest barriers to access to treatment have been chronic underfunding in health: "It's attractive to say that patents is the main issue in India, but it's not. . . . The issue is we spend so little on health care, less than 1% of GDP, which is one of the lowest in the world. Seventy-five percent of healthcare expenses are paid out-of-pocket. The barriers are structural issues that determine access."[208]

At the level of civil society participation as well, there is now recognition of the importance of an integrated approach. The executive director of the Stop TB Partnership recommends:

We should look into integrating what we do. We all run after civil society. HIV has more [NGOs] than malaria and TB. Wouldn't it be logical to pull forces together? Say, for example, in this country, malaria is a bigger problem than HIV and TB, [so] civil society should focus on malaria. [We need] an integrated approach of partnership. We are hosted all over the place. We become vertical. This [group] is a partnership for mother and child; another one [focuses] on TB; and another on malaria. How can we put all this together? . . . For this to happen, four or five donors need to sit together. Another approach is bottom-up. . . . Can we do it together? The Ministry of Health says, "We have the HIV lobbyists coming. [For] TB, they don't come." We have made ourselves vertical. It is totally not integrated.[209]

The shift toward health system thinking has already begun in certain AIDS NGOs. The Global Fund Watch, China, for instance, has started to look at broader health issues, such as TB, with the same focus on civil society governance, transparency, participation, and capacity building.[210]

Despite the slogans of country ownership, country-driven responses, the Three Ones, and a national enabling environment, Geneva continues to be in the driver's seat. The switch back to national structures arises from the fact that perhaps enduring changes at the national level are what matter. The director of the International Harm Reduction Program of OSF says:

> People who used to focus on HIV are diversifying into TB and where the money is. I feel like the era of bilateralism and multilateralism in health funding is contracting sharply. National governments are critical. If I think about some of the most important things that have happened, such as [the] success in South Africa to get universal HIV treatment, the filing of patent challenges in India, [the] Section 3(d) provision that allows India to block patents, and [the] Supreme Court decision in the US in healthcare reform, they are all national changes. The locus has started to move to national and subnational decision making. When we started, the Global Fund didn't exist. But when the Global Fund came, things became much more fragmented. An organization like UNAIDS also has to dispatch more people to the country level. . . . When you are talking about something like health, there is no way that the government is not involved in shaping the services. Health is a public good. The government is responsible for allocating and funding the public good. . . . I also think that HIV is not the only cause of AIDS. Prison is also [a] cause of AIDS. A lot of structures that shape HIV/AIDS are not health structures.[211]

In areas such as health human resources, which continues to be a critical bottleneck in the AIDS response, the role of the government is paramount. A senior advisor at the Global Health Workforce Alliance reiterates: "The key actors are countries. Much of the policy discourse should shift from the global to the national level. The situation is so different and nuanced in different countries that it is difficult to draw any universal lesson. Ensuring [that] the state . . . take[s] responsibility [for] the health of its citizens as a right, not as [a] commodity, is the biggest policy reform we as advocates can do in the twenty-first century. International institutions can play a role, but states are indispensable."[212] Many African AIDS NGOs have taken up domestic and regional health financing as their priority and mobilized their leaders around the Abuja commitment. The Ugandan government, for example, has a partnership coordination mechanism that carries out national assessments in terms of sources and types of AIDS funding. It emphasizes a demand-driven approach to sensitize the community and to empower the people to demand that their government step up funding.[213] UNAIDS' new investment framework also emphasizes synergies with national development sectors to ensure that funding corresponds to local priorities.[214]

Weak national leadership continues to undermine an effective global health response. According to a senior technical advisor at the ILO, national AIDS programs have had enough opportunity to learn how to engage with different ministries and civil society over the past twenty-plus years. It is time for them to step up and lead: "The coordination issue is more at the country level, to strengthen national AIDS programs so that there are clear opportunities for the role of other stakeholders. Very few national AIDS programs have worked with trade unions, and they tell us trade unions have no capacity. Like funding NGOs, you can build [the] capacity of a trade union. You are funding long-term institutions."[215] When asked about the biggest barrier to a malaria-free world, the executive director of the Roll Back Malaria Partnership replies:

> My honest answer is government commitments to deliver health care to people, not just malaria prevention and treatment. They are not serious. Only a few countries whose presidents want to get elected take health seriously, based on the fact that people who get health care will reelect their presidents. There are very few. We can't eradicate malaria without providing good health care to people. It is not like polio where you deliver the vaccines only once. This is about 365 days a year, but malaria control is possible. Malaria is a hook for strengthening civil society. We are traditionally not activist people, but our dialogue is completely aligned [with] the right-to-health agenda. . . . In most countries, the elimination agenda is only taken up at the subcountry level, e.g., in Indonesia it works only in Bali [because of] tourism. The response is defined by narrow economic interests rather than social ones. If there is economic advantage, governments push the agenda. . . . Political commitment and leadership [are] important because that can overcome other things.[216]

Intellectual Property and the Role of the Private Sector

Despite over a decade of yelling and screaming by activists at every WTO ministerial meeting, at national patent offices, and in domestic courts, an international IP regime enshrined in TRIPS remains a key structural barrier to universal access. The problem of having two approaches guided by opposing principles— public health by human rights and intellectual property by private interests— within the same UN system has never been resolved. A human rights regime exists in parallel to the trade regime, colliding not just in health, but also in development, the environment, gender equality, labor, water, education, and cultural diversity. There is no dispute mechanism in the UN to settle conflicts when they arise.

In AIDS, the work of UNAIDS (and its co-sponsors) has been greatly impeded by the TRIPS agreement of the WTO. As a Brazilian lawyer laments, "We have hundreds of human rights conventions and instruments that we can use when IP violates our rights to health, and yet we have no power to overcome one

TRIPS."[217] A Canadian human rights lawyer argues for the abolition of the WTO: "The most fundamental flaw in current global governance is the entire system, with the WTO at the center of globalizing corporate rule, creating a global constitution for capital. That is the rot at the core of global governance today. It is a rot that infects every area of life around the globe. I would suggest the abolition of the WTO. What we need is a global fair trading agreement."[218]

Another structural issue is the failure of the private sector to provide for global public goods, including health. Diseases such as elephantiasis, river blindness, and African sleeping sickness, which affect mostly the South, often fail to attract research and development funds due to unprofitable markets. As a result, drugs, diagnostics, and vaccines often remain unaffordable or unsuitable for populations who need them. Pediatric ARV is a great example of a global public health good that has been underserved. There is only a tiny pediatric ARV market in the North, and R&D remains grossly insufficient. Activists led by KEI have been lobbying for over a decade for various mechanisms to monitor and coordinate R&D flows, to secure sustainable financing, and to promote new incentives to manage innovation and access to meet health needs in developing countries. In April 2012, the WHO report of the Consultative Expert Working Group on Research and Development outlined several concrete proposals, including a WHO convention on global R&D. But the issue is polarized between the North and the South, with the United States, the European Union, Switzerland, and Japan leading the opposition and the private sector dragging its feet due to lack of incentives. According to a KEI campaigner:

> Some companies don't agree on the idea of global public goods, and this is a significant ideological difference. This report recognizes that the reason why the current system fails is that there is no incentive for certain areas of research. One of the publications of MSF rightly points out that if you have sustainable financing and you match it to priorities, it is going to fund consistently, [but this] currently relies on foundations and the largesse of . . . other limited initiatives. This issue isn't just related to HIV. The same questions apply to the Climate Fund: Who pays? How much?[219]

While almost all major actors, including donors, UN agencies, foundations, national governments, and civil society, have stepped up to the AIDS challenge since the 1980s, the private sector remains conspicuously absent except for a few isolated, well-publicized examples, like Chevron and Anglo American, which provide company-based prevention and treatment programs. Repeated UN attempts to more systemically engage with the private sector, such as the Global Compact, have failed to yield any tangible results. "I think the most robust structure is the private sector," says the International Harm Reduction Development Program's director. "The fact that the pharmaceutical industry can still make enormous profits out of ARVs is still a huge issue. Most of the groups I work with have hepatitis C. The same companies that manufacture AIDS drugs sell some of the hepatitis C drugs at $70,000 a year. It is immoral, and it continues. It is not totally unremarked, but is still largely in place."[220]

Why is it so difficult to involve the private sector? The Russian vice president and regional director of the Global Business Coalition for Health, which involves over 200 companies in the mobilization of resources for health through the concept of core competence, responds:

The private sector is all about profit and money. Even if it spends money on social issues, they calculate how profitable it will be for them. For example, if they take care of the environment, it contributes to their health profile. If they invest in community, it contributes to their workplace. . . . Our private sector history is young. It is still learning to make business and still learning about charity. . . . The joke here is that there are three popular topics for charity: first, children: everybody likes children; second, sports, like the Olympics and world football championships; and the last one, the Bolshoi theater. Russia is a cultural country. If you look at the list of sponsors of the Bolshoi! . . . We have a lot of education to do. What we explain to employers is that adults spend a lot of time at work. They will be thankful to you as you provide them with ready knowledge because to take care of risk behavior is easier than to treat [diseases later].[221]

In 2011, the Global Business Coalition for Health adopted its current name from the previous Global Business Coalition for HIV/AIDS. "Many international companies didn't find interest in HIV and TB," the Russian vice president explains. "With a widening mandate, it is an opportunity for us to attract new companies [that] might start their attention on diabetes, then on HIV and TB. The approach might be different. Diabetes is for everyone, in developed and developing countries. HIV is more for so-called Third World countries. The programming we developed works with diabetes as well."[222] A senior program officer with the Global Campaign for Microbicides also confirms the business approach to AIDS: "There has been more industry involvement in recent years. I am not sure whether it has to do with the outcomes we have seen in clinical trials. I suspect that it [does]. . . . Whatever they invest in has to be commercially viable. If you can prove to them that this will work, they may invest in development. We all know that they are running commercial businesses."[223]

The private sector is too important to be ignored, and its role is changing. Before, the private sector appeared mostly in the role of the US trade representative. Today, it also sits on the boards of various institutions.[224] There are many different ways to approach and engage the private sector. The existing ad hoc approach—for example, a donor gives money to an NGO to work with a company on a project—is not sustainable. The issue of private sector advocacy remains critical. A Global Fund Civil Society and Private Sector Partnerships manager believes that some fundamental changes in attitudes and communication between civil society and the private sector need to happen:

> More generally, we fail to understand that the corporate sector needs to make a profit. We have not been able to be comfortable with it. Every time civil society has a meeting with the private sector, we want to beat them up. I can understand. We need to change the nature of that debate, whether we like it or not; we need to face the real world. The private sector is going to make obscene profits. If you can accept that [then it can work] . . . otherwise, it is deadlock. The changes happen both ways. The corporate sector needs to change its attitude towards civil society. The corporate sector needs to understand that it cannot continue to screw people over; it eventually will harm their profits. The US system is [the] best example of consumer power. The consumer lobby is hugely strong and influential when people start to buy products. So what is the role of the WHO? Why is the WHO not facilitating the dialogue? It straddles both worlds. It provides technical assistance on drugs and is also approachable to civil society. They should be a catalyst.[225]

Civil Society Engagement and Capacity Building

Despite a civil society rhetoric that is by now enshrined in all high-level commitments, the engagement of this traditionally marginalized sector continues to be plagued by ideological, political, and material barriers. Civil society gains at the global level are undeniable. A senior UNAIDS bureaucrat confirms, "There is huge support through the board and also through General Assembly processes in the yearly debate on AIDS. For the first time ever, and it is from AIDS, civil society is always included in national delegations. There is also huge support in the Global Fund; UNAIDS was a main advocate to push for civil society to be members of the board. We are so interdependent."[226]

In addition to representation on the Global Fund Board, the CCM structure itself provides unprecedented civil society engagement at the national level. Funding streams and mechanisms such as community system strengthening, dual-track financing, and grants on the ground have also contributed enormously to civil society development.[227] A wide range of global health partnerships has also recognized and facilitated civil society participation through various structures. In the Stop TB Partnership, civil society is represented on both the board and the Community Task Force within each working group, and AIDS NGOs such as the Treatment Action Group have been driving a lot of civil society engagement.[228] In the Roll Back Malaria Partnership, there are two civil society constituencies: northern NGOs that are recipients of development aid to deliver services, and the civil society in southern countries, which is involved in resource mobilization. In malaria control, the context varies so much that community engagement takes different forms. Its executive director explains:

> We tried to improve community competence to reduce malaria. To give an example, a new health system in Ethiopia . . . focuses on [the] model family: families that are able to deal with common problems and share with neighbors. Today, that is the focus of the health system. They can achieve health results that are stupendous. They just took it to [a unique] step in their cultural context. I would have expected civil society to take it up. But households are taking control of malaria. We are still developing strategies, learning from PLWHA networks. In Cameroon, we use HIV networks to do community mobilization around malarial control. We use HIV networks [working with] PMTCT to deliver bed nets because it is stupid to keep women and bab[ies] healthy, but then they die of [other] diseases. We have worked so far with HIV-related organizations. There is hardly any malaria civil society in rural communities. It is a fact of life. Today, they have learned that you can do something about it. But only bed nets are given. Not campaigning. We are still not there yet.[229]

In AIDS prevention research, community advisory boards (CABs) in clinical trial sites have played an indispensable role in ensuring community participation, which had been slow to build due to skepticism because of bad experiences with previous clinical trials. Often, education and research literacy are the keys to more effective community involvement. According to the senior program officer of the Global Campaign for Microbicides, "We have seen trial sites where there is a lot of community mobilization, recruit well. Maybe there was a notion in the past that they would take part as guinea pigs and that when products became available, there was only access by the wealthy. CABs really try to reassure them."[230] Community participation in the global process also takes place through mechanisms like UNGASS. An advocacy officer of ITPC, Eastern Europe and Central Asia, explains:

We have an agreement with UNAIDS that once they have a draft of the national report of Russia to UNGASS, we would get hold of [a] copy and distribute [it] to our members and receive comments. . . . In 2008, the official report was such bullshit. People were pissed off and decided to make [an] alternative report. We published the first shadow report [about] Russia. The following year, the government started to prepare all UNGASS processes way earlier. Already in the summer of 2009, the government said it would like to involve NGOs, and we established a meeting. The team [that] was responsible for HIV at that time inside the Ministry of Health was more professional than the current one. What they did was to ask ITPC to help them gather research and info from NGOs to include in the UNGASS report. That's what we did. We gathered twenty-five research pieces and fifty comments from NGOs [that were included] in the official version of the report. This was . . . when authority inside the ministry changed. We prepared the report with one team and it came out with a different team. We lost everything. The new team deleted everything that was politically incorrect [from their viewpoint]. This is when the hard times started.[231]

When we talk about civil society in AIDS, it is important to remember whom we are talking about or working with and why. The International Harm Reduction Development Program's director explains:

We are not just working with civil society. We often work with the marginalized subsectors of civil society. Drug users, people living with AIDS, sex workers. Even within civil society, these are groups with relatively little political power and public sympathy. You could make the argument—and we wrestle with this—that what we do is creat[e] islands of empowerment without restructuring the sea. [We] just creat[e] these pockets but [don't change the] overarching structures. In Russia, you might say, if you most want to shake it up, fund [the] opposition leader. In our discussions around prisons, we don't want to just improve HIV treatment in prisons, we want to have people not in prison. For public health and harm reduction programs, the overall question is: What do you hope to get done?[232]

The funding of civil society for systemic change is easier said than done. The fundamental tension in international funding agencies between the traditional support for government and a new civil society imperative remains firmly in place.

"The conventional wisdom is that, without government, you can't take any-thing to scale," continues the OSF director. "But without civil society, [which] has direct experience in AIDS and human rights, you also cannot take anything to scale. Certain technical agencies like the UN see their first responsibility as en-gaging with governments. We see our first responsibility as support for civil society. . . . Activism is when people take risks and invite people to join them. We have enabled that to happen."[233] Further, he says, the competition for funding also means that governments' commitment to civil society may be mere lip service:

> We have mistaken participation [for] equality. So the Global Fund is incredibly ef-fective in ensuring [the] representation of people living with AIDS, MSM, IDUs, etc., on CCMs. But the fact that you sit [there] does not mean you have equal power [in] discussion and decision making. It is clear that the GIPA principle serves to mask the process [of] includ[ing] people without increasing agency. I have seen governments recapture Global Fund money and processes from NGOs as soon as they see money at stake.[234]

The country coordinator of UNAIDS-Egypt confirms a structural issue in the UN system:

> The problem with all of [the] UN in general is that we are an intergovernmental or-ganization. We have to work with governments, but also with civil society. But the problem is [that] government is not always supportive of civil society. How to find balance between supporting civil society and not the government is a challenge. UN agencies are silent about certain things because sometimes we are forced to be si-lent. In 2007, we were not silent. We were the only UN agency speaking about the issue [arrest of MSM]. But we have to be careful about not making the at-risk pop-ulation more at risk. . . . In 2007, we had to do something. We issued a press state-ment. We did it in a way that did not threaten the government. Otherwise, we will be considered as an enemy.[235]

Often, civil society's inclusion as a stakeholder is tokenistic. The openness of the board structure is not necessarily followed by a change in organizational cul-ture. An activist turned UNAIDS staff member recalls: "I think the challenge was that many of my colleagues in different departments and teams weren't particu-larly inclusive. The way of working often was that when there was an event, they would cherry-pick a friend from an NGO [at the] last minute. We really tried to advocate a more inclusive approach."[236] Full recognition continues to be impeded by a lack of understanding of the value of what civil society contributes: "the energy of civil society has to some extent been bought off by sitting on [the boards of] these institutions. Some of the anger is gone. The potential is there, waiting to be reached."[237]

There have also been material barriers against the meaningful involvement of civil society. The 2007 independent review of UNAIDS raises several issues regarding civil society participation and representation, including the demand for chairing, speaking, and full voting rights; the institutionalization of support for the NGO delegation in UNAIDS; and improvements to the communications and consultation infrastructure for the NGO delegation.[238] The challenge for the unpaid civil society members to respond to all these ideas is real. As a UNAIDS staff member admits: "If you ask governments and UN agencies, people are paid to work on these issues. When we seek the inputs of networks of people who use drugs and ask a person to stop work for one week and come to Geneva, they are much less resourced. There is the whole question of capacity building."[239] In response to the critiques, UNAIDS created a communications facility to support the PCB NGO delegation, but the larger issue remains: "We want their input, but it comes as a cost to civil society."[240] Further, the civil society delegations to UNAIDS, the Global Fund, UNITAID, the Roll Back Malaria Partnership, the Stop TB Partnership, and GAVI have been mostly disconnected with little coordination.

Civil society engagement at the national level presents even more challenges. Many institutionalized mechanisms are at the global but not at the country level.[241] The Civil Society and Private Sector Partnerships manager of the Global Fund acknowledges:

> The limit is that we have no field presence. We worked through partners like CSAT [Civil Society Action Team] and AFRICASO [African Council of AIDS Service Organizations]. There are very few dedicated funds for civil society unless they get [money] through proposal[s]. . . . I would engage more [with] civil society. I say that not because it is the standard thing I should say. The way to help governments make solid decisions is to engage civil society. . . . Country ownership is not about government, but about people. For politicians, it is just a job. [But] their knowledge isn't greater than mine. Unless we shift things [they will stay] that way. . . . That is a long-term thing.[242]

The majority of my interviewees report a lack of government support in terms of funding or legal framework, if not outright hostility. In many countries, civil society is seen as an opponent instead of as a dialogue partner. In Egypt, the executive director of Friends of Life, a PLWHA network, describes the relationship between the civil society and the government as "a dog and a wolf." The dog is always protecting the lambs from the wolf, and the wolf is always scared of the dog.[243] In such difficult political environments, where the NGO culture is not strong and there are few means to build capacity, civil society is both vulnerable and unsustained. "Many organizations are not thinking outside of the box," continues the executive director. "They have funding from [a] UN agency. They expect the project to go on forever. They are not taking the initiative to think about [a future] fundraising strategy. . . . There are also expectations by PLWHA that this NGO will be a savior."[244] This also raises the question of funding AIDS NGOs in the context of the funding needed for human rights and democratic governance. As a veteran European AIDS activist puts it, "Civil society is a respected partner only in countries where there is established democracy. In other countries, civil society is not listened to. We are getting back to human rights. Civil society can only be effective if human rights are established."[245] In the current financial context, however, any commitment to civil society is uncertain. A former Civil Society Team officer of the Global Fund concludes:

> We reached the point when we were successful. When we wanted more representation, the establishment woke up . . . and clawed back. Civil society is under pressure. Its representation is being diluted. It is under pressure to comply. . . . There is a whole move toward refocusing on governments. If the Global Fund works with governments, where is civil society involvement? The bastion is slowly shifting. Civil society was very successful in pushing for funding. The establishment of the Global Fund absolutely relied on civil society. Take the UK experience. NGOs put huge pressure on DFID to establish the Global Fund. How the Global Fund maintains that loyalty to civil society is beyond me. Civil society is reluctant to give up their [toehold]. It is likely to continue to be that way.[246]

In summary, AIDS activists recommend the following global AIDS governance reforms:

Recommendations for Donor Coordination, Accountability, and Transparency
1. Rethink AIDS beyond a charity development paradigm.
2. Create global and national donor coordination and accountability mechanisms.
3. Encourage South-South cooperation.

4. Fund beyond programmatic interventions to foster governance based on democratic principles and human rights.

Recommendations for Governance Harmonization, Inclusion, and Alignment with Human Rights
5. Expand beyond a state-centric global governance system.
6. Harmonize and rationalize existing UN structures on AIDS, including revisiting the mandate for UNAIDS.
7. Replace distant global structures with regional and national ones to enhance responsiveness.
8. Mandate transparency requirements in strategic development, human resources recruitment, funding, management, and evaluation.
9. Align all global governance structures with international human rights principles.
10. Put in place a wide range of mechanisms to ensure equal civil society participation.

Recommendations for Health System Integration and National Leadership
11. Reconceptualize the AIDS response from health system perspectives.
12. Increase health system funding streams and domestic resources mobilization.
13. Strengthen multisectoral responses to AIDS and strengthen the health system.
14. Institutionalize the right to health in national constitutions and laws.
15. Support horizontal civil society activities, especially South-South participation.
16. Fund and build mechanisms for democratic governance.

Recommendations for Intellectual Property and the Role of the Private Sector
17. Institutionalize a clear and consistent TRIPS flexibilities strategy across all UN agencies working on AIDS.
18. Mobilize against new TRIPS-plus measures.
19. Support governments to amend existing laws to make use of TRIPS flexibilities.
20. Fund legal activism to promote access to generic medicines.
21. Adopt mechanisms, such as the proposed global health R&D treaty, to correct market failures in the global provision of public goods.
22. Identify private sector champions of AIDS and global health and massively scale up industry involvement.

Recommendations for Civil Society Engagement and Capacity Building

23. Recognize civil society's contributions in knowledge building and community mobilization.
24. Mandate, institutionalize, and fund diverse mechanisms in governance, management, funding, reporting, and monitoring for different forms of civil society participation in the UN agencies working on AIDS, in global health partnerships, and in governmental AIDS bodies.
25. Remove the structural barriers for civil society participation through legal and political reforms.

The suggested recommendations share the basic principles of equity, transparency, accountability, parity of participation, and justice. Two factors cut across all of the reforms: an emphasis on human rights and the inclusion of civil society. The suggestions aim toward a more equitable distribution of power in both AIDS and global health governance, away from the traditional state-centric and market-based structures. In the fourth decade of the epidemic, the time has come for all stakeholders to pause and reflect on the hard lessons learned and the challenges that are still unmet.

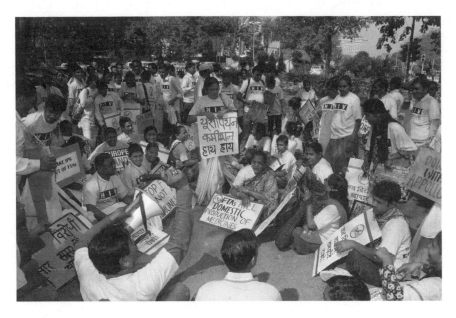

Access to Medicines: The Delhi Network of Positive People's Protest against
the EU-India Free Trade Agreement

Photo © Médecins Sans Frontières Access Campaign / Rajesh Kumar Surya

CHAPTER FIVE

Against Community and the Expertization of Activism

"Who are you?" said the Caterpillar.

This was not an encouraging opening for a conversation. Alice replied, rather shyly, "I—I hardly know, sir, just at present—at least I know who I was when I got up this morning, but I think I must have been changed several times since then."

"What do you mean by that?" said the Caterpillar sternly. "Explain yourself!"

"I can't explain myself, I'm afraid, sir," said Alice, "because I'm not myself, you see."

"I don't see," said the Caterpillar.

"I'm afraid I can't put it more clearly," Alice replied very politely, "for I can't understand it myself to begin with; and being so many different sizes in a day is very confusing."

> —Lewis Carroll, Alice in Wonderland

Hardly anybody is an AIDS activist any more. They are kind of providing services, but mostly doing whatever the funders tell them to. . . . We go to AIDS workshops and rarely have any time to challenge the power.

> —Global Campaigns Director, Health GAP

You cannot force change in the name of civil society. Civil society is not a substitute for democratic governance. Civil society is not accountable to anyone. The mere presence of civil society does not make an institution more democratic.

> —Member of the People's Health Movement

In the process of getting scientists to rethink their biomedical definition of AIDS, Pharma to loosen its grip on intellectual property, and intergovernmental organizations to be more inclusive, activists created their own AIDS wonderland with millions of dollars of grant money, a vast network of jobs in AIDS organizations, and recognition by the scientific and global health policy establishment. Through its own science, economy, and political system, AIDS activists have in effect built a community regime of power that is as vast, instrumentalizing, and influential as the other three I have discussed so far—science, market, and governance.

While acknowledging the role AIDS activists have played in organizing and empowering communities, giving voice to marginalized populations, and building alternative knowledge bases, it is important to ask: Who comprises this AIDS community? To whom is it accountable? Is it a different "community" when it presents itself to local groups, NGO peers, governments, international AIDS conferences, UNAIDS, the Global Fund, PEPFAR, or the Gates Foundation? Has part of it morphed into dominating power structures? What does it mean and do when AIDS activists invoke the community "we"?

The traditional notion of community implies boundaries marked by geography, identity, profession, or other affinities. With globalization and technology, however, community is no longer limited to one's immediate neighborhood and social networks. Instead, diverse communities spring into being through loosely defined interests. They may take the form of an online group, ad hoc coalition, or regional network. While technology has seemingly enabled people from far-flung places to come together around a cause, it also opens up complex questions about the meaning of community. Do 3,000 Facebook friends constitute a community? Are the subscribers to an online petition platform a community? Where does community begin and end?

The construction of a community's subjectivity and its effects on accountability are the focuses of this chapter. I am interested in the politics of "speaking on behalf of" community, and in how diverse kinds of community stories emerge and circulate. How does the AIDS community derive its identity, power, and legitimacy? In what ways is the community constructed and conditioned by other power systems? Who decides who counts as a member of this community? Can the AIDS community exist outside the disciplinary structures of science, market, and governance? As a newcomer among the traditional elite structures, the community needs constantly to relegitimize itself to prove its value, but it cannot do so without relying on frames of reference from the dominant power systems. How can the community sustain its oppositional consciousness?

This chapter proceeds in three sections. I begin with snapshots of different kinds of community organizations, governance and funding issues, and a typology of different advocacy models in AIDS activism. The second section analyzes power struggles in the AIDS community through external and internal techniques of power. I discuss the emergence of five community subjects—the volunteer, grantee, expert, delegate, and partner—before examining divisions in the AIDS community: the GIPA principle, North-South tensions, race, class, gender, age, and ideology. I then evaluate AIDS activists' role in community organizing and empowerment, voice and advocacy, and knowledge building. I conclude this chapter by discussing the limits and challenges of AIDS activism.

Who Are We? Community Organization, Governance, and Strategy

> Some of our partners ask: Really, do we need a new network?
> —*Project Coordinator, Coalition for Children*
> *Affected by AIDS*[1]

> As a community organizer, you have to ask what kinds of things
> you want to lead to. Provide the platform. Provide the knowledge.
> —*Global Campaigns Director, Health GAP*[2]

> Small activism is beautiful.
> —*Regional Advocacy Team Leader and*
> *Advocacy Officer, AIDS and Rights*
> *Alliance for Southern Africa*[3]

AIDS community responses emerged out of necessity and political urgency when governmental and intergovernmental organizations failed to respond to the epidemic rapidly and effectively.[4] Among diverse actors, including AIDS service organizations, community-based organizations, civil society organizations, NGOs, networks, coalitions, and movements, two core constituencies—based on the traditional criteria of community membership—are the networks of people living with AIDS and other affected populations. Part of AIDS exceptionalism comes from the fact that, for the first time in national and global public health, patient communities have organized themselves to be at the center of the response to an epidemic.

The 1983 Denver Principles on nondiscrimination and right to participation became the foundational ethos for the involvement of the HIV-positive community in all aspects of the AIDS response. Besides GNP+ and ICW, local, national, regional, and global PWA networks spread throughout the world. The Asia

Pacific Network of People Living with HIV/AIDS was established in 1994 at a
meeting in Kuala Lumpur by forty-two PLWHA from eight countries "in response to the need for a collective voice for PLWHA in the region, to better link
regional PLHIV with the Global Network of PLHIV (GNP+)."[5] The Delhi Network of Positive People was spearheaded by three drug users from Manipur,
India, who went to rehabilitation in New Delhi. "There were about a hundred
people in the rehab group; a few of us were HIV-positive," its president recounts.
"We just met each other, sat together, and drank tea in the park. We couldn't talk
openly about AIDS; the stigma and discrimination were so severe. The group
formed naturally. The work started in 1999 and grew to become the DNP+ in
2000."[6] In 2003, the National Empowerment Network of People Living with
HIV/AIDS was established in Kenya to provide "leadership for the visibility and
voice of PLHIV and affected communities."[7] In Shanghai, China, the PWA network, Beautiful Life, was founded by Zhou Yi in 2005 after he was diagnosed
with AIDS. He looked for other people living with AIDS and found a large community online. "There are so many of them. But they all keep themselves hidden," he says.[8] In Alexandria, Egypt, Friends of Life was created in 2008 after a
group of Egyptians living with HIV met with HIV-positive networks in Morocco. "Friends of Life is not just an NGO for PLWHA, but it is also led by
PLWHA," its executive director explains. "Seventy-five percent of our board
members are living with HIV and 40% are women. . . . Ninety percent of our
staff is living with HIV. But we accept anyone who supports us to be our advocates and do not discriminate against people who are not HIV-positive. We col-
laborate with physicians who care and defend for PLWHA. This collaboration
gives most strength to our NGO."[9] The Tajik Network of Women Living with HIV/
AIDS formed in 2011 after a small group of Tajik HIV-positive women attended a
meeting in Geneva. Like other PWA networks, its objective is to improve the
quality of life for HIV-positive women and children, and it focuses specifically
on the reproductive and sexual health and rights of women with HIV.[10]

Overlapping with these HIV-positive networks are identity-based community
organizations of gay men, drug users, sex workers, and migrant workers affected
by AIDS. The overall success of the community response to AIDS has much to
do with the gains of various social movements prior to the epidemic. As Altman
documents, the strong gay response to AIDS in the United States was directly
linked to the gay liberation movement in various cities with an organized gay base,
a gay press, and access to political channels.[11] Sedgwick recognizes that "[f]emi-
nist perspectives on medicine and health care issues, on civil disobedience, and
on the politics of class and race as well as of sexuality have been centrally enabling

for the recent waves of AIDS activism."[12] The gay community was united in anger due to a history of oppression, which spurred the creation of ACT UP. Moving away from the stigmatizing connection of AIDS to gay identity, some community activists preferred to call themselves MSM. Like PWA networks, MSM organizations are now found in every continent. In 2006, the Purple Sky Network was created with over eighty MSM groups in the Mekong in the context of nascent gay organizing in the Asia-Pacific region.

Similarly, sex worker and drug user responses to AIDS are situated within the larger community mobilization for decriminalization. For example, the Asia Pacific Network of Sex Workers was formed in 1994 at the International AIDS Conference in Yokohama against the backdrop of wider sex worker organizing in Australia, New Zealand, Thailand, and Japan. In Latin America, RedTraSex, a regional network that won the Red Ribbon Award for outstanding community work in AIDS, was established in 1997 as a result of sex worker organizing across the region to fight against police brutality and to lobby for legal reforms.[13] Drug users from Central and Eastern Europe felt the need for a united AIDS response and formed the Eurasian Harm Reduction Network in 1997 as part of a worldwide harm reduction movement.[14] That same year, migrant workers in Southeast Asia created the Coordination of Action Research on AIDS and Mobility in the context of a larger advocacy movement to address migrants' human rights.[15] For these affected populations, the community response to AIDS is only part of their larger struggles for human rights. As the former program director of the Eurasian Harm Reduction Network explains:

> Harm reduction is about healthy drug users. HIV is part of it, but it is not the main goal. There has been a ton of support for HIV in this region, but it's dangerous to support harm reduction work [that is focused] too narrowly on HIV and neglect other issues. For example, overdose[s] kill more drug users than HIV. In a lot of places, when harm reduction focuses too much on HIV prevention, it ceases to meet the needs of drug users, and that's damaging to HIV work.[16]

The youth community response to AIDS also has drawn on a growing global youth movement in ecology and sexual and reproductive health. The Global Youth Coalition on HIV/AIDS was founded after the 2004 International AIDS Conference in Bangkok to empower young leaders as agents of change. It builds on the strengths of existing national and regional youth movements through a focal point structure.[17] Other affected populations, such as prisoners and children, however, do not have an organized community base. In such cases, the "community" response comes from advocates and other stakeholders. Since 2005, the

Coalition for Children Affected by AIDS has engaged with UNICEF, the Global Fund, community-based organizations, academics, and healthcare providers to put all children affected by AIDS on the agenda to ensure that children's voices are heard.[18] In Ukraine, the Penitentiary Initiative, a Red Ribbon Award recipient in 2010, is a community-based organization that advocates for HIV prevention in prison settings and provides access to treatment and diagnostics for prisoners living with HIV.[19]

As we extend from this core of PWA networks and affected populations, the definition of community becomes conceptually fuzzy and politically contentious. While the majority of AIDS NGOs describe themselves as "community-based," many are based on neither geographical proximity nor identity.[20] Besides membership (who you are and who you represent), three other criteria can be considered: function (what you do in service and advocacy to support the core constituents), linkage (how close you are to the community), and efficacy (how well you advocate on its behalf). To what extent can nongovernmental professional medical, legal, and other networks that provide support to affected communities be considered as part of the community? What is the difference between the Penitentiary Initiative and MSF—both of which are advocacy organizations that serve affected populations—that qualifies the former as a community-based organization and the latter not? From a functional perspective, one could argue that physician networks like MSF and legal networks like the Lawyers Collective have done more in AIDS—by incessantly keeping up the pressure on Pharma to reduce ARV prices and by striking down discriminatory laws—than many CBOs, even though they do not have a traditional community membership base.

An advocacy function alone, however, does not automatically make one part of the community. Certainly, one cannot and should not equate "speaking on behalf of" with the community. Open Society Foundations, for example, advocates for drug users but is clearly not part of the community. Which advocacy support organizations, then, can be considered (and by whom) to be an integral part of the community? For example, is the International HIV/AIDS Alliance part of the AIDS community? Set up in 1991 by a group of donor agencies and international organizations to support community groups in developing countries that were carrying out work around HIV, the original vision of the alliance was to "put communities at the center of the response" by enabling them through funding. Soon, it shifted to focus on "building capacity, enhancing quality, learning and disseminating lessons, and using our influence to make more resources available, rather than simply channelling funds," in the broader context of a greater recognition of the role of civil society.[21] But despite its advocacy function, the International

HIV/AIDS Alliance has been criticized for being a business rather than a community organization.[22] Many AIDS activists raise concerns about the ability of the alliance, which is a secretariat-run INGO out of Brighton, England, to represent the community. But who holds the power to evaluate an organization or movement's relationship or proximity to the people?

Besides patient communities, affected populations, and professional organizations and NGOs that provide support to communities, a fourth kind of community member cuts across all of the above: thematically focused coalitions. The availability of treatment, in particular, has spurred the creation of many treatment advocacy networks and IP-focused groups. While some, including the Treatment Action Campaign, are clearly community-based, others, such as Health GAP, are not. Like MSF and the Lawyers Collective, Health GAP works with communities. Its role in AIDS activism is undeniable: pushing for cheap ARV drugs and lobbying for PEPFAR funding.[23] Yet it has only a couple of individual campaigners doing most of the work out of Washington, DC, and Nairobi, and many doubt whether Health GAP is supported by and represents people on the ground.[24] A member of ACT UP sees a clear difference between the community-based activism of ACT UP and the more professionally run campaigns of Health GAP: "By 1995–96, when new drugs came, a huge chunk of that constituency had access to these medicines and moved away. AIDS activism was no longer a primary movement of people affected by what was going on. The second wave became largely driven by people for whom HIV was not a matter of life and death personally. A lot of the people who went on to form Health GAP were not part of the first movement. There was a generational shift and positional shift as well."[25] Above all, with the help of technology, community networking no longer relies on traditional structures of membership or organization. ITPC, for example, considers itself a movement driven by community needs.[26] According to its co-founder:

> It was largely the ability to create a web of communication and information between activists doing their own things around the world, but who could easily engage with and alert others on different issues, such as drug [shortages] in Madagascar [or] advocacy around methadone on the Essential Drugs List. It was sort of a distributed network of people working in their national, local, or regional movements that had pieces of [a] common agenda. . . . It doesn't have to have the brand identity of ACT UP. People saw themselves as "members" of ACT UP, whereas for ITPC, people feel themselves "affiliated."[27]

A wide range of AIDS and human rights educational groups, social development networks, and cross-sectoral organizations make up the bulk of CBOs on the ground. As the Brazilian scholar and activist Herbert Daniel says, "AIDS in-scribes itself upon each culture in a different way. Each culture constructs its own particular kind of AIDS—as well as its own answers to the disease."[28] The form and shape of community responses are often determined by historical and politi-cal realities. In Brazil, for example, besides PWA networks, one of the earliest com-munity groups, ABIA, was created in 1986 as a cross-sectoral response to AIDS and as part of pro-democracy struggles:

> ABIA was founded at a time when the epidemic in Brazil was an emergency. We had a growing number of AIDS cases in big cities like Rio and São Paulo. The situ-ation was really severe, and there was no response from the government. The his-torical context is important. Brazilian civil society was trying to organize itself to come back to democracy after twenty years of military dictatorship. Lots of social movements, like the women's movement, gay movement, black movement, and trade unions, that had been oppressed by the dictatorship were reorganizing them-selves. This is what we call an aperture, an opening, in trying to find some ways back to democracy. The spirit in this context influenced ABIA's inception. ABIA was created not to replace the state in their responsibility. It was created to mobilize dif-ferent sectors to create a broad, interdisciplinary, intersectoral response from civil society to respond to the challenges posed by the epidemic and [to] put pressure on the government for its responsibility. We didn't have an organized national AIDS program until 1992. Among our founders were people from the gay movement, [the] scientific establishment, people from the church, [the] university. Our mandate was to mobilize by linking . . . different sectors to create a methodology and concept that could help the articulation and mobilization of a social movement concerned with the AIDS problem, to put pressure on the government, and to defend the civil rights of people living with AIDS.[29]

In Egypt, the weak community response to AIDS continues to be exacerbated by a difficult political situation, including the 2011 revolution and the post-revolution turmoil. The earliest AIDS community work in the late 1990s by or-ganizations like Caritas focused almost exclusively on raising awareness through youth education; the legal and rights elements were altogether absent. Organiza-tions working with high-risk groups are still rare.[30] A second generation of com-munity activism began with groups like the Al Shehab Foundation, which in 2001 took up a human rights approach in its social development agenda and included AIDS work from this broader perspective.[31] It was only after 2005 that PWA net-works like Friends of Life came into being. In China, "community" is subject to political definition and manipulation, as evidenced in the freezing of the Global

Fund grants to China in 2011 due to insufficient civil society engagement. When the Chinese government received its first Global Fund grants in 2004, it had pledged that 35% of the grants would be given to "NGOs." Seven years later, less than 11% of the grant money had been allocated to them.[32] For the Chinese government, community does not necessarily mean community-based organizations or NGOs. The former executive director of Chain, an AIDS information and knowledge exchange platform in China, explains:

> In China, there are three kinds of NGOs: GONGOs, NGOs, and the China offices of INGOs. The advantages of GONGOs are that they are close to the government, have a lot of staff, and are well received by the government. An example of this would be the Chinese AIDS Prevention Association that has offices nationwide. Like the Women's Federation, it is quick to mobilize resources. In that sense, GONGOs play a big role. But their advantages are also their weaknesses: they are too close and do not challenge government rules. They can only do certain things but not others. A big role that GONGOs play is service, e.g., in mobilizing volunteers and resources, a function that they do much better than NGOs or INGOs. In contrast, for local NGOs, they do not have much money or qualified staff and have no legal registration. These limit the scope of [their] activities and the number and duration of projects. The advantages are that they are not subject to government interference, especially in rights protection. They are not bureaucratic. Unlike GONGO structures and responses, they are flexible and [can] change according to needs. In addition, a lot of grassroots NGOs . . . consist of not only positive people, but also members of vulnerable communities, such as MSM, injecting drug users, and commercial sex workers. They best understand the needs of these communities. Their service often focuses on peer education, which is different from GONGOs. INGO advantages are that they relatively well funded and have experts. For example, the Clinton Foundation did a lot of training for doctors and collaborated with the government in, for example, providing pediatric ARVs for children. A lot of INGOs have experience in evaluation, monitoring, reporting, [and] financial management that neither GONGOs nor Chinese NGOs have and from which GONGOs and NGOs can learn. In this area, INGOs play an important role. But there is a barrier against INGOs. The Chinese government particularly does not like foreign NGOs. It is afraid of their close links to foreign media and worries about [the] exposure of anything bad.[33]

In such contexts, who constitutes the community becomes a question of ongoing political negotiation. Dramatic increases in AIDS funding and the legitimation of GIPA brought community politics to the forefront.

Governance and Funding

The governance, organization, and funding structures of PWA networks, MSM groups, sex worker organizations, harm reduction coalitions, professional community support groups, treatment movements, and other community-based educational centers vary according to each group's size, membership, donor requirements, and degree of institutionalization and professionalization, and the maturity of the movement or civil society development. Some are member-driven networks while others are secretariat-run NGOs. Some are primarily volunteer-based while others are managed by professionals. Some board members barely participate while others are too involved in daily operations. Some organizations are part of a national or regional network or global movement and face specific governance challenges. Where do these groups obtain funding? To whom are they accountable? Many community-based organizations and networks are formed by a few passionate individuals. What mandate do they have, and whom do they represent?

AIDS activism is divided between the haves and the have-nots. Those that do not have access to external funding either lack the capacity or are ineligible to apply and thus remain volunteer-based. For example, the Israel AIDS Task Force raises most of its funds through an annual art auction sponsored by Bank Hapoalim. The majority of other CBOs, NGOs, and networks are funded through six main sources: multilateral organizations, bilateral agencies, foundations, the private sector, governments, and INGOs.

Among the principal recipients and subrecipients of the Global Fund are local CBOs like the Shanghai AIDS Prevention Center; national PWA networks like the National Empowerment Network of People Living with HIV/AIDS in Kenya; regional networks like RedTraSex and the Asian Harm Reduction Network; and global coalitions like the Global Business Coalition for Health. Many small or nascent CBOs and national networks, for example, the China Sex Worker Organization Network Forum, 7 Sisters, and Youth Lead, receive seed, project, or event funding from UNAIDS. UNDP, UNFPA, and UN Women fund groups like the AIDS Access Foundation, the Al Shehab Foundation, the Global Youth Coalition on HIV/AIDS, the Tajik Network of Women Living with HIV/AIDS, and the National Community of Women Living with HIV/AIDS in Uganda.

USAID and PEPFAR lead in bilateral funding for groups such as TASO and the Asia Pacific Network of Sex Workers. DFID, the Australian Agency for International Development (AusAID), the Swedish International Development Cooperation Agency (SIDA), and the Canadian International Development Agency (CIDA) have been principal funders of Aidspan, the Asian Network of People Who Use Drugs, and the Russian Harm Reduction Network.

Among the most significant foundations that fund AIDS community work are OSF, the Ford Foundation, the Gates Foundation, and the AIDS Foundation East-West, each with its own characteristics and agenda. OSF tends to fund advocacy work, for example, ABIA; the Action Group on Health, Human Rights, and HIV/ AIDS; the Eurasian Harm Reduction Network; the Andrey Rylkov Foundation; ITPC; and the World AIDS Campaign. The Ford Foundation has a tradition of funding work on human rights and democratic transition, for example, the Working Group on Intellectual Property of the Brazilian Network for the Integration of Peoples, the Egyptian Initiative for Personal Rights, Friends of Life, the Freedom Project, and the Tamkin Project, Egypt. In contrast, the Gates Foundation is more known for its work in community AIDS prevention through the Avahan program. AIDS Foundation East-West only funds AIDS work in newly independent states in Central Asia. The private sector, mostly Pharma, and large INGOs, such as Christian Aid, Oxfam, MSF, the Interchurch Organization for Development Cooperation (ICCO), Hivos, and American Jewish World Service, also provide some funding. Occasionally, AIDS groups receive some government funding.

The financial challenge for all AIDS CBOs and NGOs is enormous. Most operate on grants that provide only project funding, making it difficult for them to pay for structural expenses like salaries, offices, and training. In a few cases where a funder has provided uninterrupted core funding over an extended period of time, the benefits of sustainability are clear. For example, ICCO supported the AIDS Access Foundation in Thailand with 8 million baht (roughly $250,000) for twelve consecutive years from 1991 to 2003, enabling it to put in place a hotline and support and care services, and to engage in advocacy work to change the Thai government policy on treatment.[34]

As many donors leave middle-income countries or shift their priority to other areas of global health, many AIDS CBOs and NGOs struggle for alternative funding. The dearth of government funding in most countries continues to be a great challenge while private sector and Pharma funding raises issues of undue influence. According to a researcher with the European AIDS Treatment Group, Pharma funding has not changed the organization:

> I think we are the only disease area that . . . got away with industry funding without any trouble because we don't shy away from attacking [the pharmaceutical]

industry when we think they are wrong. Some groups have been very aggressive against [the] industry and got industry funding nevertheless. The industry funding has no impact on what we do. Without industry funding, we couldn't do our work. The European Commission wouldn't fund us, and no country would fund us as a regional network. My advice is that if you get funding from [the pharmaceutical] industry, what you need to be aware [of] is potential critique and you need agreed[-upon] working methods, i.e., the dos and don't dos need to be encrusted in the organization. What you cannot do is join . . . press conferences organized by [the] industry for drug approval. We can say we always welcome new drug approval, but we do not endorse and should not do direct marketing. In the US, some patient groups work closely with [the pharmaceutical] industry, and they need to be careful. I know of national AIDS groups that receive funding from the government and are in constant fear of losing funding, and this is problematic. Wherever your funding is coming from, you need to have clear ideas about the circumstances in which you receive the funding and how free you are from the funding.[35]

The co-founder of the Treatment Action Group cautions: "Any funding comes with invisible strings attached. Our strategy is to accept money for our mission. . . . We have a reputation, and that makes it easier for us to stand up."[36] When it comes to the Gates Foundation, he admits, influence can take subtle forms:

At the International AIDS Conference in Rome, the WHO was supposed to release the guidance on couples HIV testing and counseling, including antiretroviral therapy for treatment and prevention in serodiscordant couples. The Gates Foundation got the WHO to pull the guidelines without [a] proper process. So the WHO presented the guidelines but did not release them until the spring. . . . The Gates Foundation partly funds the WHO. It has strong views on treatment [and] prevention and is much more interested in prevention, which I think is wrong. This is a good example [of] how the Gates Foundation . . . use[s] its power.[37]

In terms of governance, most medium- to large-size CBOs, NGOs, and coalitions are supposed to have a tiered structure with a board for oversight, a general assembly for decision making by constituents, and an executive secretariat supported by an administrative staff. In reality, governance issues concerning membership, the role and representation of the board, and funding are omnipresent. One of the challenges across PWA networks and affected community groups is how they count their members and claim their representation. Just as a national HIV-positive organization cannot automatically claim all people living with AIDS in a country as its members, a regional sex worker network cannot count all sex workers in the region as its default members. Many of these organizations and networks struggle to come up with a board structure and other representation mechanisms that reflect their constituents. The Asia Pacific Network of Sex Workers, for example, is unsure exactly how many organizational members it has. "Hundreds," its executive director says. "We started with a bunch of individual organizations. As the countries form national networks, our members are national and local networks, e.g., [the] All India Sex Worker Network has 500–600 member networks that cover 300,000 sex workers. If you count 300,000 in India plus 100,000 outside of India, including Thailand and Burma, we represent close to half a million sex workers in the region."[38] Similarly, the Asian Network of People Who Use Drugs, created in 2009, does not know how many drug users it represents. Its electronic list includes only people who speak English and who have a computer. Unless country networks are formalized, "English-speaking networks will always drown the others."[39] While its priority is to help establish country networks so as to ensure that every voice is counted, the trouble is that in many countries, like Thailand, Nepal, and Indonesia, factions make it difficult for drug users to be organized under one roof.

The Asian Harm Reduction Network was created in 1999 after participants at the 1992 International Harm Reduction Conference in Melbourne felt the need to build a regional mechanism for information sharing and technical capacity building. There was and is no formal membership structure although it had over 2,400 subscribers on its listserv at its height. The problem of representation was further accentuated by a balance-of-power problem: AHRN has a strong executive director and a rubber-stamping board. Its former communications manager says:

> Unlike other networks or coalitions like the International Drug Policy Consortium that has a constitution and [a] membership with clearly defined voting rights, AHRN did not have formal membership. AHRN was a loose network. We came under fire so many times from donors, civil society groups, partners, the government, and pretty much everyone for having "network" in our name. We were saying we represent IDUs, but we don't have IDUs [represented] in our decision-making process. Because of our governance structure, the internal decision-making structure was autocratic, with one person calling the shots and getting the rubber stamp from the foundation board. It wasn't the constituency . . . that was guiding the decision-making process. . . . . It was extremely difficult to mobilize [the support of] civil society with the name . . . "network" but a structure that has nothing to do with a network. If we were only delivering technical support, there wouldn't have been any

issue. From my point of view, AHRN's strength was civil society mobilization. Our governance structure was totally inappropriate for that.[40]

Three external evaluations of AHRN from 2006 to 2009 confirmed the severity of the situation: a lack of participation by constituents, a nonexistent network structure, and thin governance. Despite different attempts to rectify the situation, the new executive director failed to deliver much service or to augment participation, further undermining AHRN's credibility and alienating donor support.[41]

Other organizations, like CARAM, had to open up their membership structure to be more inclusive. A 2006 evaluation pointed out that CARAM was a closed circuit. Subsequently, it changed its constitution to allow for open partnerships; now, any organization that is aligned with CARAM's vision and activities can be a member. Today, it has thirty-eight members in eighteen countries.[42]

The issue of membership and representation is even more acute for coordinating networks and large global networks and movements. How does a convening body speak on behalf of affected populations? How do faraway international secretariat offices and global board structures govern and ensure good communication with 10,000 members? What can be done to increase the legitimacy of a global network when regional member networks disagree or outpace the global governance structure? For cross-constituent coordinating coalitions like 7 Sisters, the only network of affected communities in the Asia-Pacific region, representation issues can be daunting because of its limited convening role. "When we represent and talk about certain issues, we have to rely on our member networks," its regional program coordinator emphasizes. "If we talk about sex workers in Cambodia, for example, we have to rely on the Asia Pacific Network of Sex Workers."[43]

Global networks such as ICW grapple with the issue of regional autonomy. In 2010, its Board of Trustees decided to close its international support office in London in order to strengthen regional offices.[44] A Steering Committee member explains:

> One thing we did do that I thought was smart is that each region is autonomous. It didn't have to go through the main people in order to make decisions. That is what it should be. They know what their issues are in the region. A main thing for a network to be doing is to get the ideas out to the people and ask if they are willing to do it and get their voices and inputs. Communication in itself is an enormous challenge. We do have a members list, but we haven't used it well. We didn't connect our members enough to the issues. We speak different languages. In some cases, the issues are different or have a different emphasis at a particular time.[45]

The Global Youth Coalition on HIV/AIDS, a youth-led global network of over 7,000 youth leaders in 170 countries was created in 2004 and shares the same concerns about effective communication, coordination, and governance. According to its co-founder, "One challenge is how to govern such a diverse network. There is no bar to enter our coalition. In fact, [we] want different kinds of persons, such as those without [a] college education, to join. Out of our 7,000 members, some email us everyday, and there are others whom we don't know. Trying to govern a decentralized network is difficult. It is great if they use us as a platform for their region. People don't communicate their successes. There needs to be better coordination."[46]

In the new tightened funding environment and the complex AIDS landscape, many global networks have been forced to revisit their governance structure and strategic direction. As an organization claiming to represent people living with HIV, GNP+ has to constantly reflect on how it can best speak on behalf of 32 million people. A 2010 comprehensive strategic review found that it remains a northern-based organization led by gay men, lacking the voices of women and failing to reflect the diversity of people living with HIV on the ground. The secretariat was criticized as being too involved in programmatic work instead of global advocacy. It also has not done enough on access to treatment and engagement in Africa.[47] Further, the review says:

> GNP+ describes itself as a network of networks, governed by six autonomous regional PLHIV networks. Yet many respondents describe the "broken" relationship between the Secretariat and regional networks. While some of the networks see the Secretariat as disrespectful and unsupportive (including in times of crisis), some staff members see some of the networks as uncommunicative and unaccountable to their constituents.[48]

In response, the 2011–2015 Strategic Plan for GNP+ identifies several priorities, including moving to a member-based organization, strengthening regional networks, and defining a clear competitive advantage in a crowded civil society scene. It recommends that GNP+ focus on three core pillars—global advocacy, knowledge management, and community development—and an additional fourth pillar: internal organizational support and strengthening.[49]

In contrast to the representation deficit of GNP+, ITPC prides itself on being a region-driven movement. Formed in 2003 by 125 activists who came together in Cape Town to scale up treatment for people living in the South, ITPC started as a movement with a fluid governance structure of an international steering group supported by regional advisory committees and regional coordinators. The regional advisory committees that emerged out of meetings to get the HIV Collaborative Fund in each region going felt they had a governance role but did not understand what it was. Regional coordinators were responsible for the coordination of these different regional bodies, grant implementation, and regional advocacy. Its executive director explains:

> ITPC is a very different way of doing a network. In HIV, there are lots of networks by name, but they are not networks that are linked to the grassroots through the regional structure. I think ITPC's strength is . . . the way the Collaborative Fund works. The uniqueness of ITPC is its global community. GNP+ is a PLWHA network, but it does not have such a close affiliation with regional networks. Most GNP+ regional networks are not functional. The North American network disagrees with the GNP+ secretariat. We support our regional networks. . . . The ITPC secretariat is a coordination [and] support body. If you look at the power of a network, think of us as your spinal cord. The arms and legs are still you. We are here to make sure that your respiration and perspiration are working properly. We funded all our African coordinators to go to AFRICASO. It's very important for their own growth. No other network really does that.[50]

Like so many other networks, ITPC now has to transition its governance structure from the initial creative phase to the mundane phase of institutionalization. The executive director continues:

> One of the things we failed to do is to register because of the lack of ownership. This is a great thing about community activists; they don't want to be institutionalized. They love big principles. The people who formed ITPC never registered it. My strategy is to register the administrative and development [aspects] in New York and then register all the regional networks we have partnerships with. It's going to be a fluid movement. It should be like that. I am not going to register the secretariat with anything linked to the executive director. That should be a decision by the board as to where the secretariat will be registered.[51]

The People's Health Movement, which came into being in 2000 after activists, health workers, academics, and civil society organizations gathered for the first People's Health Assembly, is conscious of its huge challenge to shift from a global network to a more country-level structure covering over eighty countries. An Indian member of the PHM cautions:

> When you create a global movement that is issue-based, it is virtually impossible to build from the ground. All global movements are built from the top by a few in-

dividuals. They may be extremely well-meaning and democratic. But structurally, they are built from the top. You can't get away from it. It does not mean that [the] people who built the movements do not work with the community. I am not arguing against global movements. The best you can do is to try to put as many checks and balances in place to make sure that global movements understand their own limitations, that you have an extremely limited mandate to do a small number of things, which means it requires a certain level of humility not to be asserting on behalf of 7 billion people. Within PHM, we have this debate about PHM uppercase and "phm" lowercase. PHM uppercase is global leadership; phm lowercase is the different organizations on the ground. The whole challenge is to build a relationship between the uppercase and the lowercase where the uppercase is at least open to what the lowercase is saying and doing and puts in place processes that are open.[52]

Concretely, this means creating a flat rather than a hierarchical governance structure as much as possible. The PHM has moved in such a direction with a steering council, a coordinator rather than a president, shorter service terms to ensure renewal of energy and ideas, and certain principles of inclusiveness. "Global movements seek legitimacy from the community. That is the gold standard," continues the PHM member. "For me, it is not about how much time I work in the village. The bigger question is how open I am [to] involving different kinds of people with different experiences [in] the global PHM movement, which also means being sensitive to local reality. What happens is that in the process of representation, you create gatekeepers. The process of inclusiveness needs to be carefully negotiated."[53] Although certain NGOs, like Health GAP, specifically have an article in their constitution about being anti-authoritarian and nonhierarchical, how to build flat governance structures in order to stay close and true to the community remains a permanent challenge of all CSOs.

Besides membership and representation issues, a second major governance challenge concerns the board's structure and role vis-à-vis an organization's mandate. The co-founder of the Treatment Action Group, for example, is mindful of the shift in his organization's mandate beyond HIV to include TB and hepatitis C since the 2000s: "One of our challenges is to be accountable to our donors and stakeholders that include people living with HIV, TB, and hep C. Our board is not like a PWA advisory board where a substantial number of members live with HIV. There are a lot of representation issues, and we don't claim to speak on behalf of people living with AIDS in the US and globally."[54]

Sometimes, governance issues arise when the board misinterprets or oversteps its functions. A researcher at the European AIDS Treatment Group comments:

"The challenges I have witnessed . . . over and over again is that our board is too operational, wanting to intervene too much with the office. The board should be strategic, and this tension is not [re]solved. I was on the board until two years ago. I still think the board is doing too much. It is both a structural issue and a conflict in style."[55] This is reminiscent of the High-Level Independent Review Panel's report for the Global Fund, which criticizes the board for being too involved in the fund's management rather than focusing on strategies. In other cases, the direction of the board is a struggle between different stakeholders who believe in different strategies and tactics. In the Russian Harm Reduction Network, which includes experts like doctors, lawyers, social workers, and academics, as well as representatives of the community, including people living with HIV, IDUs, MSM, and commercial sex workers, one of the challenges is reconciling the different approaches used by the experts and those used by the community. Its executive director explains:

> [The] community would like to see quick results and are oriented to . . . the problems [that] the people [have] about getting treatment. Experts are mostly thinking about systemic change, e.g., to make the government system change to have better treatment protocols and indicators. Sometimes these two approaches create contradictions. People affected by [the] epidemic may make campaigns in the mass media or come out to the street to fight for their rights. Other people like the experts may say it's counterproductive because the government should have the guiding role.[56]

Having governmental or intergovernmental representation on the board and/ or in the membership structures of CBOs and NGOs may or may not cause problems. In the case of the Russian Harm Reduction Network, the membership of government AIDS centers has not jeopardized the organization; rather, it continues to speak out on things that are not quite accepted by the authorities. Occasionally, a network or partnership may also include intergovernmental organizations on its board. The Asia Pacific Coalition on Male Sexual Health (APCOM), created in 2007 after a regional risks-and-responsibility consultation on MSM and transgender health, created a multisectoral governing board with four members from UN agencies (UNDP, UNAIDS, UNESCO, and WHO), two donor representatives, two government representatives, twenty community representatives (two from each of the ten subregions in the Asia-Pacific region), six to ten sectoral advisors, and three technical experts (mostly from INGOs). While this governance structure enables donors, governments, intergovernmental bodies, and the affected communities to sit at the same table as equals, it also means that APCOM has to accommodate the different organizational cultures that various stakeholders bring. For example, the WHO has traditionally been not very open to community input. Similarly, when an activist writes a critique of the government, a government representative may tell the APCOM board that it should not publicize it.[57]

A whole new set of organizational and governance challenges arises when AIDS CBOs and NGOs are represented through broader national or regional coalitions. The Thai Nongovernmental Coalition on AIDS (TNCA) was established in 1991 with 168 NGOs (now 215) and aims to improve the quality of life of people living with HIV/AIDS in Thailand by advocating for better health care and human rights. Depending on the issue, different NGOs lead and use TNCA to negotiate with the government. This can be a problem, according to the executive director of the Thai Network of People Living with HIV/AIDS, a cluster of over 1,000 PWA groups with 20,000 to 30,000 members:

> TNCA . . . consist[s] of many NGOs covering different issues. It takes time for all
> members to understand an issue and arrive at a consensus. While we try really hard
> to make sure [we] all have [a] similar position, sometimes when we have to touch
> upon issues related to politics, some NGOs do not feel comfortable [and] fear . . . los-
> ing government support. An example would be protests against FTAs. Some mem-
> bers feel that it's about trade, not about health. I also suspect that some Thai NGOs
> get funding from the US government and fear losing that funding.[58]

In Latin America, affected populations are organized in regional and identity networks: the Latin American Network of People Living with HIV (Red LA+), ICW Latin America (for HIV-positive women), Red de Trabajadoras Sexuales de Latinoamérica y El Caribe (RedTraSex) for sex workers, Asociación para la Salud Integral y Ciudadanía en América Latina (ASICAL) for MSM, Red Latinoaméricana y del Caribe de Personas Trans (REDLACTRANS) for transgender people, and the Latin American Harm Reduction Network (RELARD). Together, these networks lobbied for a regional political platform called the Grupo de Cooperación Técnica Horizontal (GCTH, the Horizontal Technical Cooperation Group on HIV/AIDS) that consists of the AIDS departments in twenty-one Latin American and Caribbean countries. The aim is to devise a new politics for the entire region.[59] This initiative has made significant gains in access to prevention, treatment, care, and support through ARV drug price reductions and strategic planning in AIDS policy.[60] But governance challenges also multiply with each additional layer of representation and collaboration.

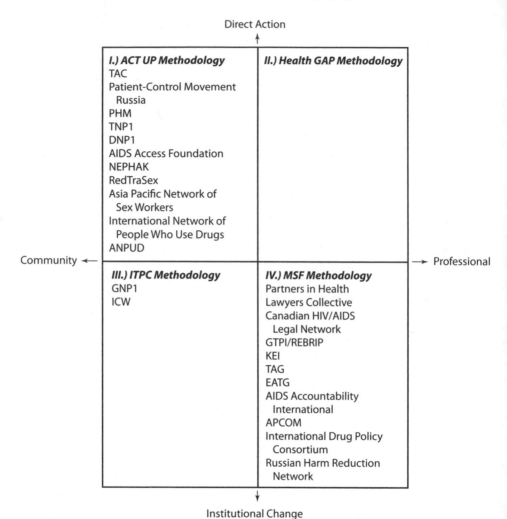

Direct Action

I.) ACT UP Methodology
TAC
Patient-Control Movement
  Russia
PHM
TNP1
DNP1
AIDS Access Foundation
NEPHAK
RedTraSex
Asia Pacific Network of
  Sex Workers
International Network of
  People Who Use Drugs
ANPUD

II.) Health GAP Methodology

Community

Professional

III.) ITPC Methodology
GNP1
ICW

IV.) MSF Methodology
Partners in Health
Lawyers Collective
Canadian HIV/AIDS
  Legal Network
GTPI/REBRIP
KEI
TAG
EATG
AIDS Accountability
  International
APCOM
International Drug Policy
  Consortium
Russian Harm Reduction
  Network

Institutional Change

AIDS Community Advocacy Models

Advocacy Strategies

Despite a wide-ranging repertoire of activism, most AIDS community-based networks and movements can be grouped into four main advocacy models depending on their bases of expertise (community versus professional) and strategic orientation (direct action versus institutional change).

In the figure, the first strategy (quadrant I), which I refer to as the ACT UP methodology, draws on community membership and knowledge, and uses direct action. From large-scale demonstrations and Stop the Church to occupying the New York Stock Exchange, die-ins on Wall Street, and taking over the NIH and the FDA, direct action by ACT UP marked the beginning and became a regular feature of the AIDS movement. ACT UP's approach to no-risk, low-risk, and high-risk activism was methodical, explained in how-to manuals, and passed on through organized teach-ins.[61] Under this methodology fall a great number of HIV-positive networks and affected community organizations, such as the Treatment Action Campaign, the Thai Network of People Living with HIV/AIDS, the AIDS Access Foundation, the Delhi Network of Positive People, RedTraSex, the Asia Pacific Network of Sex Workers, the International Network of People Who Use Drugs, and the Asian Network of People Who Use Drugs. Larger, more informal movements, such as the patient-control movement in Russia and the People's Health Movement, also fit in this category. Their ability to mobilize direct community support and knowledges defines their identity and legitimacy. They organize marches to parliaments, hold demonstrations, take over government and Pharma exhibition booths at international AIDS conferences, disrupt plenary presentations, and engage in hunger strikes and other civil disobedience to protest the lack of access to ARV drugs.

The second advocacy strategy model (quadrant II), used only by Health GAP, relies more on professional knowledges but retains direct action as its preferred mode of intervention. In contrast to ACT UP, which had a large gay movement base, Health GAP was formed in 1999 by an American physician and civil rights activist, Alan Berkman, who brought together fair trade lawyers, international health and development advocates, economists and other academics, and AIDS and human rights activists.[62] The main targets of Health GAP are the US government and the drug lobby. It mobilizes grassroots support in the Global South, but by itself does not have a large community support base at home or abroad. Health GAP continues the ACT UP tradition of direct action and has staged some of the most successful actions in AIDS social movement history, including protesting the presidential campaign of Al Gore ("Gore's Greed Kills," "AIDS Drugs for Africa"), opposing a US Pharma lawsuit against the South African government, and organizing a letter-writing campaign to the US trade representative to protest US trade sanctions against Thailand after the Thai minister of public health announced its decision to issue the first compulsory license for efavirenz in 2006. In March 2012, Health GAP helped organize a big die-in in front of the European Commission's office in Nairobi to protest donors' retreat from their Global Fund commitments.

The advocacy strategy model in quadrant III, the ITPC methodology, is driven by community needs but focuses primarily on institutional change. ITPC grew out of a gathering of 125 activists from sixty-seven countries at the International Treatment Preparedness Summit in Cape Town in 2003. It immediately created the HIV Collaborative Fund to support local, national, and regional HIV treatment literacy and advocacy; the World Community Advisory Board to enhance the capacity of the most affected populations to engage with pharmaceutical companies; and the Treatment Monitoring and Advocacy Project to assess HIV treatment policies and programming and to hold governments and international institutions accountable for the treatment gap through its Missing the Target reports.[63] An early example of successful institutional change is ITPC's leadership role in lobbying for the 3 by 5 Initiative of the WHO, the goal of which was to provide ARV therapy to 3 million people living with HIV in low- and middle-income countries by 2005. The goal was realized in 2007. The ICW and GNP+ also fall under this category of community-based networks that prioritize institutional change over direct action. The latter is recognized for its lobbying efforts for institutional change, including the WHO guidelines on antiretroviral therapy, and its technical advocacy tools, such as the Global Criminalization Scan and the Stigma Index.[64]

The last strategy model (quadrant IV), the MSF methodology, includes the bulk of nongovernmental networks involved in medical, legal, and media activism, and research-oriented groups that draw on professional knowledges to target institutional change. Typically, these doctors, lawyers, economists, IP experts, and journalists are advocates who bear witness to various aspects of the AIDS crisis and use evidence-based approaches for their advocacy. MSF doctors speak from their professional standpoint about issues in drug access and the impact of Pharma monopolies and funding shortages on patient communities. The Lawyers Collective takes up cases where people living with AIDS are being denied basic human rights, including access to affordable medicines, and advocates for change through the courts. Similarly, the Working Group on Intellectual Property in the Brazilian Network for the Integration of Peoples uses policy and juridical channels, along with patent oppositions and civil public actions, to push for accessible ARV drugs in Brazil. The Access to Medicines Research Group, China, founded by lawyers, contributes its rare technical capacity to feeding information and knowledge to the rest of Chinese civil society and to building alliances with academics and like-minded officials. According to its founder, the group's role is to serve as "an intellectual bridge. . . . We are not in the front mobilizing people; grassroots NGOs are [on] the front line. But when it comes to analyzing a law, we are in the front. We are a driving force at the systemic level to identify stakeholders, match the right people, and bring them together in some platform."[65] The global public interest advocacy work of Knowledge Ecology International draws on its highly technical research capability on IP and other knowledge governance issues. The Treatment Action Group and the European AIDS Treatment Group, both of which focus on treatment research, also fit under this category. Although both groups do a lot of community training, their scientific approach focuses on new drugs and clinical trials.

The reality of social mobilization is too complex to be summarized under four neat models, however. Many groups, networks, and coalitions fall somewhere in between the various quadrants in this categorization of AIDS community movements. Even ACT UP is known for its "inside-outside" strategy. One of its veteran activists explains:

> It perfected an inside-outside strategy, which a lot of social movements do. The outside being the sort of dramatic takeover of the stock exchange, storm[ing] the NIH, [the] die-in at the FDA . . . all these dramatic street protests and other direct actions. But [it] also [used] an inside strategy, where others and I could go and sit down inside NIH and have a discussion. . . . ACT UP [used a] dual-power mechanism that inside you can have a fact-based discussion with people in power about how they are designing drug trials or whatever, . . . you can talk their language, so you can operate on the inside as advocates. So doctors who are interested in opportunistic infections may not have power but are linked to people from ACT UP, and so their political power increase[s]. Same for statisticians who raise questions about different kinds of trial design. The[ir] internal critique was within the biomedical framework. So ACT UP could give [a] bigger voice to critical discourses within the establishment, creating a dialogue with or raising issues and posing questions, [which] is difficult in a system that tended to be conservative, . . . while all the time knowing that people are storming the NIH on the outside.[66]

"The difference with TAG [Treatment Action Group]," he continues, "is that, for TAG, the inside strategy goes ahead without the outside strategy, which only takes you so far."[67]

Many other HIV-positive networks and affected community groups in quadrant I use a similar inside-outside strategy. The Delhi Network of Positive People is equally comfortable in mobilizing tens of thousands of Indian people living with AIDS in a street protest as in filing patent oppositions with the support of the Lawyers Collective. The same is true for the community-based networks in quadrant III, where direct actions are occasionally taken despite a general tendency to work for institutional change. On the professional side of the spectrum (quadrants II and IV), some organizations may opt for direct action tactics in addition to more institutionalized advocacy strategies, as evidenced in the MSF actions in the Drop the Case campaign against Novartis in 2012. Hence, while this conceptual typology helps us to situate and understand a diverse group of AIDS community movement groups, we should consider the various quadrants as fluid spaces and acknowledge that different groups move from one side to another, straddling and negotiating between different bases of knowledge and different strategies.

This simplified typology of advocacy models shows that the bulk of AIDS activism since the 1980s has consisted of either direct action by community-based networks of affected populations or institutional change by professional groups. Few community-driven groups have the capacity to focus on institutional change. With the exception of a few cases of collaboration (e.g., the informal trinity between HIV-positive networks, MSF, and the Lawyers Collective in India, especially on patent oppositions), there seems to be a great divide between community networks (quadrant I) and professional NGOs (quadrant IV). A common simplistic criticism is that community networks are not professional and that professional organizations lack community bases. How these two groups can move more fluidly along the horizontal axis—for example, through creating platforms where both community and professional knowledges are mobilized for advocacy—is a strategic question for the AIDS movement to consider. Tensions may arise between the need for more knowledge transfer among the various quadrants, on the one hand, and the professionalization of CBOs and NGOs driven by a complex AIDS environment, on the other. What is the impact of the increasing bureaucratization and expertization of the AIDS community on exclusion and on the identity of the movement?

Who Are We? Community Subjectivity, Difference, and Exclusion

> Many people claim a place at the civil society table. . . . Frankly, there are lots of people speaking on behalf of community. [How can we say] we are negotiating on your behalf but leave out 500,000 people living with AIDS in middle-income countries?
> —*Executive Director, ITPC*[68]

> Fly and have a party, but don't forget your roots.
> —*President, DNP+*[69]

> AIDS civil society is like a personal war.
> —*UNAIDS Consultant*[70]

The AIDS community is governed through a complex set of external (donors, funders, researchers, government authorities, and intergovernmental bodies) and internal (diverse constituents) relations. The power exerted over the CBOs, NGOs, and movements manifests as different modes of subjugation and exclusion rather than emanating from a specific structure or institution. As AIDS activists lobby for inclusion in the dominant power structures of science, market, and governance, some end up losing their identity and forgetting their raison d'être. Compromises, self-censorship, acquiescence, co-optation, and selling out are part and parcel of any social movement. The AIDS movement is no exception. Externally, funding, consultation, and partnership requirements give rise to a range of subjects, including the community volunteer, grantee, expert, delegate, and partner. Internally, the AIDS movement is divided by GIPA, North-South tensions, language, class, race, gender, age, and ideology. As activists fight against the control of AIDS by scientists, Pharma, governments, and intergovernmental organizations, their own internal power struggles often remain unacknowledged.

External Techniques of Power

COMMUNITY VOLUNTEER

A common assumption about community work is that it is "free." Volunteering is lauded for increasing social capital and strengthening community ties. The AIDS movement began and grew with volunteer-based community work. Gay Men's Health Crisis, created in New York in 1982, focused originally on AIDS research and education but quickly found itself setting up different volunteer programs for home support and care.[71] Today, many community-based organizations and NGOs still rely heavily on volunteers to help run programs and deliver services. The Egyptian AIDS Society, the Jerusalem AIDS Project, and the Access to Medicines Research Group, China, for example, are run entirely by volunteers who hold other full-time jobs. Other organizations depend on a large body of volunteers to complement a small core staff. TASO, one of the biggest ASOs in Africa, created in 1986, has over 1,000 volunteers in addition to its 900 full-time staff and 100 paralegals across eleven service hubs, four regional offices, and a staff training center in Uganda.[72]

While the use of volunteers is often regarded as cost effective by governments, a volunteer subjectivity may be seen as part of a coercive neoliberal economic regime because it legitimizes state retrenchment through "free labor." It was not coincidental that ASOs in the United States emerged during the Reagan era, which emphasized small government. Critical scholars like Patton remind us of the need to "deconstruct the revitalized rhetoric of altruism which reappears in the context of Reaganism after nearly two decades in which new social move-ments have reached community and self-empowerment. This new, rightist al-truism has engendered social policies . . . [and resulted in the] privatization of formerly social welfare practices."[73] In particular, volunteerism in most coun-tries takes on a gendered dimension because it relies on mostly female labor.

The continuing reliance on community volunteers in the AIDS movement also raises issues of fairness, recognition, and sustainability for AIDS activism. As a researcher of the European AIDS Treatment Group says: "Our relationship with the European Medicines Agency [EMA] is very professional and constructive. The challenge, though, is that they expect and you need to have extensive technical know-how, but they don't pay you. If you want to be [on] an EMA decision-making committee, it means you spend seven to eight days a month with them for free, whereas others coming from the other European regulating agencies are paid. When EMA calls us as patients, most of us are volunteers."[74] The AIDS and Rights Alliance for Southern Africa, which was formed in 2002 to promote a human rights–based response to HIV in the region, has been forced to streamline its work since it does not have the capacity to do everything from handling cases to pro-viding free human rights training for its fifty-three partners. As its regional ad-vocacy team leader explains, "We are a very small team, with a secretariat out of Cape Town. One of our greatest challenges is capacity. We have over fifty to sixty volunteers each year. They come for only eight weeks, and then they are gone. They are touching here and there, haphazardly. We need to think how we [can] best support ourselves and our partners."[75]

Unpaid board positions also pose problems of engagement. "All of our ten board members are volunteers," says the executive director of ABIA. "Sometimes it's difficult to engage them on questions [about] the institution. The challenge is how to have a more participatory board. Because of the work that ABIA devel-ops in research and outreach, it is difficult to rely on volunteers. This difficulty [of] hav[ing] funds to pay salaries is a governance problem."[76] Further, civil soci-ety participation and representation on the board structures of intergovernmen-tal organizations is also often unpaid, a problem recognized by UNAIDS as a fail-ure to properly recognize community work and contribute to capacity building.[77] As AIDS civil society in countries like China, Russia, and Egypt matures, volun-teer- and membership-based activism may move to a paid professional NGO model with tremendous implications about the meaning of activism, bureaucratization, management, and donor and partner expectations of the community.

COMMUNITY GRANTEE

While chronic funding shortages causing coercive volunteerism is problematic, the sudden availability of too much AIDS funding has also created wide-ranging issues in the AIDS community. Since the 1980s, an extraordinarily complex AIDS funding regime—populated by donors, bilateral and multilateral funding agencies, intergovernmental organizations, INGOs, and community movements—has given rise to a grantee subjectivity in which grant seeking has replaced activism as the raison d'être of community work. A multibillion-dollar AIDS budget might have strengthened civil society, but it has also profoundly changed the nature of activism and activist identity. The director of UNDP's HIV/AIDS Group says: "A big problem is that too many NGOs (I deliberately use NGO, not community, here) focus on how much money they get. I don't think there is enough self-criticism about the pros and cons in moving from activists to being subcontractees. Not that it is wrong, but it profoundly changes who you are. There is a remarkable lack of accountability around conflicts of interest. Sometimes they use money as a barometer of success."[78] Several activists specifically criticize the Global Fund for creating dependency. An ITPC advocacy officer observes the detrimental impact of Global Fund money on Russian AIDS NGOs:

> NGOs got used to big amounts of money. They got used to indicators and wrote unrealistic things. Even the government now does not take us seriously because a lot of numbers are fake. They are just for the Global Fund. There are many examples in many projects, e.g., syringe coverage and testing coverage. It was impossible to implement these indicators from the beginning. For me, writing a proposal and receiving Global Fund money does not . . . change the [overall] health system. [The] Global Fund itself said the grants should help improve the health system and get the government involved. Global Fund grants finished, but the Russian government didn't take responsibility [for continuing the work]. Receiving Global Fund money is just [one] breath of fresh air. It's one breath since it will be finished soon. . . . I don't think these NGOs can be called activists. Frontaids had no structure and had almost no funding. It was a passion. That is activism for me. ITPC is not an NGO; it's an activist movement. What has changed is that many NGOs will close as [soon as] funding comes to an end. People realize the international money will be gone, and some will try to get government money and might be less willing to speak out. There are only a few leaders ready to pick up [the work], but they are burning out. People are really tired.[79]

A Russian activist from the Global Business Coalition for Health concurs: "For a few years, everyone was busy spending money. It was quite a favorable environment then to explain to people about harm reduction. Now we have no more international funding and the political environment is different. The Global Fund projects have not been institutionalized in our national system, and the first fault is NGOs'. No one took care of the sustainability issue. We lost a lot of time."[80] The executive director of the Delhi Network of Positive People also is critical of the grant procedures of the Global Fund and the fund's impact on HIV-positive networks:

> A major challenge faced by PLWHA networks is that a lot of them don't know why they are there any more. Look at the mess of the Global Fund. It is a complicated system that confuses PLWHA networks, and they allow themselves to be confused. If they don't know who they are, where they are, and why they are there, most of them end up serving the UN or the donors. They forget that they are there for the community. Initially, they were there for the community. Along the way, they [got] the money and [forgot] they are there for the community. Worship the donor, but don't forget why you [are] there. You are here not to serve the government. You are here not to serve UNAIDS. We are here for people living with HIV/AIDS. . . . Many have forgotten the reasons for their existence.[81]

The sudden proliferation of Global Fund–supported CBOs and NGOs fostered competition, infighting, and corruption. According to a former staff member of MSF–Hong Kong:

> The Global Fund expanded the problem of factionalism within the MSM community in China. It could have actually helped to ease the problem if there [had been] a mechanism, e.g., transparency in terms of knowing who gets the fund[ing]. In the Global Fund Round 5 proposal, we put in something like the small grant structure of the Collaborative Fund of ITPC with a community review panel of ten to fifteen people, most of whom were NGOs with some GONGOs. That would have gone a long way to ease some of the tensions and conflicts. But the model was abandoned. In the absence of reliable information, people who were the most competitive got the money. The lack of transparency remains a big problem.[82]

Others question whether civil society organizations can be both a recipient and a watchdog of the Global Fund. A veteran Canadian AIDS activist turned consultant confesses: "I switched from the AIDS industry to the Global Fund industry. Tons of consultants make their living through work on the Global Fund. Big NGOs find themselves implementing programs with Global Fund money, which isn't their role. Nobody is playing a watchdog role. They are too busy implementing Global Fund programs."[83]

Besides losing their identity, credibility, and watchdog role, community organizations also risk being subjected to the discursive, bureaucratic, or ideological control of funders. According to Murray, funding agencies have begun to insert the Western discourse on sexuality and HIV/AIDS into Indonesia, while local communities have appropriated elements of this discourse into their own subcultures.[84] In China, the founder of the Dongzhen Center for Human Rights Education and Action questions the impact of international funding: "International foundations would like to hear a unified voice from Chinese civil society. This desire of international funding agencies might turn into enforcement. You have to network; it is considered . . . an achievement. Some organizations may become part of a national network purely for funding rather than for voice."[85] Above all, grantees are required to prove their "value for money" according to the rules of international funding agencies.[86] The Civil Society and Private Sector Partnerships manager of the Global Fund argues that AIDS civil society has failed "to show evidence" of its value: "The World Bank and UK Consortium on AIDS and International Development undertook a large piece of research to prove the value of civil society. We need to show evidence. The evidence is there, but we haven't gathered it. We haven't done enough. The Western NGOs haven't done enough."[87] With funding comes enforcement by the disciplinary structures of science, market, and governance.

At the national level, courting state funding may be seen by one's peers as selling out, a divide-and-rule game that governments are happy to play. As a Russian harm reduction activist recalls: "At one point, I left the All Russian Network of People Living with HIV because we couldn't agree over OST [opioid substitution therapy]. They prioritize their relationship with the government in such a way that they refuse to put OST as a priority."[88] A fellow Russian AIDS activist agrees: "Unfortunately, the All Russian Network of People Living with HIV is pro-government. They receive funds from the Ministry of Health that we fight against, e.g., the ministry put out a last-minute tender earlier this year that asked NGOs to implement a project within thirty-eight days! No NGOs except the All Russian Network think it's possible. They will be the only one applying for and getting the tender."[89]

The tensions in donor-grantee relationships are further exacerbated when INGOs take up the role of funding agencies, pitting large and powerful northern NGOs against much smaller grassroots groups. In the late 1980s, donors began to discuss ways to improve mechanisms to fund AIDS NGOs. By 1991, USAID

proposed plans to set up a new international NGO to serve as an intermediate donor agency to fund AIDS assistance. The Rockefeller Foundation invited representatives of major donor agencies to meet in London in August 1991 to explore
various possibilities. A subcommittee was set up to oversee the administration
of five pilot country studies to assess the needs of indigenous NGOs and the best
methods to meet those needs. The program was formalized as the International
HIV/AIDS Alliance in 1993 to "support a transference of governance from distant
donors to affected communities."[90] The alliance has provided support to over
2,000 communities in over 3,000 projects across forty developing countries and
claims to promote community development through NGO involvement in public sector initiatives, NGO self-determination, donor-NGO partnerships, and
greater attention to human rights, people living with AIDS, women, and other
vulnerable populations.[91] But many community-based organizations and movements see it as driven by self-interests and challenge its ethics in competing
against grassroots groups for Global Fund money.

COMMUNITY EXPERT

While the AIDS funding regime has created the community volunteer and the
grantee, the exigencies of consultation have produced two other subjects in the
AIDS community: the expert and the delegate. As activists fought against exclusions by science and market, they lobbied for mechanisms like community advisory boards (CABs) to ensure the proper consultation of communities. ACT UP
was successful in getting AIDS patients involved in the design of clinical trials
through CABs. By the early 1990s, biostatisticians, medical ethicists, and treatment researchers called for greater patient participation in the planning of AIDS
clinical trials and for the routine use of community consultation.[92] In 1991, European activists adopted the ACT UP treatment agenda, which emphasized patient
participation, and created the European AIDS Treatment Agenda.[93] The European AIDS Treatment Group (EATG) was created the following year to focus on
access to treatment, standards of ethical conduct, and treatment education. "What
is unique is our focus on scientific research and patient participation in research,
which was based on the 1983 Denver Declaration and 1991 European AIDS Treatment Agenda," an EATG researcher explains. "Our scope and foci wouldn't be
there without these two earlier documents." He continues:

> There are challenges in collaborating with industry. Very early CABs worked. There
> were different types of CABs. Some were designed for a specific design trial. Others
> were set up for specific research sites. Some others [were] to guide specific compa-

nies. What was common is that there was no agreed working method (this was an emergency situation). People just tried to work alone without really having thought very much about how to do things. All this led to a number of clashes and difficulties. In 1997, the EATG met with research ethicists to think about how to formalize the collaboration with industry. They came up with the creation of the European Community Advisory Board [ECAB], which is a working group within the EATG. The ECAB decided when it wanted to meet and on what issues, and the industry had to follow. Also it wanted to be involved in [the] planning stage[s], not [after the] protocol was ready. The big discussions for many years were about inclusion and exclusion criteria because the companies wanted to have ideal populations, but patients wanted them to include the real population. This was achieved. It became a very productive and useful tool for EATG over the years.[94]

While engagement with science and Pharma has brought undeniable gains in accelerating AIDS clinical trials and a broader democratization of research beyond AIDS, it has also divided the movement. "Some people thought we were getting too close to the enemy," recalls an ACT UP activist. "They asked for a moratorium, and we thought it was an inappropriate strategy."[95] The treatment activist committee within ACT UP, which had pushed for an inside strategy to engage with science, then split off to become the Treatment Action Group. As Epstein asks, "Can one be both activist and scientist?"[96] The cleavages reflected a politics of knowledge, pitting a minority of scientifically bent activists against the majority lay group. Michelle Roland, a former member of ACT UP San Francisco, explains: "I've seen a lot of treatment activists get seduced by the power, get seduced by the knowledges, and end up making very conservative arguments. . . . They understand the science and the methodology, they can make intelligent arguments, and it's like, 'Wait a minute. . . . okay, you're smart. We accept that. But what's your role?' "[97]

Activists who have turned themselves into "experts" can be bridges to their communities or they can be gatekeepers. Some transform into consultants or AIDS career bureaucrats. Those who have remained behind in the trenches legitimately ask: How much change goes back to the community? An expertization of AIDS activism not only causes divisions in the community; it also risks legitimizing the cultural hegemony of science and Pharma when outsiders participate in distributing and therefore perpetuating the knowledges formerly monopolized by the establishment.[98]

COMMUNITY DELEGATE

Parallel to the community expert who serves on community advisory boards of science and Pharma, the community delegate sits on the boards or board-like structures of intergovernmental bodies. The delegate's role is mainly twofold: to represent the community and to hold the organization accountable to its mandate. AIDS activists fought hard for such representation on governance structures as the materialization of GIPA. Forcing more openness and transparency in an international system dominated by state structures, their inclusion has been hailed by other social movements as a major victory.

The NGO delegation to the PCB of UNAIDS, the first of its kind, is tasked with the mission of bringing to the PCB "the perspectives and expertise of people living with, most affected by, and most at risk of, vulnerable to, marginalized by, and affected by HIV and AIDS, as well as civil society and nongovernmental entities actively involved in HIV and AIDS in order to ensure that their human rights, and equitable, gender-sensitive access to comprehensive HIV prevention, treatment, care, and support are reinforced by the policies, programmes, strategies and actions of the PCB and UNAIDS."[99] The NGO delegation does so by seeking broad input from civil society; increasing participation of PLWHA; helping to set the agenda; preparing and strategizing; lobbying other PCB colleagues; recruiting and mentoring new delegates; collaborating with observer NGOs; participating in working groups; actively participating in PCB meetings; and reporting back to civil society. The delegates are bound by a code of conduct to "respect diversity, foster a culture of inclusion, take leadership and . . . be considerate of those for whom English is a second language."[100]

The reality of community delegations, however, often looks quite different from stated principles and elaborate codes of conduct. Scholars and practitioners alike are concerned about the problematic representation of AIDS civil society by large INGOs, which has marginalized the voices of affected communities.[101] Far from being diverse and representative, most community delegates tend to be experienced veteran activists who come from bigger northern NGOs, the elites among AIDS activists. The external relations officer of UNAIDS observes: "For the first five to six years, there were only five NGOs on the PCB of UNAIDS: three from Germany and two from the Netherlands. So there were only European representatives on the board. I remember asking the lady from Germany: 'Tell me in reality, whom do you represent here?' She said, 'Honestly, I represent only three organizations.' Now, we . . . ask for alternates."[102] A veteran activist from the North, the co-founder of the Health and Development Network, is extremely critical of this small corps of international civil society elites clinging to power:

> If you are going to have an international elite civil society, there is an opportunity cost in relation to genuine national representation and participation by affected communities in countries around the world. I think at the beginning of the response to the epidemic, it was necessary for this international elite to fill that space, but what they didn't do was to hand over [control] fast enough. They didn't get out of the way. I was in Geneva recently. It was the Global Fund board meeting. I happened to be in the canteen. I have known these people for a long time. I was just amazed that the civil society delegat[e]s were still the same people in the room, except that they are twenty years older. Yes, some other people and communities have been involved, but I still see the same individuals. I just got a list of twenty people that the civil society office of UNAIDS suggested [that I] talk to about the investment framework. They are still the go-to people, living in Brighton, Amsterdam, or New York. You can't tell me there is no one in Thailand, Panama City, or Ghana. You can't tell me in fifteen years that no one's capacity has been sufficiently built. I think there is a natural life cycle in leadership. If you stay for more than ten years, you become part of the problem. Many of the civil society leaders have now lost sight of what they were trying to do fifteen years ago, and they should have gotten out five years ago. These people in their late twenties and thirties when they started to be involved in AIDS activism are now in their fifties. Being twenty-five and being fifty is very different. These elites go in and out. They work for UNAIDS and UNDP. It is not civil society any more. These are international diplomats. It's their life. I see them more in airport business lounges than anywhere else.[103]

The problem is not only the lack of self-reflection among northern AIDS activists, but also the failure of most intergovernmental organizations to provide the proper resources and structures to build the capacity of smaller southern NGOs. A 2007 independent review of NGO and civil society participation in the PCB of UNAIDS specifically pinpointed the issues of support, better communications, and improved consultation infrastructure for NGO delegations.[104] Further, it recommended measures for more meaningful civil society participation and representation through full voting, speaking, and chairing rights. In response, UNAIDS set up a Communications Facility in 2008 to address PCB NGO delegation communication and logistics needs in order to achieve effective engagement.[105] But the issues of the North-South NGO capacity gap, transparency, and representation are likely to require much more time and institutional changes before they are resolved.

Can one be both an implementer and a critic? Many argue that sitting on the boards of multilateral organizations makes one too close to be a watchdog. The Civil Society and Private Sector Partnerships manager of the Global Fund sees the pitfalls of civil society delegations to the fund:

> I should mention the role of civil society delegation[s] on the board because they forgot their role. Their role on the board is two-fold: . . . (1) they channel the needs of broader civil society in the country on the debates of the Global Fund, and (2) [to ensure] the Global Fund stays true to its founding principles and multisector involvement. When the debate on national strategy application—a new system whereby [a] government can put an application to the Global Fund based on national strategy without involving civil society—happened, the civil society delegation didn't raise its voice. How can the Global Fund justify its founding principles when it approves grants without civil society involvement? The civil society delegation again dropped the ball when it came to health system strengthening. It is clear that a health system doesn't function without a robust community system. How come we allow the Global Fund to seek partnership with the World Bank that views civil society as consumers? Instead of raising [its] voice, civil society on the board tried to make it work. It allowed the creeping in of more government focus and the civil society team to be taken away. It is very seductive to sit on the Global Fund Board. Out of the three civil society delegations, you have some [of the] same people for the past six years for the developed country NGO delegation. These people are very good, but they have been around for too long. They have almost become Global Fund employees. They [have] been at times brave, but not brave enough. They were always willing to be compromised to have consensus. . . . I wrote to the executive director of the International HIV/AIDS Alliance about a number of issues. He said, "We are going to fight only battles that we will win." I said, "You have to fight battles that need to be fought. If you don't, nobody else [will]."[106]

A Global Fund observer blames the failure of the civil society delegates on the board for the "revolution" in the Global Fund toward a "value for money" framework. "I don't understand why civil society didn't cry foul more," he said. "My impression was that they were mesmerized. They were told that this was [a] critical juncture and they were just dragged into going along. Everything was done so quickly that I don't think they had much time to react."[107] How community delegates can serve on the governance structures of powerful intergovernmental organizations without losing their identity and mission remains a major challenge for AIDS activists.

In addition to funding and community consultation, partnerships have emerged as a new regime of power in which community organizations are subject to various disciplinary controls through the differential resources, expertise, and management cultures of other, more powerful stakeholders. In the UN, public-private partnerships as an alternative to traditional bilateral development assistance increased after the 1992 Rio Summit and Agenda 21.[108] Since the 1990s, multisectoral and multistakeholder partnerships—in vaccine research, drug development, policy, advocacy, and financing—have become the norm in AIDS and in global public health generally. The GAVI partnership, for example, includes the Gates Foundation, UNICEF, WHO, the World Bank, civil society organizations, developing and developed country governments, developing and developed country pharmaceutical companies, and research and technical health institutes. Its model draws on each partner's comparative advantages—from WHO's scientific expertise and UNICEF's procurement system to the financial know-how of the World Bank and the market knowledge of the vaccine industry—and aims to deliver more than each can do individually. Further, by working with in-country partners with widespread field presence to deliver its programs, GAVI is able to keep its organization lean.[109]

While partnerships supposedly offer synergies, resources, new platforms for voice and action, and a potential power gain for community organizations, critical questions need to be raised: Who is in control in the partnership? What is the level of engagement of the different stakeholders? Are adequate resources being provided to smaller and less powerful partners to ensure their effective participation? Does the partnership exist in name only, so that dominant stakeholders can check the box of "community engagement" for the sake of legitimacy? A study of nineteen global health partnerships reveals that the corporate sector by far dominates the representation in these new partnerships (26% of total membership), followed by academic institutions (17%), foundations (11%), and intergovernmental organizations (11%). NGOs remain a minor actor (6%) compared to Pharma and giants like the Gates Foundation and the World Bank. The participation of low- and middle-income countries is also low (20%).[110] The dominance of the corporate sector in private-public partnerships has raised alarm bells among global public health researchers and activists: " 'New partnerships' are leading [us] down a slippery slope toward the partial privatization and commercialization of the UN system itself."[111]

The issue of power differentials exists even in NGO partnerships. As a Burkina Faso activist criticizes: "I don't believe in partnership between NGOs of the North and South. . . . Partnership is too pretty a word to be true. The forces in play are not equal, the partners so different that it is difficult to find a consensus, and those who execute them are so rarely equal that it is difficult to go forward without some organization feeling left out. The hand that receives a gift is always under that which gives."[112]

Ideological conflicts among different constituents can also make partnerships problematic. For example, the Steering Committee of the World AIDS Campaign, formed in 2004 to develop thematic areas for World AIDS Day through consultations with key affected populations, is made up of twelve diverse organizations representing people living with AIDS, faith-based groups, youth organizations, and INGOs like the International HIV/AIDS Alliance. In one instance, according to the executive director, WAC facilitated a dialogue between faith-based organizations and sex workers: "Our faith-based organizations were not ready for that kind of discussion. While they see sex workers as humans, their religion would not advocate sex work, which they consider as sinful. Similarly, we developed posters that looked at human rights [which depicted] two men holding hands. Our faith-based organizations refused to take the posters even though the majority of our partners wanted them."[113]

Partnerships with the governmental sector are also likely to be seen by one's peers as "collaboration." A Russian activist says, "It's easier to point the finger at the government. I haven't seen a government system where a person can go in and not be part of the system. The only way to bring change is to be outside the system. Civil society plays that role. It should be outside. Once you get inside, step by step you play [by] the rules. The system grabs the people inside, and they become part of the system."[114] Activists in China share similar concerns: "The Chinese government is willing to support grassroots NGOs as service organizations but not advocacy NGOs. I think the Chinese government wants to take over AIDS as a medical issue, not as a rights issue."[115] When CBOs and NGOs partner with the government, they have to reflect on and negotiate the terms of engagement. Does partnership enhance their effectiveness or compromise their identity?

Seeking and complying with funding, consultation, and partnership requirements have caused profound changes in AIDS activism over the past three decades. Several interviewees lament that the majority of community-based organizations are "worthless" and there are few AIDS activists left.[116]Access to knowledge, resources, and power has made some lose their identity and forget their role and has caused bitter divisions in the AIDS community. Professionalization and NGO-ification have brought new challenges to the AIDS movement.[117] A Russian activist thinks that by becoming more and more like multilateral organizations, NGOs have discredited themselves: "They have become huge bureaucratic mechanisms. I don't think they play the role they [should] play, which is advocacy. They have become part of the system. They go to meetings, chair platforms. I don't see practical results."[118] An ACT UP activist reflects, "ACT UP didn't have grant funding. Every Monday night, we [went] to the meeting. I am not being nostalgic. I am just saying that we made a political choice in continuing our work in an NGO structure. We didn't invest in movement building. We thought we could effect changes in Geneva while ignoring the sort of stunted, nonexistent, or decaying national movements."[119]

Since the 1980s, civil society has been directing where the AIDS response should be going from community perspectives. Now, the AIDS movement itself has become an industry, reliant on grant funding and busy with its own survival. "If it does not 'play its cards well,' an Indian activist warns, "and forgets the fundamental reasons why it is there, it can succumb to the seduction of power," further legitimizing the existing regimes of science, Pharma, and governance.[120]

Internal Techniques of Power

Internally, members of the AIDS community police its borders according to serostatus, location in the global economy, language, class, race, gender, age, and ideology. Major differences and exclusionary tendencies in the community were already evident at the 1990 Paris NGO Conference. The two formal co-sponsors of the conference—Comité France SIDA and the US National Minority AIDS Council—could not agree on the organizational structure with the former preferring a more formal structure with presentations and dignitaries and the latter favoring a more skill-building and training emphasis.[121] Representatives of sex workers felt that they were being treated as a problem. The gay and lesbian caucus alleged that the plenary sessions failed to address their specific concerns sufficiently. The women's caucus voted to exclude men from its meetings, leading to a partial walkout of other women from the remaining caucus sessions. The African caucus voted to exclude White Europeans from its meetings.[122]All such protests, manipulation, and lobbying among activists reflect ongoing struggles for control over identity and power. Who really is the community here?

GIPA

Since the heyday of the AIDS epidemic, people living with AIDS have fought for self-determination and meaningful participation. The principle of greater involvement of people living with AIDS, adopted in 1994, has now become a standard and is incorporated in the major policies and practices of most intergovernmental, governmental, and community-based organizations. While generally regarded as a progressive development to ensure the leadership of people living with HIV in all areas of the AIDS response, GIPA in practice opens a can of worms about identity, credibility, exclusion, and boundaries.

A politics of recognition based on HIV serostatus has many implications. When a prominent person living with AIDS called for all those who were not HIV-positive to leave the room so as to create a "PWA space" during a session at the 1992 Australian National Conference on AIDS, it was other HIV-positive people who were most angered.[123] At the institutional level, GIPA plays out "in arguments about the need for open PWAs to be represented on all committees; in pressures to create affirmative hiring policies for PWAs; or in disputes over the allocation of resources between, say, treatments information and preventive education. [It] also play[s] . . . out at a level of unacknowledged anger and guilt between those who are and are not infected."[124] In the current tightened AIDS funding environment, one can imagine resentment against GIPA, which is used as a criterion in doling out limited resources, and it can be seen as unfair and discriminatory by those feeling excluded.[125]

Some activists criticize the detrimental impact of GIPA on the AIDS movement:

> It always strikes me as conspicuous. When you look at civil society organizations working in TB, they are specialists. But within HIV civil society organizations, there aren't many specialists. Many of the individuals who have been critical players in AIDS civil society don't have a background in public health or science or medicine or even social science. The limits of HIV civil society come from this fact that it just doesn't have depth that other areas have. Some activists have retrained themselves. Other people would say living with HIV in their blood give[s] them unique qualifications. It does, but it is not sufficient for a balanced civil society. You need specialists.[126]

The president of the Delhi Network of Positive People believes the responsibility lies with HIV-positive people themselves: "I blame the PLWHA community. They have so much money and they produce so many reports, but what change have they brought? Just because you are positive does not mean involvement. Involvement requires two-way communication, knowing the issues to be discussed, consulting my constituency, conveying it, and reporting back to my community.

That's real involvement."[127] A Russian ITPC activist sees GIPA as little more than vested interests:

> The idea of GIPA is great. But now people understand it as taking someone living with HIV and putting him into the CCM or other government positions. The promotion of GIPA at the high level in this region has made many people living with HIV feel themselves unique: "Look, I have HIV, you have to involve me. Bring me to Vienna or Rome." It's like a privilege. It's reverse discrimination. GIPA has made the community more divided. In Russia, the All Russian Union of People Living with HIV is being challenged by other community groups that they don't represent people living with HIV. The government said, "We are fulfilling the GIPA principle." Yes, you have the All Russian Union of People Living with HIV participate in decision-making structures, but do they represent their clients? I don't have HIV; my wife has. I know the issues in the region. I have sufficient skills to talk about it. When it comes to representation on international mechanisms, we need a person living with HIV. The person who is positive but who does not have technical skills will be qualified. The way I understand GIPA is that it's not about people living with HIV, but people affected by HIV. At the highest level, the understanding of GIPA goes to representation. It makes you feel uncomfortable. We have to stop GIPA. It has to be reexplained with a broader interpretation.[128]

The contentious politics of GIPA mean that coalition work between HIV-positive and nonpositive communities cannot be assumed. The executive director of ITPC explains:

> ITPC is not an identity network. We don't ask people about their status. What we want is just a commitment on issues about access, treatment, and social justice. Many in this movement are upset about nonpositive people getting involved, to whom they say: "What do you know about this?" It has been a fine balance for us because we do want to provide economic opportunities for people living with HIV, but that's not our mandate. Our mandate is providing treatment.[129]

NEO-IMPERIALISM, RACE, CLASS, GENDER, AND AGE

Besides serostatus, the AIDS community is also divided by a number of other identity markers and social locations. North-South tensions were already apparent at the 1990 Paris NGO Conference when North American and European activists prioritized access to treatment on the conference agenda while delegates from the developing countries were primarily concerned with basic healthcare information.[130] A North-South split also emerged over the ratification of ICASO. The Africans took the lead in opposing it. The only African member of the ICASO planning committee, Noerine Kaleeba of TASO in Uganda, claimed that she had never been consulted during the drafting process and yet was asked to endorse it as the African representative. Three-fourths of the African participants claimed that they had never heard of ICASO. In particular, delegates from francophone African countries were more reluctant to agree than were those from anglophone countries, who had perhaps more opportunity to participate in previous discussions.[131]

Many interviewees comment about the ongoing dominance of northern INGOs in AIDS civil society. A European activist reflects:

> There were up until about ten years ago a small number of organizations which in my view incorrectly represented AIDS civil society: ICASO, GNP+, and ICW. They were invited to everything. They were the precursors to civil society delegations. About ten years ago, they broadened out to include some other big INGOs. I read somewhere once an analogy between the major AIDS NGOs (and their compliance with the UN and donors) and the acquiescence of the privileged layers of postcolonial society. You [have] to have somebody to cooperate with the decision players. They participated. They couldn't be influential because they were very poorly funded, but they were because the tail was wagging the dog. They were told what to do. So there was this layer of acquiescent INGOs until around the Durban conference, when smaller NGOs could [finally] participate in the dialogue and advocacy.[132]

Even though more southern NGOs have appeared in the global AIDS political scene, unequal resources and power relations mean that the South is still usually the underdog. A South African activist says:

> The Global North tends to speak on behalf of the Global South. That is not the voice we want. . . . The Global North needs to listen to us with respect, trusting that we know what we are talking about. We know our issues. The challenge is that some of them would say, "We are helping you." They may be filled with good intentions, but it is dysfunctional helping. Sometimes, it gets to a borderline feeling of being undermined even when they are genuine in what they want to do to help. Often it is unconscious. For example, someone would say, "What [she] is trying to say is . . ." And I would say, "No, no, no, I just said it." It is colonializing for them to think, "We know your problem." It's their attitude: "We have the knowledge, equipment, and resources. We have the experience. We can help you fast-track your thing." No. We

want to go through our own process. Actually, give us our space to do the things we want to do. . . . "The child" has grown.[133]

The North-South divide plays out in different ways in agenda setting, linguistic dominance, cultures of communication, and NGO management styles. For example, in setting the health-financing advocacy agenda, civil society in Africa has been focusing its efforts on government financing while northern NGOs continue to push for international funding. "The tension is about who sets the agenda," says the executive director of the World AIDS Campaign. "For example, if WHO says you need to provide treatment for anyone below [a] CD4 count of 450, civil society of the Global North will be responding, whereas our reality is very different here. Our government provides treatment only for people with [a] CD4 count below 250. Our colleagues in the Global North talk about third-line treatment and treatment as prevention. We would say: 'Let's take care of first-line treatment for those waiting in line first.' "[134] The same concerns are echoed by an Indian activist of the People's Health Movement: "AIDS activism started in the North. The global visibility that it got is related to the fact that very endowed organizations like Oxfam and MSF made a difference. There, people in the North, including HIV-positive people, made an impact on their governments and through their governments on global governance. But it also means that there is a lack in their ability to attend to the needs of the South. . . . Even today, many more people die of TB than [of] HIV in India."[135]

Numerous southern activists in Thailand, China, Russia, Egypt, Malaysia, Latin America, and Africa say that English-language dominance is a major challenge. Participation in global AIDS "assumes knowledge of western-style meeting procedures and rhetoric, and the ability to operate in English, which has become perforce the language of the international AIDS world."[136] Conflicts also arise over the definitions of "activism" and "professionalism." "There are loads of tensions in terms of how we do advocacy and how we communicate," the South African executive director of the WAC continues. "Writing letters may be effective in the North but not necessarily here. At other times, northern colleagues would say the Global South is very silent about a certain issue or not communicating with them. How do you define silence? We may not have done a media campaign or written reports, but we were on the streets all the time."[137] A Chinese activist also finds the hegemonic Western NGO management styles ill adapted to the budding civil society scene in China:

International training on NGO management that focuses on mission, objective, and plans, etc., is not so useful in China. Most Chinese NGOs are so small. In the West,

NGOs are experienced in their field and can work according to mission statements. In China, since NGOs are new, we face a lot of changes in terms of our work. For example, a network might require a CBO to have a constitution in order to become its member, but most CBO staff members don't know about their constitution, even if there is one. Some may lie to international donors that they have a constitution, but in reality, it is never referred to. Often donors require a governance structure with a board, executive committee, and a finance department, etc., but most Chinese NGOs have only one or two paid staff. International or domestic trainers not from the CBO sector do not know about this situation. For example, after the Global Fund grants were frozen in China, there was a budget of a few million yuan for CBO capacity building in February 2011. There was no needs assessment prior to the training. We started talking about our needs only after the training. We still don't know what Chinese NGOs' needs are.[138]

Other divisions along class, race, gender, and age are directly inherited from the early AIDS movement, which was led by adult, middle-class, White gay men, and often overlap with North-South tensions. The class issue in the AIDS movement is paramount not only in terms of the composition of the movement's constituents. While AIDS activism today is certainly much more class diverse than ACT UP was, NGO leadership is still primarily composed of elites, who do not represent the majority of people living with AIDS in the world. More important, the class divide in AIDS treatment is regarded by many as morally repugnant. Robert Munk, a European activist, phrases it well: "It's like we're quibbling over the choice[s] on the menu in the West, while 95% of the world can't even get into the restaurant."[139]

The treatment divide has been further aggravated by changes in the Global Fund funding model, which is based on the World Bank's classification of countries based on gross national product. As of 2013, community groups in lower middle-income countries can only apply under the "special groups" and "interventions" categories of funding, which is a significantly reduced pool of money (50% of proposed budgets for applications to the General Funding Pool versus 100% for applications to the Targeted Funding Pool). Those in upper middle-income countries are eligible only if they have a high, severe, or extreme disease burden. A similar economic criterion is used by Pharma in its tiered pricing for ARV products. In the Medicines Patent Pool agreements with Gilead, for example, over half a million patients in more than forty-three middle-income countries were excluded from the agreements, accentuating a long-standing North-South division by adding a South-South treatment gap. This new funding criterion, which is based on aggregated national economic data, masks income disparities within countries and ignores the reality of unfunded community-based AIDS work in most middle-income countries, such as China, Russia, Egypt, and almost all of Latin America. It could very well be the kiss of death for many nascent CBOs and NGOs in these countries.

In many ways, race intersects with class and neo-imperialism in AIDS politics. As "a disease of disadvantage,"[140] AIDS is disproportionately distributed in African and Asian countries and, within these, the poorest and the most disenfranchised communities are hit the hardest. As WHO attests, this is not just a matter of how the epidemic unfolded, but has to do with poverty, poor surveillance systems, and the limited access of large segments of the population to healthcare facilities where the diagnosis of AIDS can be established.[141] In national contexts, epidemiologists understood early that ethnic communities were at greater risk. In many countries, a person of color is more likely to contract AIDS, less likely to access health care, and more likely to die earlier. When (mostly White) ACT UP activists were raging on Wall Street and at the NIH in the late 1980s, Black men were three times more likely to contract AIDS than White men, and women of color accounted for 71% of all women with AIDS. In 2010, African Americans had the most severe burden of HIV of all racial/ethnic groups, accounting for 44% of all new HIV infections among adults and adolescents despite representing only 13% of the US population. A Black man is seven times more likely to contract HIV than his White counterpart.[142]

Despite the reality of a racialized epidemic, however, the concerns of populations of color are not always reflected on the agendas of AIDS organizations or movements. In ACT UP, Latino Caucus members, who were simultaneously involved with Black and Latino grassroots movements that were "like a world apart from ACT UP," began to raise issues affecting their communities, which "historically had a very tough time with biomedical research, had a very tough time accessing good health care, and were already confronting not just AIDS but other diseases, like drug abuse, tuberculosis, and things like that."[143] One of these activists, Moisés Agosto, remembers being disappointed by others' response ("We can't fix everybody's life") when he tried to bring race into the White-dominated movement. In the ACT UP Oral History Project, he recounts to a fellow activist, Sarah Schulman:

> MA: I always say, when you're a person of color here, it's like you have to prove yourself twice and three times. In the treatment and research area, you have to prove yourself like five times.

SS: To the scientists or to the T and D [Treatment and Data Committee in ACT UP]?

MA: Both.

SS: Why was that?

MA: Because. First, you come with a thick accent. People think that if you have an accent, you're stupid. I got that a lot of times. How can I say? I was going toward politics that fit within the grassroots movement that already happened before, or at the same time that ACT UP was happening, [which] was happening within the Latino community in New York, was happening in the African-American community in New York. That was where I wanted to go—communities where this was an item added to the list, communities that already were disenfranchised. I was doing activism and having a great time with it with people that never experienced that kind of discrimination. Well, some of them, but you know what I mean. Like access to care was not that much of an issue for the majority of the members who had access to [Anthony] Fauci, who had access to trials. They could go into the trial because they had a good doctor, while all these people that I felt more identified with didn't.[144]

Racial and ethnic tensions always have an economic dimension. In 1993, straight Black men and gay White men accused each other of discrimination in a bitter dispute over city funding for HIV in Washington, DC. The director of the city's HIV/AIDS agency was fired after allegations of a pro-gay bias in his allocation of contracts.[145]

In a completely different national and historical context, race also is a factor in the bitterly divided South African AIDS movement. On March 30, 2004, the South African AIDS Consortium—dominated by two heavyweight community groups, the National Association of People with AIDS (NAPWA) and the Treatment Action Campaign (TAC)—held a meeting in Johannesburg. The very first comment by a NAPWA member was a racial attack on a White member of the AIDS Consortium's Executive Committee: "[W]e are sick of white people sitting at the front of the meeting; it causes us pain."[146] At the end of the meeting, the national organizer of NAPWA confronted Mark Heywood, one of the TAC founders: "We are sick of you fucking white racists taking advantage of black people with HIV/AIDS."[147] Race in South Africa also mixes with politics and economics. Funding competitions exacerbate racial tensions between NAPWA, which sides with the African National Congress, and the TAC, which is aligned with the Congress of South African Trade Unions.

The AIDS community is also plagued by gender disparities. Women AIDS activists charge that their experiences and needs are not prioritized in HIV-positive communities and in affected population groups. The first US CDC definition for AIDS, developed in 1987, specified twenty-three AIDS-defining conditions but excluded gynecological conditions, such as cervical dysplasia, pelvic inflammatory disease, and recurrent vulvovaginal candidiasis, which occur more commonly in HIV-infected women than in other women.[148] The CDC definition was used not only by physicians and in research protocols, but also in the allocation of federal funds under the Ryan White Comprehensive AIDS Resources Emergency Act of 1990 and as a measure of disability in benefit programs administered by the Social Security Administration.[149] Women activists in ACT UP had to convince the gay male leadership about the issue before successfully lobbying for a new CDC definition of AIDS in 1991, which made HIV-positive women eligible for disability claims.

Women's vulnerability to AIDS is often related to broader cultural, economic, and religious factors. The Global Fund Grants Program manager at UNDP-Kyrgyzstan agrees:

> Women are one of the most vulnerable groups in this region. It is linked to stigma and the submissive role of women in society. Also culturally, a woman cannot have many sexual partners. But men can have as many sexual partners as they want to. Everyone knows about it. He has more or less the freedom of choice. This is more or less the same for all five countries in this region. It may be linked to Islam, even though Islam is not very strong here. I think it's an issue, but it is not really on the agenda. I attend a lot of conferences and meetings here, but I don't hear women [being acknowledged] as a separate group that requires attention. No one is raising the issue. Everyone is playing hide and seek.[150]

In the activist community, women living with AIDS continue to face the "gay men syndrome." As a Steering Committee member of ICW puts it: "We do a lot of partnering with GNP+. It is clear that they want to be leaders. It is about their chair, their ED, their somebody else to deliver the awards or do the presentations. They are aggressive and they take everything on."[151] Without close attention to gender equality, the representatives of people living with AIDS and of affected populations on various governance structures may all be men. Such is the case for the Chinese CCM. In 2008, the Global Fund adopted a Gender Equality Strategy that recommends: "CCMs must strive to achieve sex parity among their membership and leadership. Tools provided by the Global Fund will include terms of reference for gender experts and other CCM members."[152] Research by the China Global Fund Watch, however, finds that none of the twelve delegates (one member plus two alternatives for each PWA sector and the same for the NGO sector) for two CCM terms were women.[153] Further, given the diversity among women, it is important to pay attention to the double or triple stigma and discrimination faced by women in various affected populations, such as young women, drug users, migrants, and prisoners.

Last but not least, age remains very much a barrier for AIDS activism. Youth AIDS issues are little understood by adult-dominated science, Pharma, governance, and community. As the coordinator of Youth Lead, a nascent Asia-Pacific network, says, "When we talk about youth, we often talk about youth in general. But in the Asia-Pacific region, 95% of new HIV infections come from youth. There is an urgent need to address the needs of young key affected populations."[154] "In terms of [the] youth agenda, we used to focus almost exclusively on abstinence," says the co-founder of the Global Youth Coalition on HIV/AIDS (GYCA). "Now we are looking more at systemic issues, like economic empowerment, gender equality, and integrating family planning and reproductive health. HIV can't be looked at in isolation any more."[155]

The focus on youth leadership and participation in the AIDS response is recent and came about only after the vehement protests of young AIDS activists. GYCA's co-founder continues:

> Those [who are] managing programs tend . . . to be men and over fifty. In the UN, they never get fired. There is no opportunity for fresh blood. It also has to do with colonialism and imperialism. The whole response has been driven by the North. . . . The global AIDS response so far has very much overlooked young people. What we do is positioning for young people to have a place.[156]

A particular challenge is "reaching most-at-risk young people who may not have internet or speak English, and [who are] not tied to or identifying with communities of sex workers, MSM, and injecting drug users; and rural and urban young poor people."[157]

The representation of adolescents and younger children on governance structures also has proved to be difficult. As the project coordinator of the Coalition for Children Affected by AIDS observes:

> If you look at the youth contingent at IAS [International AIDS Society], every two years, youth will make a lot of [noise] about how terrible the adults are. My opinion is that the same group of people made the same noise two years ago. Some of it is legitimate, some of it is not, because they don't know what has been done at the global level. What is problematic is that it is one of the largest subgroups and visible subgroups at IAS [that] keeps saying, "There needs to be more youth." The UN

has recommendations [and] guideline[s] about increasing youth representation. The problem is how to find youth that [are] representative of their peers. It is unfortunate that the children they find are often not that representative of their peers: they tend to be the more articulate, brightest, most outgoing, probably speak English, and their parents are engaged in international movements. They are elites. Are these kids representative?[158]

IDEOLOGY

The AIDS community is also fraught with all kinds of ideological tensions over drug use, sex work, homosexuality, abstinence, sex, AIDS education, and behavior change. Prejudice gives rise to the stigmatization of affected populations. One of the most marginalized groups among the vulnerable populations is drug users. For a long time, they were left off everybody's radar screen. As the former program director of the Eurasian Harm Reduction Network sees it, "A lot of the people involved in AIDS work still stigmatize drug users. Think of the stereotypical MSM and think of the stereotypical drug user. These are very different communities. Their personal hygiene is opposite. They are in the same room, and they might hate each other. But then later on they are supposed to work together."[159] On the other hand, MSM may feel that they are being discriminated against by other affected populations.[160] Stigma in the HIV community is evident in the differential recognition and acceptance of the various affected populations. While it is common to see people living with AIDS on various board structures, the presence of heroin users on a board of directors may raise eyebrows and objections.

Above all, ideological differences mean that coalition work among HIV-positive communities and other affected populations cannot be taken for granted. For example, while needle exchange is generally understood and accepted by people living with AIDS, the legalization of drugs and opioid substitution therapy remain contentious. The former program director of the Eurasian Harm Reduction Network explains:

> Sometimes you see on our listserv discussions, e.g., on OST. A lot of people living with HIV might be involved in [a] twelve-step program and oppose OST. Many of them who deal with their addictions in a certain way believe that others should deal with theirs in the same way. . . . In Russia, two national networks of people living with HIV will not come out [and] say they support OST. The issue has become so politicized that if you want to maintain a good relationship with the government, you can't come out to support OST.[161]

Who Are We? Community Empowerment, Voice, and Knowledge

True diversity is time-consuming.
> —*Founding Member, Asia Pacific Coalition on*
> *Male Sexual Health*[162]

The only way to bring change is to be outside the system. Civil
society plays that role.
> —*Advocacy Officer, International Treatment*
> *Preparedness Coalition*[163]

After more than three decades of grassroots organizing, billions of dollars
spent in service and advocacy, and unprecedented political mobilization at the
highest levels, what are the successes, failures, and challenges of the AIDS movement? A broad question such as this cannot be meaningfully answered in any
single study. With the exception of a few large INGOs and global networks, the
majority of AIDS CBOs and NGOs do not have enough resources to go through
a formal review exercise. Evaluation is also plagued by a number of other issues,
including changing mandates due to the evolving epidemic, the difficulty of as-
certaining causal linkages in complex policy and operational environments with
a multitude of actors, and the long time frame that many advocacy actions require.
As the former communications manager of the Asian Harm Reduction Network
puts it: "AHRN contributed to civil society mobilization, engagement, and participation. We were a focal point for advocacy. But the problem was that we didn't
have a focus. We were investing a bit everywhere. We didn't have three clear areas. We were too diffused, and it is very difficult to measure the impact. In that
sense, I don't think we can claim anything."[164]

The evaluation of larger, more diffused networks proves even more challenging. The executive director of ITPC acknowledges: "It is hard to measure
ITPC's role. The activists wanted to start a movement surrounding the idea of
treatment preparedness: taking complete control over treatment, increasing knowledge about treatment, and being able to do advocacy on treatment scale-up. As
such, there was no real ownership of ITPC as a network."[165] Despite these difficulties, some preliminary remarks can be made based on AIDS activists' own
evaluations of their triumphs, pitfalls, and challenges.

The impact of AIDS activism since the 1980s has resulted from three central
roles taken up by civil society: (1) organizing and empowerment, (2) voice and advocacy, and (3) knowledge building. While institutional change in terms of new
laws, policies, and programs may not always happen as a result of advocacy, one

clear, visible triumph of AIDS activism has been community organizing and empowerment. AIDS created a timely political opportunity for diverse communities, including gay men, sex workers, drug users, migrants, and youth, to organize themselves, often beyond AIDS. As an activist puts it, "Yes, we try to stop infections. But because we started as a human rights movement, ultimately what we are trying to do is also about empowerment."[166]

Community Organizing and Empowerment

The drive for self-organization and empowerment started with the 1983 Denver Principles on the rights of people living with AIDS to self-determination and participation. "HIV/AIDS made the community organize itself," an MSM activist says. "HIV made the West[ern] gay community organize itself. It wasn't organized except around sex and gay bars and saunas. Suddenly, it organized into a community that took care of itself. That's what HIV did and does."[167] Drug user organizing has also come a long way, in part thanks to AIDS. The notion of empowerment for people who use drugs has finally gained global purchase. "This is where the legal network has made a major contribution," according to the executive director of the Canadian HIV/AIDS Legal Network. "Our report *Nothing about Us without Us* [2005] . . . borrows from the slogan of the disability movement. It has now been taken up globally."[168]

Sex workers are now regular participants at international AIDS conferences not only as attendees but also as plenary speakers. RedTraSex has been recognized for its power in organizing sex workers throughout Latin America. "We have to empower the worker so that she may dialogue and demand her rights and enforce the role that UNAIDS is expected to play in the strengthening of civil society," says its executive director.[169] In South Africa, the Sex Workers Education and Advocacy Taskforce considers sex worker organizing to be one of its greatest impacts: "In 2011 alone, we made 24,000 contacts and interventions. We have come a long way in terms of organizing sex workers nationally and their advocacy in South Africa. We are not just a sex worker technical organization. We have a very good human rights defense model, and we use the evidence generated to support our decriminalization campaign."[170] In Egypt, one small community group, the Al Shehab Foundation, spearheaded a sex worker peer network in Cairo. Its cofounder recalls:

> A group of young people started to work on different issues in our neighborhood in the late 1990s. Then we started to be more organized as an NGO in 2001 to have more impact. Our overall objective was and still is to develop human rights in the

slum areas. . . . One of our core programs is the economic empowerment of women. We also assist them by providing them with lawyers [since] they cannot easily access the justice system to address issues of violence and discrimination. . . . We started our project with female sex workers in 2006 as we observed that many women in the slum areas are involved in sex work. . . . We looked [to see] if there was any information on female sex workers in Egypt, e.g., population size. There was no information, so we started by conducting a qualitative study with a small group of thirty-five female sex workers and a small group of gatekeepers, like taxi drivers, about their socioeconomic background, risk factors, and problems that they face. The study shows [that] most of the women come from poor families. Most of them are uneducated, and they face a lot of legal issues and a lot of issues with police because sex work is illegal. They have medical issues and are afraid to go see a doctor for fear of stigma. They have psychological issues because of violence from clients or family or community. We started to design a comprehensive project where we trained and established a female outreach team to identify the gathering points of female sex workers in Cairo, conduct mapping exercises about places and prices, and share basic information on HIV and sexual rights.[171]

He continues:

Then, in 2006, we created a drop-in center as a pilot project (funded by UNDP and UNAIDS) to provide legal and medical help. After one year, we scaled up to provide psychological service[s] as the second phase of the project. We increased the number of outreach workers to eight and . . . added male outreach workers. One of the main activities is condom use. But we found out that most of the time sex workers don't use condom[s]. We thought maybe we needed to start work[ing] with clients. We trained four male outreach workers to work with clients. We opened another drop-in center in downtown. That phase worked for two years. Now another two years later, we added one more NGO and trained yet another NGO to conduct outreach activities. We are training a third NGO. . . . When we work with female sex workers, we don't work from a moral point of view. We work from an empowerment point of view. Based on their needs, we started to provide skill workshops to 100 female sex workers from performance classes to cooking, hairdressing, and literacy classes. [Every] six months, we also train a group of sex workers to be peer educators (so far, a total of 120 [have been] trained) to transfer knowledge related to HIV prevention, testing, condom use, and to promote [the] drop-in center and [our] service[s]. We have reached out to more than 5,000 female sex workers and over 2,500–3,000 male clients.[172]

From Egypt to China, Thailand to Russia, Kenya to India, Israel to Malaysia, communities organized themselves to respond to AIDS before governments stepped in. In direct care, support, testing, peer education, and advocacy, AIDS CBOs, NGOs, networks, and movements involving HIV-positive people and affected populations took the lead.[173] In Russia, "civil society grew tremendously. Actually all techniques and tools that local NGOs use were brought from abroad. . . . Activists brought expertise in prevention and outreach, in work with MARPs. The government didn't work with marginalized populations. [It] simply didn't reach them. The only organizations were CBOs and NGOs. This is a very important contribution."[174] In Thailand, "the biggest success of the Asian Harm Reduction Network is bringing the Thai community to form a national network called 12D to advocate for itself, even though we may not be able to take credit for it. We only provided the platform for Thai IDUs to come together. There were existing platforms already, but AHRN was critical."[175]

Empowerment—being informed, strengthened, enabled, and filled with confidence and the capacity to make choices and assert them—can occur at the individual, organizational, community, national, regional, or global level and can encompass social, political, and economic dimensions. The regional program coordinator of 7 Sisters, composed of seven regional networks of people living with AIDS, sex workers, transgender people, drug users, and migrants, comments: "We are an advocacy network. It is extremely difficult and time-consuming to see progress. . . . But maybe in the area of empowerment, we can speak with confidence. For example, some members of the coalition may [have felt] uncomfortable speaking to the Ministry of Health. Now they are part of a group [or] community and that has changed the way they approach the government. We can clearly see this difference."[176] The co-founder of the Asia Pacific Coalition on Male Sexual Health also finds that "personal empowerment for people involved with APCOM" is one of its most important achievements. Further, he has witnessed more community organization at the regional level: "In the region, there is a lot more community work going on, a lot of empowerment of local people doing something for the drug user community. It's new, but not brand-new. A lot of it has been there in some fashion before. But it's been organized better and heard about better. HIV/AIDS became an opportunity for that."[177] According to the executive director of CARAM, one of its main successes is the "empowerment and capacity building from the bottom, involving not only migrants, but also other groups such as drug addicts, sex workers, and people living with AIDS in the Asia-Pacific region who understand the issues of migration."[178] In China, the Chi Heng Foundation continues to foster community self-help among children affected by AIDS and other vulnerable populations. Its executive director explains: "In a traditional charity model, there is a clear boundary between service providers and recipients. We have tried to go beyond that by recruiting the AIDS orphans we have supported to be staff members. . . . Through our social enterprise projects, we also provide employment, training, and self-empowerment of our clients. This is an area that I would like to work on more, based on the triple bottom line: economic, social, and environmental."[179]

In some cases, community organizing in response to AIDS is so successful that the government ends up adopting the community model in its national health system. Mothers2Mothers (M2M), for example, is an organization based out of Cape Town, South Africa, that is focused on the peer prevention of mother-to-child transmission. Created in 2001, it provides psychosocial support by hiring and paying HIV-positive mothers to mentor newly diagnosed mothers. Despite any formal evaluation of the organization, the assistant communications manager feels confident that M2M has played a role in ensuring that mothers adhere to their medication regimens and receive accurate information in addition to the support it provides to healthcare workers on the ground:

> M2M speaks a lot about empowerment. The women we employ are women living with HIV. Each is employed for only a year and then they move on to another role, to work somewhere else. Yes, she got all the information and she has been empowered financially. We are still doing . . . internal monitoring to see what happens after they leave. The other thing we are currently doing is capacity building to help the government to implement the M2M model in the national health system. The first one is Kenya. Since 2008, there are sites where we are the primary implementers, and there are sites where the government has taken over.[180]

In other cases, AIDS community organizing has spilled over to other areas, strengthening community life as a whole. In Thailand, the local and national organizing of people living with AIDS has completely changed the identity, perception, and self-acceptance of PLWHA. "Previously, HIV meant death. Today, PLWHA can lead a life and show their ability to the community. This network started [with] work on the AIDS issue. Now, with increased capacity, we think about other issues [and are] develop[ing] into a people's movement on health. Our movement is the biggest and strongest people's movement in Thailand," says the executive director of the Thai Network of People Living with HIV/AIDS.[181] "The spin-off of HIV mobilization has transformed community mobilization permanently," the co-founder of the Health and Development Network adds. "The community mobilization around the financial crisis in 1996–1997 was really informed by the HIV mobilization, [which] has forged new ground in terms of community care, such as health workers task shifting, that is part of every response to local health priorities now. That is permanent change."[182]

Community Voice and Advocacy

Based on the grassroots mobilization of patient communities and affected populations, AIDS activists have been able to project their voice for advocacy.[183] Undeniably, the social and political visibility of AIDS worldwide has to do with the effectiveness of community voice and representation. They give a face to AIDS. Whether it is in gender, sexual orientation, harm reduction, sex work, PMTCT, human rights, or public health, the AIDS communities have played a crucial role in setting the global agenda. People living with AIDS and representatives of civil society have been sitting on the decision-making structures of science, Pharma, and governance because they fought for it. As discussed at length in chapters 2, 3, and 4, AIDS advocacy has brought institutional changes in access to treatment; the right-to-health framework; the IP regime; decriminalization of homosexuality, drug use, and sex work; and funding for civil society and marginalized populations, and it has resulted in a certain democratization of governance in science and global public health beyond AIDS.

AIDS activism made community voices heard at the global level. As the former program director of the Eurasian Harm Reduction Network confirms:

> I have seen it happen and I have seen it responded to. I have seen that civil society first and foremost made that happen. I would sit and talk to drug users about what their issues are, and the following day I would talk to the director of an important organization or WHO-Europe. This sort of thing does happen and I have seen improvement over the years. We constantly have to fight to get, for example, MSM and drug users on the international agenda, and there is political resistance. But there are successes, and civil society has been driving them.[184]

GNP+ thinks that it has been most effective in voice and representation, in "demanding and ensuring universal access. We don't believe in prioritization, whether it is by medical criteria or between men and women, urban and rural, poor and rich, etc. We believe in universal access."[185]

For civil society voices to be heard, training and consultation need to be organized and coordinated. The former regional program coordinator of 7 Sisters notes:

> 7 Sisters has been able to coordinate to make sure voices are heard. We hold regular consultations around the Global Fund processes. We do one-on-one training,

gender assessment, and a lot of skill building. We work closely with the UN Regional Support Team. They call us for . . . meetings when our voice is required. The Youth Team works with UNICEF and UNFPA. You can observe that [when] there is any regional consultation, e.g., the last [meeting of] ESCAP [the Economic and Social Commission for Asia and the Pacific]. We [had] our own consultations prior to ESCAP, and we brought more than 50–60 people as participants. We have been that medium where civil society voices are heard.[186]

Agenda setting and representation at the regional, national, and local levels are equally important. The Asian Network of People Who Use Drugs has been involved in all of the major regional consultation mechanisms, working to put drug users on the agenda: the WHO five-year regional strategic plan on IDUs for the Asia-Pacific region; the ESCAP Declaration, which was part of the regional implementation of the Political Declaration on HIV/AIDS; and the regional meetings for the Global Commission on HIVAIDS and the Law.[187] The executive director of the Asia Pacific Network of Sex Workers says: "There is no way the UN would not consult us." But he acknowledges: "The real struggle is at the country level. It depends on the policing structure at the local level because the police are the ones that control sex work. Sex workers might be given condoms but then [get] arrested by police. You can have [a] comprehensive HIV policy, but it is up to national governments to work with the police. We need to have champions to drive policy forward."[188]

Institutional changes lobbied for by AIDS civil society at the national level are innumerable. In country after country, from Brazil to Thailand, South Africa to China, Uganda to Kenya, national governments finally rolled out ARV treatment programs after AIDS activists protested, smuggled generic drugs in underground networks, took governments to court, and told their stories to the media. The situation is still far from being perfect. There are still drug shortages and expired ARV shipments. Some drugs, especially for second- and third-line treatments, are priced out of reach. Patent issues have not gone away. With the retreat of donors and the Global Fund in the majority of middle-income countries, governments have to come up with alternative financing to meet the next phase of the epidemic as HIV-positive people live longer, treatments get more expensive, and scientists push for treatment as prevention. But AIDS activism has not only saved lives, but also radically altered the terms of the AIDS treatment debate. It is no longer acceptable to let people die of AIDS because of their inability to pay, as was the case just ten or twenty years ago when intergovernmental agencies and some governments preferred to focus on prevention. Other successes in policy change in different countries include anonymous and rapid testing, nondiscrimination, prevention services and education, increased funding, and above all, government recognition of and mobilization around the disease.

At the global level, the four most significant institutional changes brought by the AIDS movement are treatment advocacy, human rights and decriminalization, increased funding, and the democratization of science and health governance, all of which have been discussed in the preceding chapters. AIDS activism has had a visible impact on the access movements of patient communities in TB, hepatitis C, and cancer as well. These groups too want their own community advisory boards, inclusion in clinical trials, full participation in medical and political decision making concerning their constituents, and representation. Medical and legal activists like MSF and the Lawyers Collective, in conjunction with HIV-positive communities and other NGO advocates, have helped to unlock the IP regime in the WTO, denounced Pharma obstructionism whenever necessary, worked with generic companies to bring drug prices down, run parallel procurement and treatment programs, supported national governments to issue compulsory licenses, written national ARV guidelines, fought against discrimination, and changed laws. The executive director of ITPC says:

> ITPC has provided an opportunity for advocacy on issues that normally people would not be advocating for, e.g., FTA, data exclusivity, MARPs. In Russia, we have become the entry point for them to talk about hep C. A lot of activism went into community strengthening. Many have lost the treatment focus, I think. One thing is to bring back treatment into their focus, and that's why we are here. They will age, they may get diabetes, etc. In three years' time, if I can get them [to] align with noncommunicable disease groups to give them movement strength, it would be a real advocacy community movement, parallel to the MSF Access Campaign. The MSF Access Campaign is done by professionals. There are not many from the community like us.[189]

It was community groups and NGO networks that introduced and operationalized a right-to-health framework in AIDS. In Russia, the Andrey Rylkov Foundation uses a human rights approach to advocate for the right to health and the right to access to treatment for drug users.[190] In China, the Shanghai AIDS Prevention Center's peer outreach among MSM is based on the belief that "everybody has the right to information, right to health, and right to treatment."[191]

A right-to-health approach often requires the collaboration of different stakeholders. As a representative of the MSF–South Africa Access Campaign realizes, "access to treatment never stands alone as an issue; it is related to the right to health and the broader health movement."[192] The AIDS and Rights Alliance for Southern Africa also sees the application of a human rights framework to health and beyond. Its regional advocacy team leader says: "We have dealt with HIV as a numbers game. We don't look at the individuals. That's why so many rights are violated. How to mainstream . . . a rights approach is our challenge, to push countries to prioritize health with both first-generation and second-generation rights. It is an agenda beyond health."[193] In Egypt, networks of people living with AIDS cooperate with developmental NGOs and human rights organizations. The Health and Discrimination Project manager of the Egyptian Initiative forPersonal Rights says: "In the litigation area, we are very prominent and pioneering. We started this and did some very good cases. We were helpful in going to court with people living with AIDS."[194] In South America, the work of the International Drug Policy Consortium, an evidence-based and human rights–centered network of ninety-four NGOs and professional organizations, has led to significant changes, including decriminalization in Mexico and the pardon of over 2,000 IDUs by the national district attorney in Ecuador.

The raised voices of civil society and marginalized populations brought an unprecedented level of funding. According to the information manager of the Andrey Rylkov Foundation, the "Global Fund's Community System Strengthening Framework came from civil society advocacy because we realized [that] just supporting AIDS services is not enough. So much more needs to be done to expand the capacity of community organizations. It's a vertical system right now, and it's not integrating."[195]

AIDS activism also has brought about some democratization of governance in science and global public health. Civil society has played the role of check and balance in driving accountability. "Some of the inclusive governance mechanisms like the Global Fund Board and the PCB of UNAIDS are very specific, and they are small victories. Now it is hard to imagine not . . . includ[ing] civil society in board structures," says the co-founder of the Health and Development Network.[196] An ACT UP activist says, "The presence of civil society has helped to bring different players together, not just activists, but also faith-based groups and academics, etc. I think civil society involvement has created pluralism while, at the same time, certain doors are closed because of civil society. Civil society community is defined not only by who is included but also by who is excluded. This has always been a double-edged sword, two sides to every coin."[197] A veteran HIV-positive woman activist sums up the role of AIDS activism: "We have continued to put . . . feet to the fire. We are the guardians of the things they have done. We pointed out the ethical side of the research that they do, the way they make decisions and set their priorities. We have not been always successful, but we continue."[198]

Community Knowledge Building

Behind and beyond the sit-ins, kiss-ins, and die-ins, the disruptions of presidential campaigns and plenary presentations, the marches and demonstrations, the hunger strikes, boycotts, grant oppositions, and court challenges, what AIDS activists have built is continuous social learning, which feeds into advocacy actions. "Social learning cannot be mandated by the pre-emptive action of central political authority. Nor can it be programmed by bureaucratic procedures," according to the economist and political activist David Korten. "It is a product of people, acting individually and in voluntary association with others, guided by their individual critical consciousness and recognizing no organizational boundaries. Its organizational forms are found in coalitions and networks, which become aggregated in large social movements, driven by ideas and shared values more than by formal structures."[199]

Often unconscious and mostly undocumented, social learning in the AIDS movement takes place in the day-to-day activities and interactions among activists when they learn the ropes of direct action; attend IAS and grasp the science and politics of AIDS; get inspired by and replicate actions by activists in other countries; do research into marginalized populations, ARV drug prices, drug shortage scandals, and frivolous patenting; and organize teach-ins, seminars, and presentations to their peers, the public, governments, police, judges, businesspeople, and UN officials. A young Russian ITPC activist recalls:

> The first time I went to an international meeting and met great activists like David Barr and Greg Gonsalves, I learned how they presented their positions and how they . . . demanded their rights. Here in Russia, we are not used to that. Maybe it's related to my drug use background, [but] we don't know how to assert our rights. Here, people keep silent. I also learned how to use a multistakeholder approach, how to work with the UN system as equal partners, that we should be heard, that we could present our positions. I learned mostly from activists whom I met. I also read a lot in the ITPC global listserv. I learned from lots of different kinds of training on, e.g., treatment literacy and resource mobilization. One of my first training[s] was on OST and harm reduction in Moscow by a Ukrainian doctor. That really opened my eyes. Before, I thought only rehab would help. Today, I understand that drug users should have choices. After my treatment literacy training, I could answer questions from my friends about treatment, e.g., side effects. Now I know how to present myself

and talk to donors, etc. When I made my presentation at the GF [Global Fund] Board, I felt so ashamed because my government didn't want GF money. I talked to [the] Norway ambassador to the GF board, who told me not to be ashamed. [Now,] I share these experiences with activists who didn't have the same opportunity to travel. They don't have confidence. I bring what is going on at the global level back to Russia. When a new colleague joined ITPC, I shared with him. This is an important part of activism. Each time you share these knowledges with others, you are repeating them for yourself. The challenge is that the more you know, the more you realize you don't know![200]

Some AIDS groups were conscious of their epistemic role from the beginning, while others have more recently incorporated it as one of their core mandates and strategies. ABIA in Brazil, for example, has consistently used a knowledge production approach in its advocacy work: "Cross-cutting all three axes of our work in outreach, research, and advocacy is the production of knowledge and information dissemination for the population. We have been developing social research on AIDS, always . . . linking with the university. We produce documents and information that could orient and inform the advocacy work not only of ABIA but also of other Brazilian social movement groups on AIDS."[201] The Israel AIDS Task Force as well bases its service and advocacy work on knowledge building: "Knowledge is a very important term in our work. It is our base. One of our goals and strategies has always been that we are the most updated body in AIDS, even more professional than the government. Each board member plays a role in collecting, criticizing, translating the knowledges to different communities and audience[s], and adapting their relevancy to our sociopolitical contexts."[202] Knowledge Ecology International borrows the concept of sustainable ecology from the environmental movement and applies it to the knowledge economy. It engages in extensive research, provides technical advice to different stakeholders, and monitors key actors in order to manage knowledge resources in more fair and efficient ways.[203] GNP+ has more recently refocused its strategies on knowledge management to "expand its research agenda, building upon the proven success of action research; decentralize research management where possible through the engagement of further PLHIV networks; [and] communicate findings more broadly so that partners and other stakeholders can use findings for advocacy."[204] In its own evaluation, MSF acknowledges that in addition to being successful in getting generic drugs to its patients, it has played a big role in knowledge transfer.[205]

What has emerged out of more than three decades of activism is an enormous corpus of alternative knowledges on AIDS, health, sexuality, drug use, stigma, discrimination, and human rights, or, in short, a democratization of knowledge and power. As a veteran ACT UP activist who later co-founded ITPC sums it up, "What used to be the provinces of physicians, PhDs, and elites were invaded by ordinary people, these fags in ACT UP, and poor people from different parts around the world."[206] By being present and highlighting differences, what AIDS civil society has achieved is "opening the minds of governments, Pharma, scientists, international bureaucrats, and anyone else who has nothing to do with HIV and who has never seen a positive person, that is, opening a new world to the traditional way of thinking."[207]

Pitfalls and Challenges

For every achievement, however, there has been a setback. AIDS activists are cognizant of their own limits. The availability of extensive funding has generated much complacency, fragmentation, and co-optation in the AIDS movement. "Tensions among local NGOs are largely personal conflicts," says a former MSF–Hong Kong activist. "Slightly below the surface is competition for funds. Maybe competition for power comes first. Above everything else, it is the need to be the *laoda* [boss] that causes the factionalization among the MSM community in China."[208] According to the social mobilization advisor of UNAIDS-China, "Activists' attitude towards each other is a major obstacle. They are combative rather than collaborative. There are a few people who try to change that, but the change has been limited. The government probably likes that, to divide and conquer."[209] An activist turned Global Fund bureaucrat thinks that AIDS CBOs and NGOs have become too preoccupied with their own survival: "Where we failed is not being self-critical and self-reflective about avoiding entitlement problem[s] and taking care too much of ourselves. Civil society is closer to reality on the ground than [the] vested interests of the government. But civil society has vested interests too. We do have pushy advocates that call the shots, not unlike losing an election. How do we get accountable for that?"[210] AIDS activists have largely not dealt with the problem of co-optation as they became entrenched.

Others pinpoint the failure of AIDS activism in holding governments accountable. "Civil society did a lot, but the goals were not reached. There is a gap between civil society at the global and national level[s]. At the global level, we know everything, but we failed at the national level. Governments signed things at the highest political level, but on the ground they did nothing. I think civil society should be stronger at the national level," says a Russian activist.[211] AIDS activism has also been uneven in terms of impact. According to a Thai activist living with AIDS: "We did a good job in terms of access to treatment. But in terms of stigma and discrimination, it's quite hard to change people's attitude in the society. Discrimination in the workplace and in schools is still going on."[212] Despite all the rhetoric, stigma remains a major barrier in the world's response to AIDS.

Above all, many activists lament the fact that their work has not brought about systemic and sustainable change. In many countries, AIDS activism remains a pocket of relatively well-funded activities, but it has failed to change the health system and it has failed to build a mass movement to engage all of society. "PLWHA groups were not able to be involved with groups with larger interests. Mainstream movements have not done a very good job of working with people living with HIV and that includes the People's Health Movement. The problem lies [on] both sides. We have struggled for years in India to involve HIV groups," says a member of the People's Health Movement.[213] The director of the HIV/AIDS Group of UNDP also thinks that "there have been real serious shortcomings in how AIDS activists have not connected with other activists. There is a lot of animosity between AIDS and gender [activists], for example. Even when alliances were built, they were not necessarily helpful."[214]

"Civil society didn't manage to change systemic issues, such as the global economic structure," adds a Chinese activist. "We need to change priorit[ies]. This is not just an AIDS issue. It's about our lifestyle, consumption, the environment, etc. But these cannot be solved by civil society. These are structural issues about the relationships between economics, politics, and society."[215] The co-founder of the Health and Development Network believes that there needs to be an analysis of the social determinants of health: "We have not really looked at that either. A couple of discourses have continued, separate from AIDS, that I think . . . are very contemporary and very relevant. We need to get AIDS into those discussions as quickly as possible, so that there is a real exchange of views. The emerging nations look at the response to HIV, [and] it is very top-down. Someone [has] to marry these cultures together."[216] Above all, a veteran activist questions whether the AIDS movement will be able to sustain its effectiveness through institutionalizing change:

> The big question within AIDS is how much of the change we push for has been institutionalized and will be lasting. The public health clause within TRIPS is critical, but it is part of the TRIPS agreement. It is institutionalized and is a big gain in one sense, but the question is how many countries use it. The Brazilians told me their government negotiated seventy voluntary licenses, and the government wouldn't even tell them about them. So the achievement of getting it into a treaty

is a gain, but the enforcement and implementation of those provisions by countries is contingent. In terms of gains, the less [we rely] upon a system that is tied to current political power, the better. I think it is too early to tell. We have to come back in ten years and see how much change remains.[217]

As with all other social movements, AIDS activists face the classic challenges of choosing depth versus breadth, single-issue advocacy versus broad-based coalition, short-term gains versus systemic change.

Despite the movement's significant achievements, the challenges facing AIDS activists are enormous. Internally, much remains to be done to build leadership and movement sustainability through governance reform, management training, evaluation, and transition planning. "HIV/AIDS has become so complicated. Sometimes it's beyond the capacity of our staff to follow [the] changing issues. We have a large number of members. Even conveying a message from the management team to the field is a challenge," says the executive director of the Thai Network of People Living with HIV/AIDS.[218] The majority of AIDS groups have little management training and no evaluation system in place. As an activist with the European AIDS Treatment Group reflects:

> The most important card civil society can play is its credibility. People are incredibly motivated and convinced about what they do. They don't necessarily use the best methods to do that though. When you look at HIV NGOs, maybe NGOs everywhere, they all have trouble with management, organization, and governance structure. This is a continuous challenge, an inherent problem in NGOs, because people working in NGOs are not bankers. They do their work for a different reason, and the reason is motivation. But passion doesn't mean expertise . . . I think an organization needs to have [the] capacity to reflect on itself, to be open to internal and external criticism. This is incredibly difficult for an organization driven by people's passions.[219]

With a complex scientific and funding scene and a huge number of actors, almost all AIDS movements and networks have been forced to reflect on organizational and governance structures and grapple with the demands of professionalization in all aspects of their work, from fundraising to evaluation.[220] A co-founder of ITPC recalls: "[The] ITPC founders had some big questions about our organizational structure. There was a split between people like David Barr, who was very invested in giving money to small groups, [and] others, [who thought] we should focus more on advocacy rather than community grant giving."[221]

Smaller CBOs and NGOs face serious issues of high staff turnover, lack of experience especially in connecting to the global level, and language and communication. The social mobilization advisor of UNAIDS-China observes:

> Chinese CBOs and NGOs are generally reactive, not proactive. Most of the responses are critical rather than constructive. Most of them are detached from global developments [because of] serious issues of language and communication. Those who are capable of [plugging] in to the international level do not share the information locally. It's an issue of competition, of keeping the information so that they [can] get the resources. The regional networks tend to rely on one or two people and don't plug into the national networks. In that sense, they don't really represent China. There are isolated examples of highly effective individuals, e.g., Thomas Cai's group, AIDS Care, [which advocates] behind the scenes about drug quality and second-line treatment. They [have] produce[d] very good reports in the field and submit[ted] them to the National Center for AIDS, and the government looked into the issues. Thomas himself is well respected and had some successes, but we can't say that for AIDS civil society as a whole.[222]

A GNP+ activist concurs: "As a global organization, we have information, and our advocacy informs our experiences at the country level. GNP+ has been great at research, but it was not sure how to get it back down to the community. The question is to what extent there is a dual flow. One of our greatest challenges is ensuring that the voices of [people] living with HIV are represented and to make sure that we are able to honestly use the data that we gather and use it to good effect."[223]

Externally, the biggest challenges are financial, social, economic, and political sustainability and democratic governance. AIDS funding is likely to continue to decrease in the context of economic crises in donor countries and HIV fatigue. One Thai activist is highly critical of the UN's tokenistic rhetoric about civil society's "capacity building":

> Thirty years into the epidemic, we are still talking about capacity building, stigma and discrimination, and issues in community settings. People should look at how capacity building has been done and look at how skills have been built. I am not sure how much assessment has been done about how civil society has actually participated. What has all this representation on PCB, [the] Global Fund, and CCMs meant? People have been used as tokens. There is still a critical gap. We are made to be present so that [the agencies] could say civil society has been consulted, but how much have we effectively participated and contributed? So much money is invested in

building the capacity of the community, but look at who the implementers of [this] skill building are: fly-by international consultants. What is the problem? What needs to happen?[224]

Besides capacity building, another broad sustainability issue concerns the ability of the AIDS movement to institutionalize its political power beyond sporadic gains over a specific law or policy. An ACT UP activist says:

> One of the biggest challenges in the work of ACT UP was understanding how to create [a] lasting framework for achieving political power. ACT UP burned brightly and burned out. . . . It was too intense for people, I think. It was too charged to take a step back to think how we were going to extend it. The right wing, to all our detriment in the US, had only one goal of extending their power, and for forty years they have been doing it. Nothing comes without a struggle. Poor people are not going to get anything unless they have political power. Elites remain as elites. It is all about political power. You can be the smartest activist, but it is about achieving political power. . . . The AIDS movement has achieved some political power, but it is episodic. It is not sustained.[225]

AIDS activism continues to be challenged by structural economic and political barriers that are beyond the scope of the epidemic. "From the perspectives of MSF, the biggest barrier to a world without AIDS is poverty," says a South African representative of MSF's Access Campaign. "It is very difficult to run HIV programs in poor areas. When you look at the massive issues that people face on a daily basis, you realize [that] poverty fuels HIV and impedes the HIV response. That's why HIV is the most severe in the poorest areas in Asia and Africa."[226] The lack of democratic governance in many countries also makes it difficult for civil society to sustain its work. Government hostility, opposition, and censorship come in different forms, including a lack of legal registration, funding shortages, and criminalization. The MSF–South Africa representative continues: "Government leadership is a huge issue. We see how governments are scaling back. Governments used to say: 'We can't invest in something if we don't know if it works.' Now we know it works. We do have the science and the ARVs. But we are still not seeing government investment. There is a great deal of apathy at the national level."[227]

The country coordinator of UNAIDS-Egypt says: "I wouldn't say civil society failed. It has to do with the political environment, the fact that civil society has so little space. It could have done so much more if [it] had more space."[228] In Russia, AIDS activists find it difficult to work with an intransigent government that maintains that it does not need any foreign money or assistance. The vice president and regional director of the Global Business Coalition for Health, Russia, despairs: "We have the impression that these people who sit at the high level in the government don't care how they look to [the] international community. This is absolutely a very bad thing about Russian policy, not just HIV. You are constantly knocking your head [on] a closed door. You spend a lot of resources and efforts with zero results. You make one step forward, but lots of steps back."[229] One of the biggest lessons that has been learned in AIDS activism is that hard-won gains in discursive, funding, policy, and legal changes can only go so far if broader issues of democratic governance are not addressed. An ACT UP activist reflects:

> There is no such thing as an international community. It is lovely to have international law, but we basically work on a nation-state model still. The international community has no obligations to its citizens; national governments do. Constitutions like the ones in Brazil and South Africa are . . . explicit . . . with the right to health. The movement for treatment access, including the Thais, Brazilians, and Ugandans, . . . all this was happening at the national level. . . . When the AIDS conference happened in Durban in 2000 with the protest against Mbeki, [the] Treatment Action Campaign had already been [around] for several years. The treatment movement was all driven by Thailand, Brazil, Uganda, and South Africa. So the Global Fund didn't just come out of some sort of beneficent grand idea in Geneva. There was already a tidal wave of support. So the international changes were born from the tidal wave of treatment activism at the country level, but they live and die by it too. A banker is now in charge of the Global Fund, and there is very little we can do about it because national movements are much weaker compared to ten years ago. The key lesson is that where we succeeded, we were able to enshrine institutional change that was not contingent on contemporary political power. So it is better if you [can] change a law, win court cases, something that is binding. If it is tied to congressional appropriations, like the Global Fund, [that] means that when you lose your political power, you lose your gains. The treatment gains in South Africa are something very concrete, but now there are attacks on the judiciary, which [has] nothing to do with AIDS. If the rule of law backs off in South Africa, everything else backs off too. So even institutional gains depend on the larger context of democratic governance.[230]

The AIDS community emerged in the 1980s out of a great urgency to meet unfulfilled needs on the ground. The global AIDS response would not have been the same without sustained community interventions. While the achievements of AIDS activists are impressive—from voice to advocacy and from representation to a knowledge paradigm shift—the power dynamics in the community are rarely discussed. Along the way to challenging the monopoly of power by scientists, Pharma, and a traditional global health governance structure, AIDS activists have created their own regime of power to control the community's identity and boundaries. The competition for resources and recognition has led to compromises, exclusions, and discrimination among the movement's constituents. How the AIDS movement can sustain its participation and legitimacy by showing evidence and yet not succumb to a "value for money" logic is an urgent question. Only critical self-reflection and mechanisms for internal and external accountability will guard against the pitfalls of an expertization of AIDS activism.

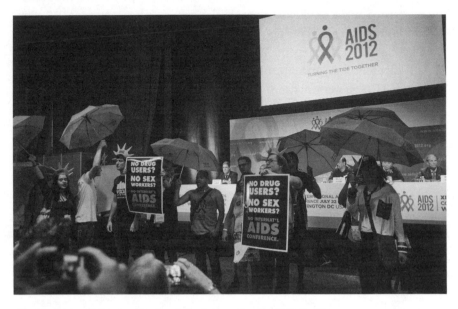

No Drug Users? No Sex Workers? No International AIDS Conference

Photo © International AIDS Society / Deborah W. Campos—Commercialimage.net

CHAPTER SIX

Conclusion

Knowledge and Inclusion in Global Governance

What does need to be questioned, however, is the mode of representation of otherness.
 —*Homi K. Bhabha*, The Location of Culture

TAC would not have been as successful without simplifying the
knowledge and giving back the power to where it belongs, which is
the people.
 —*General Secretary, Treatment Action Campaign*

We raised the bar. Civil society mobilization around HIV has done
so much to teach others and connect with health activists to deal
with other issues.
 —*Senior Researcher, AIDS*
 Accountability International

AIDS exploded into the world over thirty years ago, forcing us to respond. I began this book with vignettes of civil disobedience and direct action by activists
of ACT UP, the Thai Network of People Living with AIDS, and the International
Treatment Preparedness Coalition in Washington, DC, Bangkok, and Vienna
three decades apart, and I asked the question: What role has AIDS activism played
in reforming global AIDS governance?

I have focused on AIDS activists' interventions in four areas—science, market, governance, and community—and analyzed competing narratives of the at-
risk body, intellectual property, governance, and the community "we." I have argued for the role of AIDS activists in knowledge making, breaking open the
cultural and political boundaries of existing systems of power through a new pathway of legitimacy based on human rights. In this final chapter, I summarize their
interventions and conclude by discussing four policy recommendations: diversify

global governance, operationalize human rights standards, move beyond the existing IP regime, and decolonize community development.

AIDS as Legitimation Crises: The Human Rights Pathway to Legitimacy

Few issues troubled the medical and scientific establishment in any fundamental way until AIDS. The infamous Tuskegee experiment, a clinical study by the US Public Health Service between 1932 and 1972 on the natural progression of syphilis, involved 600 poor, rural, Black men without informing them or treating them with penicillin, and led to major changes in scientific protocols on participant protection in clinical studies. But it was AIDS in the 1980s that opened up and transformed a closed, elitist scientific system for the first time. This vast system—operating with self-referential and legitimating rules, extensive resources, and competitive reward mechanisms—named and defined AIDS, collected data, tracked down and monitored at-risk populations, conducted clinical trials, and controlled drug approvals. According to Epstein, AIDS activists were able to penetrate the tight-knit scientific community through four pathways to credibility: by teaching themselves and appropriating the languages and cultures of biomedicine; by insisting that they were "obligatory passage points" as research subjects; by adding moral arguments to methodological design; and by seizing on preexisting lines of cleavage in the scientific establishment, tipping the balance for change.[1] AIDS activists were the first patients who became as knowledgeable about their disease as the scientists were, who challenged the CDC's definition of AIDS, who won the right to an "advisory jurisdiction" in the scientific and pharmaceutical establishments,[2] who successfully expanded the inclusion criteria for clinical trials, and who dramatically sped up drug approvals.

But activists did a lot more. They had to because the AIDS crisis revealed more than credibility struggles within science. They forged a new pathway to legitimacy by injecting new knowledges: alternative discourses based on the lived experiences of marginalized populations and on larger human rights frames. This new pathway based on human rights goes beyond appropriating the existing knowledges and cultures of biomedicine; it has created a new language and culture in science, market, and governance. Patients and their advocates are not only just as knowledgeable about the scientific aspects of AIDS, thereby pushing the scientific establishment to be more inclusive and effective; they also have forced science to be open to nonscientific frames of reference based on human rights. People living with AIDS are involved in the design of clinical trials both because it makes better science, and out of the GIPA principle. Similarly, the airtight free market/

free trade regime espoused by the WTO, WIPO, the US trade representative, and the EU commissioner for trade has been influenced by the development and public health concerns of the South not because it makes better trade, but because even the WTO now recognizes that intellectual property protection has a negative impact on prices and on access to essential medicines. And the seventy-year-old statist United Nations has seen its various governance structures pried open, not because donors and governments were ready to yield power to nonstate actors, but because it is no longer seen to be legitimate to be operating without the involvement of those most impacted by AIDS. These incursions into the age-old recalcitrant power structures of science, market, and governance are no small victories for the AIDS movement.

In science, one of the most significant interventions of activists has been to challenge its organizing principles and concept of risks. The scientific classification of AIDS risks sets the parameters for surveillance and reporting, determines funding, delineates the contours of AIDS prevention education, and has been used by the court system to normalize and regulate the sexual behavior of people living with AIDS. While some scientists continue to rely on a narrow epidemiological approach to AIDS risks by singling out various "most-at-risk populations," activists continue to fight back with a human rights approach to HIV, focusing on structural vulnerability, discrimination, recognition, and equitable participation. Instead of blaming marginalized populations as being inherently risky, AIDS activists counter this limited and problematic approach by expanding the discourse to include structural factors, such as poverty, unemployment, violence, gender and racial discrimination, unequal opportunities, and other kinds of social exclusions that render these groups more vulnerable to HIV infection. A significant aspect of AIDS activism has been the fight not only for the rights of people living with AIDS, but also for nondiscrimination and the decriminalization of all marginalized populations. Gay men quickly disassociated AIDS from their stigmatized identity by proposing the more neutral term "men who have sex with men," and in some cases, like India, homosexuality has been decriminalized thanks to AIDS activism. Similarly, people who use drugs have been successful to some extent in replacing the traditional biomedical model of forced rehabilitation with an evidence-based harm reduction model, even though a forty-year-old "war on drugs" ideology remains firmly entrenched in UNODC, in the United States, and in many other countries. Sex workers too have managed to put sex work on the global agenda despite great resistance in certain UN bodies and in a great majority of member states. When the battle over the scientific definition of risk is fought in courtrooms, people living with AIDS and legal advocacy networks have fought unjust and ineffective laws built on arbitrary definitions of risk that are applied to already highly marginalized populations.

In the market, while international development activists were the first to expose the democratic deficit of a free trade regime based on the interests of the North,[3] it was AIDS and public health activists who mobilized and successfully challenged TRIPS through the 2001 Doha Declaration, which specifically allows WTO members to use a range of flexibilities, including compulsory licensing and parallel importing, to protect public health and to promote access to medicines. The AIDS community never managed to scrap TRIPS or the WTO—"the rot at the core of global governance today," according to one activist[4]—but the increasing use of compulsory licensing shows that the legal and normative shift from an IP regime to a right-to-health framework has had material consequences for the lives of people living with AIDS in many middle-income countries. Between 2006 and 2012, Thailand, Brazil, South Africa, India, Indonesia, and Ecuador issued compulsory licenses for AIDS and cancer drugs, enabling them to sustain their treatment programs. At the national level, HIV patients and AIDS advocacy networks have filed successful lawsuits against Pharma for frivolous patenting and evergreening. Governments with generic manufacturing capability, such as Thailand and Brazil, now produce generic fixed-dose combinations of ARV drugs, greatly reducing each nation's health budget. Activists in Thailand, India, Brazil, and China have filed pre- and post-grant patent oppositions not only on pharmaceutical arguments but also on public health grounds.

The IP versus right-to-health battle is far from over, however. Pharma continues to outsmart AIDS activists by filing more patent applications, taking governments to court for IP infringement, using diplomatic pressure, and lobbying for wide-ranging TRIPS-plus measures in the proliferating bilateral and regional trade agreements. Meanwhile, some activists have pushed for innovative mechanisms, such as the Medicines Patent Pool, trying to change industry norms so that generic companies can enter the market, driving down costs and expanding access to essential ARV drugs. So far, two companies—Gilead and ViiV Healthcare—have entered into licensing agreements with the MPP to expand the market's access to tenofovir and pediatric abacavir, respectively. The devil of such industry engagement is always in the details. Gilead has been criticized for excluding many middle-income countries with high disease burdens in the licensing agreements and for limiting generic production to Indian companies only. The drug-by-drug, patent-by-patent approach, while incredibly important, is too piecemeal and too slow to meet the needs of the 10 million people still in need of treatment, not counting those currently in first-line treatment who may require costly and largely inaccessible second-line and third-line drugs. The patent landscape is no doubt still largely in favor of Big Pharma.

In governance, AIDS activists were not the first to expose the ineffectiveness, democratic deficit, and legitimation crisis of the outdated UN model. Environmentalists and other development activists knocked on the doors of the World Bank to challenge its lending policies and structural adjustment programs long before AIDS activists did. But it was AIDS activists who successfully fought for representation on UN governance structures and thereby asserted their role in setting the global AIDS agenda. This is no small change, and NGOs are now more than just grant recipients and service providers who loiter in UN corridors waiting for a handout. They are legitimate actors who sit at the table next to ministers and UN bureaucrats and who bring their own knowledges and perspectives to various state-dominated intergovernmental structures. Civil society representation and participation has profoundly changed the UN response to the epidemic, cajoling it out of lethargy and complacency. The presence of civil society has moved AIDS beyond a narrow epidemiological frame into a top global security and political issue; has helped AIDS to gain more funding than any other global health issue, including maternal and child health, diarrhea, TB, and malaria, all of which kill more people each year than HIV; and has added new legal and discursive frames to understanding AIDS as a public health and human rights issue. More fundamentally, AIDS activism has changed the meaning of "governance" from a power-based to a rights-based concept. Assuming equal capacity—no small caveat—civil society's vote in principle carries the same weight as that of the United States, again not because it necessarily makes better governance, but because the human rights principles of the right to participation and equitable representation demand its inclusion. Civil society continues to advocate for tighter donor coordination; the harmonizing of governance structures; health system integration and national leadership; reforming the IP regime and engaging more with the private sector; and promoting the genuine capacity building of civil society organizations.

In terms of community, AIDS activists did not invent community development, but they did transform the landscape by bringing in funding, strengthening capacity, building and transmitting knowledge, organizing and empowering the members, networking, representing, and advocating. Along the way, as they cracked open various systems of power, however, AIDS activists turned themselves into experts, consultants, grantees, partners, and bureaucrats, creating their own scientific knowledge bases, economy, and politics and thereby legitimating a new social system in the name of community. Subtle techniques of power based on the GIPA principle, North-South divisions, class, race, gender, age, and ideology now are applied by activists themselves in order to control the borders and identity of this non-monolithic movement. A new pathway to legitimacy based on human rights principles, while demanding that science, market, and governance be inclusive, also requires the AIDS community to be accountable to itself and to other stakeholders.

In sum, what AIDS activism has achieved is more than inclusion in clinical trials, increased funding, treatment access, and a foot inside the United Nations. More fundamentally, it has revealed the deep legitimation crises of four contemporary regimes of power—scientific monopoly, market fundamentalism, statist governance, and community control—and, in very concrete ways, challenged their power by imposing rights-based rules of legitimation. The case of AIDS activism is instructive for other social movements: activism can play a role in diversifying and democratizing existing power structures by changing the representation of traditionally marginalized actors through a new pathway to legitimacy. In contrast to coercive power and traditional political authority, activists rely on four new bases or benchmarks of legitimacy: credibility, democratic principles and processes, moral acceptability, and human rights.

Lessons Learned and Policy Implications

Arguing for an agenda based on human rights is not new. Jonathan Mann laid out a vast program before his untimely death in 1998. In the conclusion of his exceedingly important analysis of health and structural violence in *Pathologies of Power* (2003), Paul Farmer forwarded six suggestions for marrying health and human rights: engage health professionals in human rights work broadly defined; work with community-based organizations to provide services to remediate inequalities of access; establish new research agendas to incorporate human rights questions; assume a broader human rights education mandate; maintain independence from powerful states and bureaucracies; and secure more resources for health and human rights. I build on these ideas and propose four further actions to realize and expand the pathway to legitimacy for civil society based on human rights. These four pillars should be considered together, since strengthening one—in particular, the first one, about getting a seat at the table—leads to greater gains in the others.

New "Tea Party": Diversify and Democratize Global Governance

AIDS activism has clearly shown that life is far too important to be left in the hands of experts, the market, and international bureaucrats. The victories in funding, treatment access, and shared governance were all possible because people affected by the epidemic had a seat at the AIDS tea party. How we ensure that this representation and participation becomes a permanent feature or, in other words, how we deal with a politics of difference in global governance is one of the greatest challenges of all global justice movements.

Since the 1990s, two parallel discourses have emerged—one based on functional grounds and the other on equity principles—to push for a democratization of global governance. On the one hand, a broad policy community on aid effectiveness, largely driven by the North, including donors, UN agencies, governments, and development activists, has argued for diversity in global aid architecture in order to improve the quality and impact of aid ("aid works when we work together").[5] The 2005 Paris Declaration and the 2008 Accra Agenda for Action, "born out of decades of experience of what works and what doesn't for development," both emphasize inclusive partnerships.[6] On the other hand, health activism has led to support for "bio-multiculturalism" and limited governance pluralism based on principles of recognition and equitable representation.[7]

While a variety of innovative health partnerships have broadened the participation of different actors from the private sector and community-based organizations, Richter cautions that these fundraising, research, or consultative partnerships are not in themselves inherently diverse, as the assumption of a shared governance structure suggests.[8] Instead, she warns that unequal power and conflicts of interest can mask the true nature and impact of these much-lauded partnerships, and she recommends specific safeguards for public interests. Rather than pushing for specific partnerships, what is needed is a set of organizing principles and institutional developments to diversify and democratize global governance. These include, first, liberation from the political privilege of sovereignty, as Agamben suggests.[9] The Westphalian model of state sovereignty is far from crumbling, but in a network model of governance, states are only one set of actors. Nonstate actors should be able to compete for power and influence with their own legitimacy based on credibility, democratic principles, moral acceptability, and human rights.

Second, "postcolonialism begins from its own knowledges."[10] Democratizing global governance entails a decolonization of the Other—whether they are people living with AIDS, TB, or malaria; sex workers; drug users; gay men; transgender people; migrant workers; youth or children; or other marginalized populations—by recognizing their knowledges and lived experiences. Third, a network of public spheres and deliberative institutions, separate from traditional hierarchical structures, needs to be developed to ensure the meaningful participation of nonstate actors. Finally, accountability mechanisms are essential to ensure transparency and effectiveness. These four principles of recognition, representation, participation, and accountability form the cornerstones of a post-Westphalian governance architecture.

Rights 'R' Us: Operationalize Human Rights across Science, Market, Governance, and Community

Recognizing civil society as a legitimate actor can only go so far if human rights standards remain high-sounding principles in thick volumes of international conventions, declarations, and resolutions. Human rights principles must be operationalized across science, market, governance, and community in concrete laws, policies, and programs. It is one thing for activists to successfully reframe AIDS (or any other global issue) as a human rights problem at the global level, and quite another for them to be able to mobilize for change on the ground if the right in question is not institutionalized in the scientific establishment, pharmaceutical companies, intergovernmental organizations, and community-based structures. The persistent stigma and discrimination surrounding AIDS, despite UN leadership on the issue and community mobilization, is a reminder that the fight against the epidemic is far from over because human rights protections for marginalized populations are still lacking in the majority of countries. Pharma's lack of concern for public health beyond bottom-line thinking is another indicator that unless all major systems of power are made accountable to human rights norms, progress remains piecemeal and temporary.

In AIDS activism, some of the most significant victories—a free public ARV access program in Brazil; universal HIV treatment and public medical insurance in Thailand; the passage of the Medicines Amendment Act in South Africa to increase ARV access; and successful patent oppositions in India—happened when the right to health was enshrined in either the constitution, laws, policies, or amended patent acts. Unfortunately, local activists cannot expect UN agencies to come to their rescue when a drug user or sex worker is arrested or imprisoned. A UN diplomat in Southeast Asia recognizes: "You need to take positions on HIV but the UN is not good at that. Everything at the UN depends on consensus. All member states have to sign up—even though, of course, some member states are more vocal than others. This makes it hard to take leadership on an issue—you can't stand up and speak out because you can't criticise any member government."[11] Ensuring that human rights principles are institutionalized in national systems will allow activists to mobilize around AIDS broadly, addressing all the risk factors that structure vulnerability, including criminalization, gender-based violence, racism, poverty, underdevelopment, and other forms of social exclusion.

One of the perennial tensions in activism is the global-local gap: how much attention should be paid to activism at the global versus the national level, and how to ensure that gains at the global level get translated into national change. Globalists believe in the strategic importance of global agenda setting and framing while local activists argue that the most material gains having the greatest impact on people's lives are overwhelmingly at the national level. The mobilization around human rights by AIDS activists has shown that both are necessary and complementary. Without global human rights norms, national governments can more easily brush off activists' claims. And yet activists alone cannot hold the United Nations accountable. Only national laws, policies, and programs can ensure their hard-won rights.

The domestication and operationalization of human rights norms is a long political process that requires educational and mobilization efforts. Here again AIDS activism has taught a great lesson: the efficacy of treatment literacy in informing and empowering the patient to demand her basic citizenship rights, including the right to health, the right to information, and the right to life. Broad human rights literacy, tied to the lived experiences of marginalized people, is the anchor of all global activism and therefore should be funded, systematized, and expanded. The history of AIDS activism shows that rights are never bestowed by governments, corporations, or UN institutions. If a rights language is now part and parcel of any AIDS discourse, it is because affected communities and their advocacy networks demanded it.

Elephant in the Room: Move beyond an Intellectual Property Regime

Even if civil society can now exercise its own legitimacy in any global arena, and even if human rights standards are institutionalized in concrete laws and policies, there remains the elephant in the room: an intact IP regime firmly entrenched in the WTO and in most national patent laws. AIDS activism has shown that it is urgent to move beyond the existing IP paradigm through a variety of financing and coordination mechanisms.

In this book I briefly looked at voluntary licensing and the Medicines Patent Pool as examples of measures to circumvent the absolute IP protection of patent holders. Other mechanisms include non-assert declarations, where a patent holder does not enforce its rights against the agreement partner. These are grossly insufficient, however. As MSF argues, pharmaceutical companies negotiate voluntary licenses as leverage over their competitors, with different geographical scopes as their "red lines." Voluntary licenses do not address the problem of access in excluded countries.[12] The MPP was set up to change industry norms by negotiating with Pharma from a public health perspective, but so far only two companies have come forward with the patents for only a limited number of ARV drugs.

Another facet of the access problem concerns the absence of market development and funding for the longer-term medical R&D needs of developing countries. This issue was thoroughly investigated by the Consultative Expert Working Group on Research and Development (CEWG), established by the World Health Assembly in 2010. The CEWG recognizes both an economic problem (the current incentives based on an IP regime fail to correct the complete neglect of developing countries' needs) and a moral one (the technologies to develop life-saving products exist, and yet millions die for lack of access to them).[13] Its 2012 report recommends six concrete measures to circumvent the IP regime: patent pools; an international convention on R&D for diseases prevalent in developing countries; open approaches to research and development in order to delink R&D costs from product prices to promote access; direct grants to companies to promote capacity building and technology transfer to developing countries; pooled funding from various sources to subsidize R&D costs; and milestone prizes and end prizes to provide incentives to researchers, especially those in developing countries. All of these measures require sustainable sources of funding, which, according to the CEWG, could include a new indirect tax (on arms trade, alcohol or tobacco sales, airline tickets, internet traffic, or bank transactions); voluntary consumer and business contributions (like Product Red); taxation on foreign pharmaceutical company profits (a proposal from Brazil); and new funds from nontraditional donors, like China and Venezuela.[14]

It is clear that unless urgent actions are taken in the next few years—more voluntary licenses covering larger territories, a lot more companies entering into agreements with the MPP and/or initiating non-assert declarations, and new funding to finance some of the CEWG's proposed incentive measures to correct market failures—a massive treatment time bomb is likely to go off in a decade or so. A 2009 study by the UK All-Party Parliamentary Group on HIV and AIDS estimates that by 2030 over 50 million people will need HIV treatment compared to just 9 million who need it today. Many of those needing treatment in the future will also need more expensive medicines, having developed resistance to basic HIV therapy. The combination of more people needing more complex treatment means that unless Pharma is willing to cut prices, the world faces a larger-than-ever treatment crisis.[15]

Access to treatment is a human rights nonnegotiable, and the existing IP regime remains a major barrier. One of the greatest legacies of AIDS activism is to have exposed the emperor with no clothes: the lie undergirding the global regime that IP is necessary so that pharmaceutical companies can recoup high R&D and production costs. Generic competition, making the same drugs available for pennies, has helped destroy that myth. The time has now come for taking concrete, bold actions.

Off the Wrong Bus: Decolonize Community Development

Community development did not begin, nor will it end, with AIDS. More than three decades of activism have only confirmed what was already known, although not yet accomplished: changes are only sustainable if they are rooted in communities. "Community development," a concept and practice developed in the heyday of the postcolonial 1960s, had already become a cliché before AIDS. While folklore, symbols, dances, stories, ceremonies, customs, and dialects once occupied only the margins of the dominant knowledge systems of the West, "community" gained political saliency with the international development regime. Suddenly, it became associated with all things positive: community participation, capacity building, sustainable development, empowerment, alternatives to the dominant economic and political systems, community learning, and transformation. AIDS did create an unexpected political opportunity for various communities to organize themselves and act collectively. But the bureaucratic and political landscape of AIDS also meant that community development quickly became a funding category, an object of knowledge for regulation and control, a checkbox for international agencies and big INGOs, and an internal technique of power for activists' self-discipline ("my mandate is to develop 'my community' because it is the outcome that donors want to see"). AIDS has helped to develop not only communities, but also a community development industry worldwide.

In the fourth decade of the epidemic, a decolonization of the concept and praxis of community development is in order. If neo-colonialism means "crushing objecthood" and a colonization of the mind through the imposition of the legal, economic, and cultural systems of the North, community development needs to be guided by a radically different set of principles for community sovereignty and cultural diversity. The great Kenyan Nobel Peace Prize laureate, Wangari Maathai, who died in 2011, analogized the problem as being "on the wrong bus." She writes:

"For five centuries, the outside world has been telling Africans who they are. . . . All local populations became perpetual students of the new knowledge and wisdom. Inherent in the very nature of being a learner and not a teacher is an inability to be master of one's own world. . . . One is forever being led, forever having to look for guidance from someone else, forever vulnerable to a master's misinformation or exploitation."[16] She questions how much good versus damage has been done in the name of community development: "As it is, Africa is like a person who's fallen into a hole. Someone is telling her, 'I'll throw you a rope so you can get out.' While the rope provided is never quite long enough for her to grab on to it, it's long enough so she has a hope of reaching it. At the same time, the person holding the rope has thrown down a spade, and is encouraging the person in the hole to dig herself in deeper." Maathai urges us to think beyond "aid effectiveness," donor-driven agendas, and a culture of dependency. She recognizes, "Nevertheless, the culture of aid is hard to change. The international community often expects fast returns from its development investments, but the problems of underdevelopment, marginalization, lack of self-esteem, fear, and cynicism didn't afflict Africa's peoples yesterday—indeed, they have accumulated over centuries. This is a reality the international community understands but doesn't always acknowledge."[17]

The community plays far too important a role for it to be left to the dictates of donors. While science continues to provide new tools to combat the disease, the keys to the removal of some of the greatest remaining obstacles to universal access lie in the community. "We should be winning in HIV prevention," the Global HIV Prevention Working Group writes in 2007. "There are effective means to prevent every mode of transmission; political commitment on HIV has never been stronger; and financing for HIV programs in low- and middle-income countries increased six-fold between 2001 and 2006."[18] Yet we are still faltering. Only massive community mobilization around stigma, discrimination, testing, treatment adherence, treatment literacy, and rights knowledge will achieve the goal of an AIDS-free generation in my children's lifetime.

To move beyond the colonialist teacher-learner relationship in which most communities live, many things need to happen, including leadership, funding, and institutionalization. Wangari Maathai pinpoints the "leadership deficit" in Africa, but notes a few successful examples of community development, such as her own Green Belt Movement and the Constituency Development Fund, where communities define their own development agenda and assume responsibilities as well as assert their rights. On the ground, numerous other initiatives are based on the principle of community sovereignty. The Collaborative Fund of ITPC is a community-driven funding mechanism that gives small grants to CBOs for HIV treatment advocacy and education projects and supports regional networks to share information, implement collaborative strategies, and provide technical assistance to grantees. It was created out of the realization that "we are our own cure, that we use our voices to educate and advocate, and that we will realize our goals."[19] The Dongzhen Center for Human Rights Education and Action, a small CBO in Beijing that encourages human rights dialogues between China and the world, runs a bookstore and café as part of a social enterprise to sustain its advocacy activities. The Tajik Network of Women Living with HIV/AIDS, based in Dushanbe, is in part financially supported by a clinic run by its founder that provides regular medical services to the community for a fee.

Above all, as they move from a creativity phase to a consolidation phase, many AIDS CBOs have to manage the mundane steps of growth and institutionalization, including legal registration, accounting and management development, governance review, and passing on the torch, all of which require a certain minimum democratic governance and broader civil society development at the country level. In this regard, community development is a holistic concept that involves not only the local, but also continuous advocacy at the national, regional, and global levels. Civil society in itself is not a substitute for democratic governance, an Indian activist cautions.[20] How to foster genuine community building while at the same time putting in place different checks and balances to hold the community accountable is one of the great challenges for the global AIDS movement.

AIDS activism raised the bar. Drawing on broad human rights frames and producing their own knowledges to legitimize their new identity and role, activists did much to change the culture, business, and politics of science, market, governance, and community. While AIDS activism did force some limited pluralism in the dominant systems of power, there are already signs of retreat. Donors are more concerned about the burning crises in their backyards than about sick patients waiting in line for treatment. Innovative funding partnerships have returned to a "value for money" model that privileges results over inclusion. Lyotard warns: "Whenever efficiency (that is, obtaining the desired effect) is derived from a 'Say or do this, or else you'll never speak again,' then we are in the realm of terror, and the social bond is destroyed."[21]

The terror of AIDS—both the morally unacceptable deaths and the corruption of power that caused them—drove my research on activism and its impact. In his magnum opus, *La Misère du Monde*, Bourdieu writes: "To subject to scrutiny the mechanisms which render life painful, even untenable, is not to neutralize them; to bring to light contradictions is not to resolve them."[22] Neither neutralizing nor resolving the complex machinations of power in the global response to AIDS, this book is a reminder of our own transient passage along the long corridor of dying.

List of Interviewees

HIV-Positive Networks and Patient-Control Movements

Delhi Network of Positive People (DNP+), President
Friends of Life, Egypt, Executive Director
Global Network of People Living with HIV/AIDS (GNP+), Technical Support Officer
International Community of Women Living with HIV/AIDS (ICW), Steering
    Committee Member
National Community of Women Living with HIV/AIDS in Uganda, Advocacy Officer
National Empowerment Network of People Living with HIV/AIDS in Kenya
    (NEPHAK), Executive Director, Finance Officer, and Assistant Program Manager
Patient-Control Movement, Russia, Activist
Tajik Network of Women Living with HIV/AIDS, Director
Thai Network of People Living with HIV/AIDS (TNP+), Executive Director

Issue-Focused Groups and Coalitions

Children Affected by AIDS

Coalition for Children Affected by AIDS, Project Coordinator

Commercial Sex Work

Al Shehab Foundation, Egypt, Co-Founder
Asia Pacific Network of Sex Workers, Executive Director
China Sex Worker Organization Network Forum, Chief
RedTraSex, Founder and Executive Director
Sex Workers Education and Advocacy Taskforce (SWEAT), South Africa, Advocacy Officer

Cross-Issue Coalition

7 Sisters, Regional Program Coordinator

Gender and Prevention of Mother-to-Child Transmission

Astra Women's Foundation, Russia, Founder and Executive Director
Center on Mental Health and HIV/AIDS, Tajikistan, Founder and Executive Director
Mothers2Mothers (M2M), Assistant Communications Manager

Injecting Drug Use

Andrey Rylkov Foundation, Russia, Information Manager
Asian Harm Reduction Network (AHRN), former Communications Manager
Asian Network of People Who Use Drugs (ANPUD), Regional Coordinator
Eurasian Harm Reduction Network (EHRN), former Program Director
Freedom Project, Egypt, Outreach and Administrative Director
International Drug Policy Consortium, Consultant
Malaysian Network of People Who Use Drugs, Executive Director
Russian Harm Reduction Network, Executive Director and Board Chair

Men Who Have Sex with Men

ACT UP, Activist
Asia Pacific Coalition on Male Sexual Health (APCOM), Founding Member
Shanghai AIDS Prevention Center, General Manager
Tamkin Project, Project Manager

Migration

Coordination of Action Research on AIDS and Mobility (CARAM), Executive Director

Transgender People

Asia-Pacific Transgender Network, Coordinator

Youth

Global Youth Coalition on HIV/AIDS (GYCA), Co-Founder
Youth Lead, Coordinator

AIDS Prevention and Treatment Research Groups

European AIDS Treatment Group (EATG), Researcher
Global Campaign for Microbicides, Senior Program Officer
Treatment Action Group (TAG), Co-Founder

Foundations

Avahan, India, Bill and Melinda Gates Foundation, Executive Director
Open Society Foundations, China, Consultant
Open Society Foundations, International Harm Reduction Development Program,
     Director

Generic Pharmaceutical Companies and Business Coalitions

Cipla, Founder and CEO
Global Business Coalition for Health, Russia, Vice President and Regional Director
Indian Pharmaceutical Alliance, Secretary-General

International Organizations and Partnerships

Global Fund, Civil Society and Private Sector Partnerships, Manager
Global Fund, former Civil Society Team Officer

Global Health Workforce Alliance, Advisor to the Executive Director
ILO, Programme on HIV/AIDS and the World of Work, Senior Technical Advisor
Medicines Patent Pool, General Counsel
Roll Back Malaria Partnership, Executive Director
Stop TB Partnership, Executive Director
UNAIDS, Community Mobilization Chief
UNAIDS, External Relations Officer
UNAIDS-Brazil, Country Coordinator
UNAIDS-China, Social Mobilization Advisor
UNAIDS-Egypt, Country Officer
UNDP, HIV/AIDS Group, Director
UNDP-Kyrgyzstan, Global Fund Grants Program Manager
UNFPA, HIV and Key Populations, Senior Technical Advisor
UNITAID, Executive Director
UN Special Rapporteur on the Right to Health
World Health Organization, HIV/AIDS Department, Senior Advisor

Medical and Legal

Access to Medicines Research Group, China, Co-Founder
AIDS Lawyer, Shanghai
AIDS and Rights Alliance for Southern Africa (ARASA), Regional Advocacy Team
    Leader and Advocacy Officer
Canadian HIV/AIDS Legal Network, Executive Director
Lawyers Collective, India, Co-Founder
MSF-Beijing, National Program Director
MSF–Hong Kong, former Staff Member
MSF–New Delhi, Advocacy Officer
MSF–South Africa Access Campaign, Representative
Uganda Network on Law, Ethics, and HIV/AIDS (UGANET), Executive Director

Other Organizations

Action Group on Health, Human Rights, and HIV/AIDS, Uganda, Executive Director
AIDS Accountability International, Senior Researcher
Aidspan, Consultant
Aidspan, Executive Director
Chain, China, former Executive Director
Chi Heng Foundation, Executive Director
Dongzhen Center for Human Rights Education and Action, Founder and Executive
    Director
Egyptian AIDS Society, Executive Director
Egyptian Initiative for Personal Rights, Health and Discrimination Project Manager
Global Fund Watch, China, Associate Director
Health and Development Network, Co-Founder
Health Rights Action Group, Uganda, Program Officer
Israel AIDS Task Force, Executive Director
Jerusalem AIDS Project, Co-Founder
People's Health Movement, India, Member

The AIDS Support Organization (TASO), Uganda, Advocacy and Networking Team
  Leader
World AIDS Campaign (WAC), Executive Director

Scientific Researchers, Consultants, and Government Representatives

Brazilian HIV/AIDS Program, former Director
Thai Center for Disease Control, Principal Investigator
Uganda AIDS Commission, Coordinator of Advocacy and Civil Society
UNAIDS Consultant, Middle East

Treatment Access, Literacy, and Advocacy Networks

AIDS Access Foundation, Thailand, Executive Director
Brazilian Interdisciplinary AIDS Association (ABIA), Coordinator
Grupo de Trabalho sobre Propriedade Intelectual (GTPI/REBRIP; Working Group on
  Intellectual Property, Brazilian Network for the Integration of Peoples), Lawyer
Health GAP, Global Campaigns Director
International Treatment Preparedness Coalition (ITPC), Executive Director
International Treatment Preparedness Coalition (ITPC), Eastern Europe and Central
  Asia, Advocacy Officers 1 and 2
International Treatment Preparedness Coalition (ITPC), Latin America, Coordinator
Kenya Treatment Access Movement (KETAM), Executive Director
Knowledge Ecology International (KEI), Campaigner
Treatment Action Campaign (TAC), South Africa, General Secretary

Chapter 1 · Introduction

Epigraph. http://filmmakermagazine.com/1775-necrorealism [accessed Jan. 5, 2013].

1. http://www.actupny.org/documents/FDAhandbook1.html [accessed Jan. 5, 2013].

2. Epstein 1996.

3. Harden 2012.

4. http://www.essentialdrugs.org/edrug/archive/199912/msg00060.php [accessed Jan. 5, 2013].

5. http://isites.harvard.edu/fs/docs/icb.topic1146995.files/Session%208%20-%20Oct%2023/Nathan%20Ford%20et%20al%20-%20The%20Role%20of%20Civil%20Society%20in%20Protecting%20Public%20Health%20over%20Commercial%20Interests.pdf [accessed Jan. 5, 2013].

6. http://www.cptech.org/ip/health/c/thailand/arv-iprdisputes.html [accessed Jan. 5, 2013].

7. Interview with the Executive Director, AIDS Access Foundation, Dec. 2, 2011.

8. Interview with Advocacy Officer 2, ITPC, Eastern Europe and Central Asia, Sept. 26, 2011.

9. http://www.aidspan.org/gfo_article/dont-compromise-your-principles-new-funding-model-global-fund-told [accessed Jan. 5, 2013].

10. Ibid.

11. Interview with the General Secretary, TAC, May 4, 2012.

12. http://www.rusfilm.pitt.edu/booklets/Necro.pdf [accessed Jan. 5, 2013].

13. Ibid.: 8.

14. Epstein 1996: 267. For visual representations of this conflict, see the films *Dallas Buyers Club* (2013); *United in Anger: A History of ACT UP* (2012); and *Fight Back, Fight AIDS: 15 Years of ACT UP* (2004).

15. http://www.citizen.org/PC-statement-on-compulsory-licensing-in-Indonesia [accessed Jan. 5, 2013].

16. UNIFEM 2010: 25.

17. Lyotard 1984 and Rabinow 1984. I draw upon the pioneering work of Steve Epstein on the politics of AIDS knowledge. According to him, the AIDS movement was the first social movement where a "disease constituency" became an alternative basis of expertise, causing science to be "impure."

18. In the 1950s, the director of the Guggenheim Museum, James Johnson Sweeney, used the phrase "taste-breakers" to describe avant-garde artists who "break open and enlarge our artistic frontiers." I borrow from Sweeney's concept to look at the role of AIDS activists in knowledge breaking. See "Art of Another Kind: International Abstraction and the Guggenheim 1949–1960," http://www.guggenheim.org/new-york/exhibitions/past/exhibit/4462 [accessed Apr. 30, 2014].

19. Buchanan and Keohane 2006.

20. Epstein 1996.

21. See Crimp 2004 for a critique of Daniel Harris, "AIDS and Theory: Has Academic Theory Turned AIDS into Meta-Death?" (1991).

22. Foucault 1972.

23. Rabinow 1984.

24. Foucault 1978.

25. Ibid.: 96–97.

26. Castells 2010.

27. Castells 2012: 9.

28. Ibid.

29. Stoler 1995: viii.

30. Bartky 1990: 80. For other feminist critiques of Foucault on resistance and depoliticization, see Ramazanoglu 1993 and Hekman 1996.

31. Sedgwick 2008.

32. Anderson, qtd. in Stoler 1995.

33. Pepin 2011: 230.

34. Ibid.

35. Pepin 2011: 202; Farmer 1992.

36. Patton 1990 and Crimp 2004.

37. For a discussion of how a dozen multinational pharmaceutical companies managed to put intellectual property restrictions into the WTO agenda, see Sell 2003.

38. Patton 1990, 1996, 2002; Treichler 1999; Crimp 2004; and Epstein 1996.

39. Patton 1990: 131.

40. Eyerman and Jamison 1991; Melucci 1996; and Conway 2004.

41. Conway 2004: 56–58.

42. Rajagopal 2003.

43. Farmer 1992: xi.

44. Farmer 2003.

45. Briggs and Mantini-Briggs 2003: 46.

46. Millen, Fallows, and Irwin 2003; and Fort et al. 2004.

47. Derrida 1981: 28.

48. See O'Malley, Nguyen, and Lee 1996.

49. Derrida 1981.

50. Foucault 1978.

51. Interview with the President, DNP+, Nov. 8, 2011.

52. Interview with the Executive Director, Israel AIDS Task Force, June 20, 2012.

53. Interview with the Executive Director, Chi Heng Foundation, Mar. 25, 2013.

54. Buse, Hein, and Drager 2009.

55. Slaughter 2005; Held 2003; and Cerny 2005.

56. Hein, Burris, and Shearing 2009.

57. Interview with the Co-Founder of GYCA, July 3, 2012.

58. Interview with the National Project Director of MSF-Beijing, Oct. 11, 2011.

59. Human Rights Watch 2013.

60. Shilts 1987; Patton 1990; Stockdill 2002; Silversides 2003; Crimp 2004; Smith and Siplon 2006; Rau 2007; Foller and Thorn 2008; Harden 2012.

61. http://www.unaids.org/en/resources/presscentre/featurestories/2011/april /20110412refgrouphr [accessed Jan. 5 2013].

62. On South Africa, see for example, Fassin 2007 and Nattrass 2004. On China, see Sutherland and Hsu 2012 and Hood 2011. On Brazil, see Nunn 2009, and for an earlier analysis, Daniel and Parker 1993. D'Adesky 2004 does focus on activism, but is restricted to treatment issues until the early 2000s.

63. See, for example, Griffin 2000 on media analysis; and Patterson 2010 on religion and AIDS in Africa.

Chapter 2 · *Against Science*

Epigraphs. Pepin 2011: 219; Waldby 1996, qtd. in Treichler 1999: 46; and Pisani 2008: 5.

1. Sontag 1990: 93.

2. See, for example, Hunter 2003, 2005; and Guest 2003.

3. Oppenheimer 1988: 279.

4. UNICEF, UNAIDS, and WHO 2002: 6.

5. Mann 1999: 218.

6. Shilts 1987.

7. Ibid.: 96.

8. Oppenheimer 1988: 277.

9. Qtd. ibid.: 278.

10. Shilts 1987.

11. Stanton 1993: 12.

12. Qtd. in Shilts 1987: 322.

13. Ibid.

14. Sellman 2010.

15. Lawson, Lawson, and Rivers 2001.

16. http://en.wikipedia.org/wiki/Single_Convention_on_Narcotic_Drugs#cite_note -unodc2-4 [accessed Jan. 6, 2013].

17. Qtd. in UNAIDS 2011c: 198.

18. Gallahue and Lines 2010.

19. Abel et al. 2010.

20. Pepin 2011: 230.

21. Pisani 2008: 19.

22. http://www.thebody.com/content/art10223.html [accessed Jan. 6, 2013].

23. Beyrer 1998: 13.

24. http://en.wikipedia.org/wiki/Anti-prostitution_pledge [accessed Jan. 6, 2013].

25. http://www.cbsnews.com/stories/2007/04/28/national/main2738173.shtml %3e"usaid%20chief%20resigns%20over%20"d.c.%20madam"%20%20randall %20tobias%20steps%20down%20after%20name%20surfaces%20in%20call-girl

%20investigation,"%20ap%20on%20cbs%3c/a%3e%3c/p%3e%3cp%3e%3ca%20href= [accessed Jan. 6, 2013].

26. http://www.nih.gov/news/pr/nov96/niaid-27.htm [accessed Jan. 6, 2013].

27. Qtd. in Pisani 2008: 28.

28. www.tac.org.za/Documents/MTCTPrevention/mtcthist.rtf [accessed Jan. 6, 2013].

29. Fassin 2007.

30. http://www.independent.co.uk/life-style/health-and-families/features/carla -brunisarkozy-mothers-babies-and-hiv-6270099.html [accessed Jan. 6, 2013].

31. http://www.cdc.gov/globalaids/Global-HIV-AIDS-at-CDC/AIDS-free.html#sidebar [accessed Jan. 6, 2013].

32. Guest 2003: 1.

33. UNICEF 2008: 4.

34. Guest 2003: 10 and 12.

35. UNICEF, UNAIDS, and WHO 2002.

36. Ibid.

37. Ibid.

38. UNICEF and WHO 2008: 4.

39. Green 2003: 8.

40. For a brief discussion on the origins of ABC, see http://www.avert.org/abc-hiv.htm [accessed Jan. 6, 2013].

41. http://en.wikipedia.org/wiki/Joycelyn_Elders [accessed Jan. 6, 2013].

42. http://www.capitolhillblue.com/node/2368 [accessed Jan. 6, 2013].

43. http://www.huffingtonpost.com/2012/12/03/chinese-wankathon_n_2232063. html [accessed Jan. 6, 2013].

44. Stillwaggon 2003.

45. Hrdy 1987: 1112–1116, qtd. in Fassin 2007: 148; Green 2003: 11; Orubuloye et al. 1994: 45, 134, and 137, qtd. in Fassin 2007: 150; Rushton and Bogaert 1989: 1214–1218, qtd. in Fassin 2007: 151.

46. Fassin 2007: 153.

47. Guest 2003: xvi.

48. Engel 2006: 311.

49. http://www.irinnews.org/Report/96941/How-to-Map-sexual-networks [accessed Jan. 6, 2013].

50. UNAIDS 2008.

51. http://www.hivtravel.org/Default.aspx?PageId=143&Mode=list&StateId=7 [accessed Jan. 6, 2013].

52. Ibid.

53. http://www.singapore-window.org/swoo/000524ip.htm [accessed Jan. 6, 2013].

54. All-Parliamentary Group on AIDS 2003.

55. http://www.singapore-window.org/swoo/000524ip.htm [accessed Jan. 6, 2013].

56. Ibid.

57. Interview with the Executive Director of CARAM, Nov. 18, 2011.

58. Ibid.

59. Beyrer 1998: 165.

60. Desmond Tutu HIV Foundation and Joint UN Team on HIV/AIDS 2011: 33.

61. Pisani 2008: 16.

62. Beyrer 1998: 164.
63. Lyttleton 2008: 6–7.
64. Interview with an Interim Working Group Member, Asia-Pacific Transgender Network, Dec. 7, 2012.
65. Gaucher 2002: 13.
66. WHO, UNAIDS, and UNODC 2008: xiii .
67. Ibid.: 11.
68. Ibid.: xii.
69. Ibid.: 51.
70. Rabinow 1984: 17.
71. UNAIDS 2011a: 12 .
72. UNICEF, UNAIDS, and WHO 2002: 6.
73. http://www.unaids.org/en/targetsandcommitments [accessed Jan. 6, 2013].
74. UNAIDS 2011a.
75. Ibid.: 18.
76. Patton 1990: 127.
77. UNAIDS 2007: 9.
78. UNAIDS 2011a: 30.
79. UNAIDS, UNICEF, and USAID 2004.
80. UNAIDS 2011a: 4.
81. UNICEF 2009 .
82. Dreifus 1994.
83. http://www.harm-reduction.org/news/2137-the-global-fund-changed-the-eligibility-and-prioritization-criteria.html [accessed Jan. 6, 2013].
84. http://www.indicatorregistry.org [accessed Jan. 6, 2013].
85. UNAIDS 2011b.
86. http://info.worldbank.org/etools/docs/library/164047/howknow/definitions.htm [accessed Jan. 6, 2013].
87. UNAIDS 2011b.
88. UNAIDS 2011a: 125.
89. UNICEF 2002: 9.
90. Cameron, Burris, and Clayton 2008: 68.
91. Kirby 1988: 25.
92. Pearshouse 2007.
93. http://www.thecourt.ca/2012/02/07/mabior-and-d-c-does-hiv-non-disclosure-equal-rape-part-1 [accessed Jan. 6, 2013].
94. Miller 2005.
95. Canadian HIV/AIDS Legal Network 1999: 5.
96. Ibid.
97. Ibid.: 6.
98. http://en.wikipedia.org/wiki/Johnson_Aziga [accessed Jan. 6, 2013].
99. Canadian HIV/AIDS Legal Network 2010: 2.
100. Ibid.: 2.
101. Ibid.
102. http://criminalhivtransmission.blogspot.ca [accessed Jan. 6, 2013].
103. Ibid.

104. Ibid.

105. http://www.hivjustice.net/news/canada-supreme-court-makes-bad-law-worse [accessed Jan. 6, 2013].

106. http://www.aidsmap.com/law-country/Western-Africa/page/1444873 [accessed Jan. 6, 2013].

107. Ibid.

108. Pearshouse 2007.

109. http://www.plusnews.org/Report/81758/WEST-AFRICA-HIV-law-a-double-edged-sword [accessed Jan. 6, 2013].

110. Pearshouse 2007.

111. For the full text of the bill, see http://www.gnpplus.net/criminalisation/country/uganda [accessed Jan. 6, 2013].

112. The exceptions are if the person was unaware of being infected with HIV; if the other person was aware of the HIV status of the accused and the risk of infection and voluntarily accepted the risk; if a condom or other reliable protective measure was used during penetration; if the other person was already infected with HIV at the time of the alleged transmission or attempted transmission; and in the case of transmission of HIV by a mother to her child before, during, or after the birth of the child. Ibid.

113. UGANET 2010: 4. Led by the Uganda Network on Law, Ethics, and HIV/AIDS (UGANET), members of the coalition include HIV-positive networks (National Forum of People Living with HIV, National Guidance and Empowerment Network of People Living with HIV/AIDS, Positive Women Leaders of Uganda, National Community of Women Living with HIV/AIDS in Uganda, International Community of Women Living with HIV/AIDS, Uganda Network of Young People Living with HIV/AIDS, National Coalition of Women with AIDS in Uganda, Uganda Young Positives); women's networks (Global Coalition on Women and AIDS in Uganda, Mama's Club); AIDS service organizations (TASO); and other human rights and AIDS organizations (Health Rights Action Group, Civil Society Inter-Constituency Coordination Committee, ActionAid International Uganda, Uganda National AIDS Services Organization, Nordic Consulting Group Uganda, International AIDS Alliance, Mildmay Uganda).

114. UGANET 2010. See also interview with the Executive Director of UGANET, Apr. 27, 2012.

115. Interview with the Executive Director of UGANET, Apr. 27, 2012.

116. http://en.wikipedia.org/wiki/R._v._Cuerrier [accessed Jan. 6, 2013].

117. http://www.opensocietyfoundations.org/publications/ten-reasons-oppose-criminalization-hiv-exposure-or-transmission [accessed Dec. 7, 2012].

118. Global Commission on HIV and the Law 2012.

119. Mann 1999.

120. http://www.egyptindependent.com//news/eliminating-stigma-aids [accessed Jan. 6, 2013].

121. Mann 1999.

122. Ibid.: 218.

123. Ibid.: 220.

124. Ibid.: 220.

125. Ibid.: 223–225.

126. UNAIDS 2007.

127. http://www.lawyerscollective.org/hiv-and-law/hiv-law-background.html [accessed Jan. 6, 2013].

128. Ibid.

129. http://www.unaids.org/en/resources/presscentre/featurestories/2011/april /20110412refgrouphr [accessed Jan. 6, 2013]; UNAIDS Reference Group on HIV and Human Rights 2011: 3.

130. http://www.lawyerscollective.org/hiv-and-law/hiv-law-background.html [accessed Jan. 6, 2013].

131. Interview with ACT UP Activist, July 4, 2012.

132. http://www.apcom.org [accessed Jan. 6, 2013].

133. Interview with Co-Founder, APCOM, Dec. 8, 2012.

134. http://www.ihra.net/what-is-harm-reduction [accessed Jan. 6, 2013].

135. http://www.nswp.org/page/history [accessed Jan. 6, 2013].

136. Some notable national and regional examples include the Lawyers Collective in India; the Canadian HIV/AIDS Legal Network; ARASA; the AIDS Legal Network and Section 27, South Africa; the AIDS Law Unit, Legal Assistance Center of Namibia; the Botswana Network on Ethics, Law and HIV/AIDS; the *Kenyan* Legal and Ethical Issues Network on HIV and *AIDS*; UGANET; and the Access to Medicines Research Group, China.

137. For the judgments on these cases, see http://www.lawyerscollective.org/hiv-and-law /judgements-a-orders.html. See also http://legal-articles.deysot.com/constitutional-law/law -and-hiv-with-special-emphasis-on-stigma-and-discrimination.html [accessed Dec. 7, 2012].

138. http://www.lawyerscollective.org/updates/188-constitutional-challenge-to-sod omy-law-in-india-2.html. See also Human Rights Watch, *This Alien Legacy: The Origins of "Sodomy" Laws in British Colonialism* (2008), http://www.hrw.org/en/reports/2008/12 /17/alien-legacy-0 [accessedJan. 6, 2013].

139. http://www.lawyerscollective.org/vulnerable-communities/drug-use/death -penalty.html#more-150 [accessed Jan. 6, 2013].

140. http://www.lawyerscollective.org/hiv-and-law/draft-law.html See also http://info changeindia.org/agenda/hivaids-big-questions/do-we-need-a-separate-law-on-hivaids .html [accessed Jan. 6, 2013].

141. Interview with the Co-Founder, Lawyers Collective, Nov. 3, 2011.

142. See, for example, Canadian HIV/AIDS Legal Network 2002, 2005a, 2005b, 2005c, 2007, 2008.

143. Interview with the Executive Director, Canadian HIV/AIDS Legal Network, July 9, 2012.

144. http://www.prisonhealthnow.ca [accessed Jan. 6, 2013].

145. http://positivelite.com/component/zoo/tag/news/Canadian%20HIV%20AIDS %20Legal%20Network [accessed Dec. 7, 2012].

146. Canadian HIV/AIDS Legal Network 2005c. See also http://www.pivotlegal.org /sex_workers_rights [accessed Jan. 6, 2013].

147. Interview with the Executive Director, Canadian HIV/AIDS Legal Network, July 9, 2012.

148. Ibid.

149. For a comprehensive archive of HIV law and human rights, see http://www.aid slex.org/english/Home-Page. For a global criminalization scan, see http://www.gnpplus .net/evidence/criminalisation-scan [accessed Jan. 6, 2013].

150. Epstein 1996: 8–9.

151. Interview with a Member of ACT UP New York, July 4, 2012.

152. Ibid.

153. Interview with a Member of Patient-Control Movement, Russia, Sept. 16, 2011.

154. Interview with the Executive Director, KETAM, Mar. 28, 2012.

155. Interview with the Co-Founder, Access to Medicines Research Group, China, Oct. 11, 2011.

156. Ibid.

157. Interview with the Coordinator, Youth Lead, Dec. 6, 2011.

158. Interview with the President, DNP+, Nov. 8, 2011.

159. Interview with the Regional Advocacy Team Leader and Advocacy Officer, ARASA, May 2, 2012.

160. Interview with the General Secretary, TAC, May 4, 2012.

161. Interview with a Researcher, EATG, Aug. 6, 2012.

162. http://joaobiehl.net/global-health-research/right-to-health-litigation [accessed Dec. 10, 2012]. See also Biehl 2007.

163. Safreed-Harmon 2008; Reis, Vieira, and Chaves 2009.

164. Safreed-Harmon 2008: 4.

165. http://www.wto.org/english/tratop_e/dda_e/dohaexplained_e.htm [accessed Jan. 6, 2013].

166. http://www.doctorswithoutborders.org/news/issue.cfm?id=2392 [accessed Jan. 6, 2013].

167. Interview with a former Staff Member, MSF–Hong Kong, Oct. 25, 2011.

168. Interview with the National Project Director, MSF-Beijing, Oct. 11, 2011.

169. Interview with a former Staff Member, MSF–Hong Kong, Oct. 25, 2011.

170. Gonsalves and Harrington 1992; see also http://www.treatmentactiongroup.org/tagline/2012/spring/tag-20-early-campaigns [accessed Jan. 6, 2013].

171. McDonnell 2007.

172. Ibid.: 4.

173. Interview with the Global Campaign Director, Health GAP, Mar. 26, 2012.

174. McDonnell 2007: 1 and 3.

175. http://www.pepfar.gov/press/107735.htm [accessed Jan. 6, 2013].

176. http://www.theglobalfund.org/en/about/whoweare [accessed Jan. 6, 2013].

177. Interview with the Executive Director, Canadian HIV/AIDS Legal Network, July 10, 2012.

178. http://www.actupny.org/documents/Denver.html [accessed Jan. 6, 2013].

179. Ibid.

180. http://www.iasociety.org/default.aspx?pageId=223 [accessed Jan. 6, 2013].

181. http://www.gnpplus.net/about-gnp [accessed Jan. 6, 2013].

182. Interview with Technical Support Officer, GNP+, May 3, 2012.

183. http://www.gnpplus.net/?s=hiv+leadership+through+accountability [accessed Dec. 7, 2012].

184. Interview with Technical Support Officer, GNP+, May 3, 2012.

185. Ibid.

186. http://www.icwglobal.org/en/about/history.php [accessed Jan. 6, 2013].

187. http://www.icw.org/twelvestatements [accessed Jan. 6, 2013].

188. Interview with Steering Committee Member, ICW, July 9, 2012.

189. http://usersvoice.org/international/letter-from-aids-activist-of-european-aids-treatment-group [accessed Dec. 7, 2012].

190. www.icw.org/files/IDUEN.pdf [accessed Jan. 6, 2013].

191. http://www.unicef.org/aids/index_iatt.html [accessed Jan. 6, 2013].

192. For a general discussion on the use and limits of GIPA by various AIDS nongovernmental organizations, see www.aidslaw.ca/publications/publicationsdocEN.php?ref=85 *[accessed* Jan. 6, 2013].

193. In his analysis of the role of civil society in UN governance, Cakmak (2008) argues that civil society's participation has been limited to providing input in international treaty making and world conferences.

194. http://www.icw.org/files/PLHIV_involvement_eng.pdf [accessed Jan. 6, 2013].

195. Interview with the Co-Founder, Health and Development Network, Aug. 15, 2012.

196. Interview with the Special Rapporteur on the Right to Health, Nov. 3, 2011.

197. Interview with the Health and Discrimination Project Manager of the Egyptian Initiative for Personal Rights, May 30, 2012.

198. UNAIDS Reference Group on HIV and Human Rights 2011: 3.

199. Interview with the Co-Founder, Health and Development Network, Aug. 15, 2012.

200. http://www.positivelivingbc.org/news/120817/government-ideology-affects-aids-funding [accessed Jan. 6, 2013].

201. Interview with Advocacy Manager, SWEAT, May 2, 2012.

202. Interview with the Executive Director, Asia Pacific Network of Sex Workers, Dec. 5, 2011.

203. Interview with the Founder and Executive Director, Dongzhen Center for Human Rights Education and Action, Oct. 13, 2011.

204. Interview with the Executive Director, Russian Harm Reduction Network, Sept. 5, 2011.

205. http://www.hivlawcommission.org/index.php/report [accessed Jan. 6, 2013].

Chapter 3 · *Against Pharma*

Epigraphs. Garnier 2003, qtd. in Desphande, Sucher, and Winig 2011: 3; http://www.actupny.org/treatment/slashprices.html [accessed Jan. 8, 2013]; D'Adesky 2004: 6.

1. UNAIDS 2011a.

2. WHO, UNAIDS, and UNICEF 2011.

3. McSherry 2001.

4. Ibid.: 3.

5. http://www.wto.org/english/thewto_e/minist_e/min99_e/english/misinf_e/05killin_e.htm [accessed Jan. 8 2013].

6. Global Commission on HIV and the Law 2012.

7. D'Adesky 2004: 8.

8. http://www.wto.org/english/thewto_e/whatis_e/wto_dg_stat_e.htm [accessed Jan. 8, 2013].

9. Ibid.

10. Moore 2004: 1.

11. Dunkley 2004: 223.

12. Johnson 1967: 44, qtd. in Jones 2004: 150.

13. Moore 2004: 69.

14. http://www.wto.org/english/thewto_e/whatis_e/who_we_are_e.htm [accessed Jan. 8, 2013].

15. Sell 2003: 2.

16. http://www.msfaccess.org/content/trips-trips-plus-and-doha [accessed Jan. 8, 2013].

17. Jones 2004: 158.

18. http://www.msfaccess.org/content/trips-trips-plus-and-doha [accessed Jan. 8, 2013].

19. www.twnside.org.sg/title2/resurgence/196/cover3.doc [accessed Jan. 8, 2013].

20. Ibid.

21. http://www.msfaccess.org/content/trips-trips-plus-and-doha [accessed Jan. 8, 2013].

22. Ibid.

23. www.twnside.org.sg/title2/resurgence/196/cover3.doc [accessed Jan. 8, 2013].

24. http://donttradeourlivesaway.wordpress.com/2012/08/31/eu-pushing-for-data-exclusivity-in-thai-eu-fta [accessed Jan. 8, 2013].

25. Ibid.

26. D'Adesky 2004: 22.

27. Ibid.

28. Desphande, Sucher, and Winig 2011.

29. http://investors.gilead.com/phoenix.zhtml?c=69964&p=irol-newsArticle&ID=908393&highlight= [accessed Jan. 8, 2013].

30. Desphande, Sucher, and Winig 2011: 13.

31. http://www.huffingtonpost.com/james-love/obama-administration-rule_b_174450.html [accessed Jan. 8, 2013].

32. http://news.cnet.com/8301-13578_3-57466330-38/last-rites-for-acta-europe-rejects-antipiracy-treaty [accessed Jan. 8, 2013].

33. http://www.international.gc.ca/media_commerce/comm/news-communiques/2011/280.aspx?lang=eng&view=d [accessed Jan. 8, 2013].

34. MSF 2012b.

35. D'Adesky 2004: 6.

36. http://www.cehurd.org/2012/04/sections-of-the-kenya-anti-counterfeiting-act-struck-down-as-a-threat-to-fundamental-human-rights [accessed Jan. 8, 2013].

37. http://www.ncbi.nlm.nih.gov/pmc/articles/PMC1119675 [accessed Jan. 8, 2013].

38. Interview with the Executive Director, ITPC, Dec. 7, 2011.

39. Interview with an Advocacy Officer, MSF–New Delhi, Dec. 9, 2012.

40. Qtd. in Desphande, Sucher, and Winig 2011: 11.

41. D'Adesky 2004.

42. http://apps.who.int/medicinedocs/en/d/Jh1461e/1.4.html [accessed Jan. 8, 2013].

43. Ibid.

44. http://www.wto.org/english/thewto_e/minist_e/min01_e/mindecl_trips_e.htm [accessed Jan. 8, 2013].

45. http://www.actupny.org/treatment/slashprices.html [accessed Jan. 8, 2013].

46. Ibid.

47. Ibid.

48. Hamied 2005b: 9.

49. Qtd. in D'Adesky 2004: 48.

50. In his State of the Union address in January 2003, President George W. Bush said, "On the Continent of Africa, nearly 30 million people have AIDS including 3 million children. There are countries in Africa where one-third of the population carry the infection, 4 million require immediate treatment. Only 50,000 are receiving the medicines they need. In an age of miraculous medicines, no person should hear 'You've got AIDS. We can't help you. Go home and die.'" Qtd. in Hamied 2005a: 3.

51. Kijtiwatchakul 2009: 1.

52. MSF 2012a.

53. MSF 2010. For Merck's Tier II list of countries, see annex 10 on p. 86.

54. Ibid.

55. Qtd. ibid.

56. Terto, Reis, and Pimenta 2009.

57. Limpananont et al. 2009: 141.

58. Ibid.: 144.

59. Ibid.: 147.

60. Interview with the Executive Director, AIDS Access Foundation, Dec. 2, 2011.

61. Ibid.

62. Qtd. in Kijtiwatchakul 2009: 95.

63. http://apps.who.int/medicinedocs/fr/m/abstract/Js18718en [accessed Jan. 8, 2013].

64. Kijtiwatchakul 2009.

65. Ibid.: 161.

66. Wetzler 2007.

67. Nunn 2009.

68. Wetzler 2007.

69. Ibid.

70. Reis, Vieira, and Chaves 2009: 26 and 27.

71. Interview with the former Director of the Brazilian HIV/AIDS Program, Feb. 29, 2011. For a detailed chronology of the EFV CL process in Brazil, see http://www.cptech .org/ip/health/c/brazil [accessed Jan. 8, 2013].

72. http://www.uschamber.com/press/releases/2007/may/brazil-takes-major-step backward-intellectual-property-rights-says-us-chambe [accessed Jan. 8, 2013].

73. http://www.economist.com/node/9154222?story_id=9154222 [accessed Jan. 8, 2013].

74. Reis, Vieira, and Chaves 2009.

75. For the statement of the Competition Commission, see http://www.tac.org.za/news letter/2003/ns10_12_2003.htm [accessed Jan. 8, 2013].

76. http://www.tac.org.za/community/node/2329 [accessed Jan. 8, 2013].

77. Ibid.

78. MSF 2012a.

79. Ibid.

80. Ibid.

81. Ibid.

82. http://www.doctorswithoutborders.org/news/hiv-aids/tenofovir_briefing_doc .cfm [accessed Jan. 8, 2013].

83. Ibid.

84. de Carvalho 2012.

85. Ibid.

86. Ibid.

87. Interview with a Lawyer from the GTPI/REBRIP, Feb. 24, 2012. See also http://www.deolhonaspatentes.org.br/default.asp?idiomaId=2 [accessed Jan. 8, 2013].

88. de Carvalho 2012.

89. Interview with a Lawyer, GTPI/REBRIP, Feb. 24, 2012.

90. de Carvalho 2012.

91. Interview with a Lawyer, GTPI/REBRIP, Feb. 24, 2012.

92. Ibid.

93. http://patentoppositions.org/drugs/4f1081fb04a7f937af000019#patent-applications [accessed Jan. 8, 2013].

94. Grover 2008.

95. George, Sheshadri, and Grover 2009.

96. Hamied 2005b.

97. D'Adesky 2004: 6.

98. http://www.doctorswithoutborders.org/news/access/background_paper_indian_generics.pdf [accessed Jan. 8, 2013].

99. George, Sheshadri, and Grover 2009.

100. http://www.who.int/medicines/areas/policy/wto_trips/en/index.html [accessed Jan. 8, 2013].

101. George, Sheshadri, and Grover 2009.

102. Ibid.

103. Ibid.

104. Ibid.

105. For a full list of Gilead's TDF patents in India, see http://patentoppositions.org/drugs/4f1081fb04a7f937af000019#patent-applications [accessed Jan. 8, 2013].

106. Ibid.

107. Interview with the Executive Director, ABIA, Feb. 24, 2012; de Carvalho 2012.

108. http://patentoppositions.org/drugs/4f1081fb04a7f937af000019 [accessed Apr. 30, 2014].

109. MSF 2012a.

110. Sutherland and Hsu 2012; and Hood 2011.

111. Interview, Chinese AIDS lawyer in Shanghai, Oct. 21, 2011.

112. Interview with the National Project Director, MSF-Beijing, Oct. 11, 2011.

113. http://www.chinadaily.com.cn/cndy/2008-08/21/content_6956414.htm [accessed Jan. 8, 2013].

114. For a critical analysis of Chinese AIDS policy until the 2006 regulations, see Balzano and Jia 2006.

115. Interview with the Executive Director of the Dongzhen Center for Human Rights Education and Action, Oct. 13, 2011.

116. http://www.unaids.org/en/regionscountries/countries/china [accessed Jan. 8, 2013].

117. Yang and Yen 2009: 1.

118. Hu 2011.

119. Chen 2001.

120. http://english.gov.cn/laws/2005-09/19/content_64918.htm [accessed Jan. 8, 2013].

121. Wang, Hu, and Jia 2009.

122. Interview with the Co-Founder, Access to Medicines Research Group, China, Oct. 11, 2011.

123. Wang, Hu, and Jia 2009.

124. Ibid.

125. Interview with the Co-Founder, Access to Medicines Research Group, China, Oct. 11, 2011.

126. Ibid.

127. Ibid.

128. http://english.sipo.gov.cn/laws/lawsregulations/201012/t20101210_553631.html [accessed Jan. 8, 2013].

129. Ibid.

130. Interview with the National Project Director, MSF-Beijing, Oct. 11, 2011.

131. Ibid.

132. http://www.reuters.com/article/2012/06/08/us-china-medicines-patents-idUS BRE8570TY20120608 [accessed Jan. 8, 2013].

133. MSF 2012a.

134. Kijtiwatchakul 2009. See also http://patentoppositions.org/drugs/4f10820404a 7f937af000021#patent-applications [accessed Jan. 8, 2013].

135. MSF 2010.

136. Interview with the Co-Founder, Access to Medicines Research Group, China, Oct. 11, 2011.

137. Ibid.

138. Jambert 2004.

139. Ibid.

140. Ibid.

141. Ibid.

142. MSF 2012a.

143. http://www.msfaccess.org/our-work/hiv-aids/article/1307 [accessed Jan. 8, 2013].

144. MSF 2012a.

145. Reis, Vieira, and Chaves 2009.

146. Interview with the former Director, Brazilian HIV/AIDS Program, Feb. 28, 2012.

147. Interview with a Lawyer, GTPI/REBRIP, Feb. 24, 2012.

148. MSF 2012a.

149. Ibid.: 41.

150. http://patentoppositions.org/drugs/4f1081f604a7f937af000010 [accessed Jan. 8, 2013].

151. Kijtiwatchakul 2009.

152. http://www.petitiononline.com/bcottabb/petition.html [accessed Jan. 8, 2013].

153. http://www.cptech.org/ip/health/c/thailand [accessed Jan. 8, 2013].

154. Ibid.

155. http://www.cptech.org/ip/health/c/thailand/thainews-janapro7.html [accessed Jan. 8, 2013].

156. Kijtiwatchakul 2009.

157. www.who.int/hiv/amds/AMDSmailJune.pdf [accessed Jan. 8, 2013].

158. http://www.citizen.org/press-release [accessed Jan. 8, 2013].

159. MSF 2010: 3.

160. Interview with the Executive Director, UNITAID, June 25, 2012.

161. WIPO Global Challenges Seminar on Licensing and Prices: New Approaches in the Pharmaceutical Sector, Geneva, June 27, 2012 [transcript by author].

162. Interview with the Acting Executive Director of the MPP, June 29, 2012.

163. Ibid. For the full text of the UNITAID Constitution, see http://www.unitaid.eu /governance-mainmenu-4/resolutions-mainmenu-34/3-news/press/341-fourteen-executive -board-meeting-adopted-resolutions [accessed Jan. 8, 2013].

164. Chan Park, presentation at the WIPO Global Challenges Seminar on Licensing and Prices: New Approaches in the Pharmaceutical Sector, Geneva, June 27, 2012 [transcript by author].

165. Ibid.

166. http://www.medicinespatentpool.org/licensing/current-licences/the-medicines -patent-poolgilead-licences-questions-and-answers [accessed Jan. 8, 2013].

167. Ibid.

168. Ibid.

169. Ibid.

170. http://www.medicinespatentpool.org/medicines-patent-pool-announces-first-li censing-agreement-with-a-pharmaceutical-company [accessed Jan. 8, 2013].

171. Ibid.

172. Interview with the Executive Director, UNITAID, June 25, 2012.

173. Greg Alton, Executive Vice President, Gilead, presentation at the WIPO Global Challenges Seminar on Licensing and Prices: New Approaches in the Pharmaceutical Sector, Geneva, June 27, 2012 [transcript by author].

174. Conversation with Greg Alton, Executive Vice President, Gilead , June 27, 2012.

175. Ibid.

176. http://www.whitehouse.gov/blog/2011/07/12/medicines-patent-pool-agreement -gilead-key-milestone [accessed Jan. 8, 2013].

177. Alton, presentation at the WIPO Global Challenges Seminar on Licensing and Prices: New Approaches in the Pharmaceutical Sector, Geneva, June 27, 2012 [transcript by author].

178. Interview with the General Counsel, MPP, June 29, 2012.

179. http://www.pharmatimes.com/Article/11-07-12/Gilead_is_first_pharma_firm _to_dive_into_HIV_patent_pool.aspx [accessed Jan. 8, 2013].

180. Ibid.

181. Ibid.

182. Interview with a Campaigner, KEI, June 27, 2012.

183. MSF 2011: 1.

184. Ibid.

185. Ibid.: 5 and 13.

186. Ibid.: 3 and 4.

187. Ibid.: 8.

188. Ibid.

189. Ibid.

190. Ibid.: 11.

191. Ibid.: 13.

192. http://www.petitionbuzz.com/petitions/mppunitaid. For the MPP's guiding principles, see http://www.wipo.int/wipo_magazine/en/2011/03/article_0005.html [both accessed Jan. 8, 2013].

193. Interview with the Executive Director, ITPC, Dec. 7, 2012.

194. International Treatment Preparedness Coalition and Initiative for Medicines, Access, and Knowledge 2011.

195. Ibid.

196. Ibid.

197. Interview with the Co-Founder, Treatment Action Group, July 17, 2012.

198. Interview with the General Counsel, MPP, June 29, 2012.

199. Ibid.

200. Ibid.

201. Ibid.

202. Ibid.

203. Interview with the Co-Founder, ITPC, July 4, 2012.

204. Interview with an Activist, ITPC–Eastern Europe and Central Asia, Sept. 24, 2011.

205. Interview with ITPC–Latin America's Coordinator, Feb. 28, 2012.

206. Interview with the Regional Advocacy Team Leader, ARASA, May 2, 2013.

207. Interview with the Secretary-General, Indian Pharmaceutical Alliance, Nov. 7, 2011.

208. Interview with the CEO, Cipla, Nov. 10, 2011.

209. http://keionline.org/node/1665 [accessed Mar. 8, 2013].

210. Nunn 2009.

211. Interview with the Executive Director, Asia Pacific Network of Sex Workers, Dec. 5, 2011.

212. Interview with a Campaigner, MSF–South Africa, May 2, 2012.

213. Interview with the President, DNP+, Nov. 8, 2011.

214. Interview with the Executive Director, ABIA, Feb. 24, 2012.

215. Kijtiwatchakul 2009: 93.

216. Interview with the Executive Director, AIDS Access Foundation, Dec. 2, 2012.

217. de Carvalho 2012.

218. Interview with the Executive Director, UNITAID, June 25, 2012.

219. MSF 2010.

220. Interview with the Advocacy Officer, MSF–New Delhi, Dec. 9, 2011.

221. Interview with a Lawyer, GTPI/REBRIP, Feb. 24, 2012.

222. http://www.msfaccess.org/novartis-drop-the-case [accessed Jan. 8, 2013].

223. http://www.lawyerscollective.org/updates/supreme-court-rejects-novartis-appeal-upholds-high-standard-section-3d.html [accessed Apr. 29, 2013].

224. UNAIDS 2011a.

225. MSF 2010: 26.

226. Ibid.: 18.

227. Ibid.

228. http://www.who.int/phi/CEWG_Report_5_April_2012.pdf [accessed Jan. 8, 2013].

229. http://www.essentialdrugs.org/edrug/archive/201211/msg00042.php [accessed Jan. 8, 2013].

230. http://www.msfaccess.org/content/stuck-time-warp-who-brokered-global-rd -action-plan-shelved [accessed Jan. 8, 2013].

231. http://keionline.org/node/1612 [accessed Jan. 8, 2013].

Chapter 4 · Against Governance

Epigraphs. Interviews with the External Relations Officer, UNAIDS, June 25, 2012, and with the Executive Director, ABIA, Feb. 24, 2012.

1. Kickbush 2007: xi.

2. Gordenker et al. 1995: 2–3.

3. Ibid.: 4.

4. Ibid.: 39.

5. Ibid.

6. Ibid.

7. Chin 2007.

8. Ibid.

9. Gordenker et al. 1995: 59.

10. Ibid.

11. Ibid.; Chin 2007.

12. Gordenker et al. 1995.

13. Braithwaite and Drahos 2000; Hein, Bartsch, and Kohlmorgen 2007: 120.

14. Gordenker et al. 1995: 83.

15. UNAIDS 2010.

16. Ibid.: i.

17. Ibid.

18. Interview with External Relations Officer, UNAIDS, June 25, 2012.

19. Interview with the Senior Advisor, HIV/AIDS Department, WHO, June 27, 2012.

20. Ibid.

21. Gordenker et al. 1995: 61.

22. Interview with the Director, HIV/AIDS Group, UNDP, July 2, 2012.

23. Ibid.

24. Ibid.

25. Interview with the Senior Technical Advisor, HIV and Key Populations, UNFPA, July 3, 2012.

26. Ibid.

27. Interview with the Country Coordinator, UNAIDS-Brazil, Feb. 29, 2012.

28. Interview with the Advisor to the Executive Director, Global Health Workforce Alliance, June 29, 2012.

29. MSF 2007.

30. http://www.ilo.org/global/publications/KD00015/lang--en/index.htm [accessed Jan. 11, 2013].

31. Interview with the Senior Technical Advisor, ILO Programme on HIV/AIDS and the World of Work, June 29, 2012.

32. Interview with the External Relations Officer, UNAIDS, June 25, 2012.

33. Ibid.

34. Interview with the Senior Advisor, HIV/AIDS Department, WHO, June 27, 2012.

35. Ibid.

36. Ibid.
37. Interview with the Community Mobilization Chief, UNAIDS, June 28, 2012.
38. Interview with the Director, HIV/AIDS Group, UNDP, July 2, 2012.
39. Interview with the Senior Technical Advisor, HIV and Key Populations, UNFPA, July 3, 2012.
40. Interview with the Director, HIV/AIDS Group, UNDP, July 2, 2012.
41. Interview with the External Relations Officer, UNAIDS, June 25, 2012.
42. Interview with the Country Coordinator, UNAIDS-Brazil, Feb. 29, 2012.
43. Interview with the Director, HIV/AIDS Group, UNDP, July 2, 2012.
44. Interview with the former Communications Manager, AHRN, Dec. 2, 2011.
45. Interview with the Senior Technical Advisor, HIV and Key Populations, UNFPA, July 3, 2012.
46. Ibid.
47. Ibid.
48. http://www.securitycouncilreport.org/monthly-forecast/2011-06/lookup_c_glK WLeMTIsG_b_7497341.php [accessed Jan. 8, 2012].
49. http://www.un.org/millenniumgoals/aids.shtml [accessed Jan. 8, 2012].
50. http://ap.ohchr.org/documents/alldocs.aspx?doc_id=4820 [accessed Jan. 8, 2012].
51. http://www.humanrightsimpact.org/rthia/resources/resolutions-and-reports [accessed Jan. 8, 2012].
52. http://www.un.org/ga/aids/coverage/FinalDeclarationHIVAIDS.html [accessed Jan. 8, 2012].
53. http://www.unaids.org/en/targetsandcommitments [accessed Jan. 8, 2012].
54. http://www.unaids.org/en/dataanalysis/knowyourresponse/countryprogressre ports/2010countries [accessed Jan. 8, 2012].
55. Interviews with the Director, HIV/AIDS Group, UNDP, July 2, 2012, and the Executive Director, Canadian HIV/AIDS Legal Network, July 10, 2012.
56. http://news.bbc.co.uk/2/hi/africa/1297474.stm [accessed Jan. 8, 2012].
57. http://www.theglobalfund.org/en/about/donors [accessed Jan. 8, 2012].
58. See http://web.worldbank.org/WBSITE/EXTERNAL/COUNTRIES/AFRICAEXT /EXTAFRHEANUTPOP/EXTAFRREGTOPHIVAIDS/0,,contentMDK:20415735~me nuPK:1001234~pagePK:34004173~piPK:34003707~theSitePK:717148,00.html [accessed Jan. 8, 2012].
59. Okie 2006.
60. Gates Foundation HIV Strategy Overview, July 2012, http://www.gatesfoundation .org/hivaids/Pages/default.aspx [accessed Jan. 8, 2013].
61. http://www.unitaid.eu/who/role-in-global-health-landscape [accessed Jan. 8, 2012].
62. Interview with the Executive Director, UNITAID, June 25, 2012.
63. http://thehill.com/blogs/congress-blog/healthcare/275677-innovation-to-fund -global-health#ixzz2H40UYbf9 [accessed Jan. 8, 2012].
64. http://www.joinred.com/aboutred/how-red-works [accessed Jan. 8, 2012].
65. http://www.unitaid.eu/resources/publications/annual-reports/9-uncategorised /360-feasibility-financial-transaction-tax [accessed Jan. 8, 2012].
66. Boler and Archer 2008: 106.
67. Human Rights Watch 2005.
68. Qtd. in Boler and Archer 2008: 104.

69. Interview with the Director of Global Campaigns, Health GAP, Mar. 26, 2012.

70. Ibid.

71. Ibid.

72. Ibid.

73. Interviews with a Campaigner, KEI, June 27, 2012, and with the Advisor to the Executive Director, Global Health Workforce Alliance, June 29, 2012.

74. https://docs.gatesfoundation.org/Documents/Avahan_FactSheet.pdf [accessed Jan. 8, 2012].

75. Ibid.

76. Ibid.

77. Interview with the Executive Director, Avahan, Nov. 25, 2011.

78. Ibid.

79. Ibid.

80. http://methodlogical.wordpress.com/2011/10/13/doubting-the-success-of-avahan. See also Rao 2010.

81. Rao 2010: i8.

82. People's Health Movement, Medact, Health Action International, and Medico International 2011.

83. McCoy et al. 2009.

84. Lancet 2009: 1577.

85. Ibid.

86. Interview with a Researcher, EATG, Aug. 6, 2012.

87. People's Health Movement, Medact, Health Action International, and Medico International 2011.

88. Qtd. ibid.: 271.

89. www.theglobalfund.org/documents/ . . . /framework/Core_GlobalFund_Framework_en [accessed Jan. 8, 2012].

90. Interview with the Civil Society and Private Sector Partnerships Manager, Global Fund, June 26, 2012.

91. Interview with the former Executive Director, Chain, China, Oct. 25, 2011.

92. Interview with the Global Fund Grants Program Manager, UNDP-Kyrgyzstan, July 8, 2011.

93. Carroll 1865: 63–64.

94. http://www.un-ngls.org/orf/UNreform.htm [accessed Jan. 9, 2012].

95. http://esango.un.org/civilsociety/displayConsultativeStatusSearch.do ?method=search&sessionCheck=false [accessed Jan. 9, 2012].

96. Gordenker et al. 1995.

97. Ibid.

98. http://web.worldbank.org/WBSITE/EXTERNAL/NEWS/0,,contentMDK:20040 873~menuPK:34480~pagePK:34370~theSitePK:4607,00.html [accessed Jan. 9, 2012].

99. Gordenker et al. 1995: 89.

100. Ibid.: 90.

101. Ibid.: 91.

102. Ibid.: 93.

103. Ibid.: 93.

104. Ibid.

105. Ibid.

106. Interview with the Senior Technical Advisor, HIV and Key Populations, UNFPA, July 3, 2012.

107. Interview with the Community Mobilization Chief, UNAIDS, June 28, 2012.

108. http://www.fundsforngos.org/latest-funds-for-ngos/robert-carr-civil-society -network-fund-call-proposals [accessed Jan. 9, 2012].

109. Interview with the External Relations Officer, UNAIDS, June 26, 2012.

110. http://www.theglobalfund.org/en/board/members [accessed Jan. 9, 2012].

111. http://www.rollbackmalaria.org/mechanisms/partnershipboard.html; http://www .stoptb.org/about/cb [both accessed Jan. 9, 2012].

112. http://webcache.googleusercontent.com/search?q=cache:FN5nr47G8mkJ:www .theglobalfund.org/documents/core/infonotes/Core_DTF_InfoNote_en/+&cd=1&hl=en &ct=clnk&gl=ca&client=safari [accessed Jan. 9, 2012].

113. Gordenker et al. 1995: 101.

114. Ibid.

115. Interviews with the Civil Society and Private Sector Partnerships Manager, Global Fund, June 26, 2012, and the Global Campaigns Director, Health GAP, Mar. 26, 2012.

116. Interview with the Global Campaigns Director, Health GAP, Mar. 26, 2012.

117. Global Fund 2008: 3, qtd. in Seale, Bains, and Avrett 2010: 3.

118. See, for example, this independent review of UNAIDS, http://www.unaids.org/en /media/unaids/contentassets/dataimport/pub/externaldocument/2007/review_ngo_par ticipation_item_3.2_en.pdf [accessed Jan. 9, 2012]. See also Fraser 2003.

119. Buse and Harmer 2009.

120. Gordenker et al. 1995: 93.

121. Interview with the Executive Director, CARAM, Nov. 18, 2011.

122. Interview with the National Program Director, MSF-Beijing, Oct. 11, 2012.

123. Interview with the Senior Researcher, AIDS Accountability International, May 4, 2012.

124. http://webcache.googleusercontent.com/search?q=cache:DHt_wwWhjaUJ:www .theglobalfund.org/documents/replenishment/2013/Replenishment_2013NeedsAssess ment_Report_en/+&cd=3&hl=en&ct=clnk&gl=ca&client=safari [accessed Apr. 30, 2014].

125. http://www.globalhealthcheck.org/?author=21 [accessed Jan. 9, 2012].

126. http://reason.com/blog/2008/01/03/too-much-money-for-aids [accessed Jan. 9, 2012].

127. http://blogs.nature.com/news/2012/07/economists-debate-paying-for-aids.html [accessed Jan. 9, 2013].

128. http://chrisblattman.com/2008/07/10/are-we-spending-too-much-money-on -aids [accessed Jan. 9, 2012].

129. WHO 2008.

130. Presentation at the 2009 Canadian Society for International Health annual meet-ing, Ottawa [transcript by author].

131. http://chrisblattman.com/2008/07/10/are-we-spending-too-much-money-on -aids [accessed Jan. 9, 2012].

132. http://icssupport.org/wp-content/uploads/2012/02/3-Investment-Framework -Summary-UNAIDS-Issues-Brief.pdf [accessed Jan. 9, 2012].

133. Ibid.

134. UNAIDS 2011a.

135. Interview with the Co-Founder, Health and Development Network, Aug. 15, 2012.

136. Ibid.

137. http://www.aidspan.org/gfo_article/financial-transaction-tax-be-introduced-11 -countries-europe [accessed Jan. 9, 2012].

138. http://www.businessweek.com/news/2012-11-14/french-transaction-tax-misses -mark-as-speculators-find-loopholes [accessed Jan. 9, 2012].

139. http://webcache.googleusercontent.com/search?q=cache:JpfaXIqIRz8J:www .theglobalfund.org/documents/performance/Performance_ValueForMoney_Frame work_en/+&cd=3&hl=en&ct=clnk&gl=ca&client=safari [accessed Jan. 9, 2012].

140. http://www.google.ca/url?sa=t&rct=j&q=&esrc=s&source=web&cd=1& ved=0CCgQFjAA&url=http%3A%2F%2Fwww.theglobalfund.org%2Fdocuments %2Fboard%2F23%2FBM23_14PICPSCJEligibilityAttachment1_Policy_en%2F&ei=fZAC U5ToA8Ho0ATIl0DwDQ&usg=AFQjCNEJ7YDjhRCPiwUAREMp5WXY8aGBXQ&bvm =bv.61535280,d.cGU [accessed Jan. 9, 2012].

141. http://www.theglobalfund.org/en/activities/fundingmodel [accessed Jan. 9, 2012].

142. http://www.aidspan.org/gfo_article/new-funding-model-will-push-lac-out -global-fund%E2%80%99s-portfolio [accessed Jan. 9, 2012].

143. Interview with the Global Fund Grants Program Manager, UNDP-Kyrgyzstan, July 8, 2011.

144. Interview with a Representative of MSF–South Africa's Access Campaign, May 2, 2012.

145. Interview with the Executive Director, ABIA, Feb. 24, 2012.

146. Interview with the Co-Founder, Health and Development Network, Aug. 15, 2012.

147. Ibid.

148. Interview with the Executive Director, CARAM, Nov. 18, 2011.

149. Interview with the Executive Director, Chi Heng Foundation, Mar. 25, 2013.

150. Interview with the former Program Director, EHRN, July 19, 2011.

151. Interview with the President, DNP+, Nov. 8, 2011.

152. Interview with the Executive Director, AIDS Access Foundation, Dec. 2, 2011.

153. Interview with the Vice President, Global Business Coalition for Health, Sept. 6, 2011.

154. Interview with the National Project Director, MSF-Beijing, Oct. 11, 2011.

155. Interview with the Director, International Harm Reduction Development Program, OSF, July 3, 2012.

156. Interview with the Country Coordinator, UNAIDS-Egypt, May 29, 2012.

157. Interview with the Social Mobilization Advisor, UNAIDS-China, Oct. 13, 2011.

158. Interview with the External Relations Officer, UNAIDS, June 26, 2012.

159. Interview with the Co-Founder, Health and Development Network, Aug. 15, 2012.

160. Interview with Advocacy Officer 1, ITPC, Eastern Europe and Central Asia, Sept. 24, 2011.

161. Interview with a Member of the PHM, Nov. 8, 2011.

162. Interview with a former Civil Society Team Officer, Global Fund, June 28, 2012.

163. Interview with the Civil Society and Private Sector Partnerships Manager, Global Fund, June 26, 2012.

164. Interview with a Researcher, EATG, Aug. 6, 2012.

165. Interview with the Co-Founder, Health and Development Network, Aug. 15, 2012.

166. Interview with the Executive Director, Roll Back Malaria Partnership, June 29, 2012.

167. Interview with the Executive Director, Aidspan, Mar. 26, 2012.

168. Interview with a Consultant, Aidspan, Mar. 27, 2012.

169. Ibid.

170. Ibid.

171. Interview with the President, DNP+, Nov. 8, 2011.

172. Interview with a Consultant, Aidspan, Mar. 27, 2012.

173. Interview with Advocacy Officer 2, ITPC, Eastern Europe and Central Asia, Sept. 26, 2011.

174. Interview with the Global Fund Grants Program Manager, UNDP-Kyrgyzstan, July 8, 2011.

175. Interview with the National Project Director, MSF-Beijing, Oct. 11, 2011.

176. Interview with the Executive Director, Dongzhen Center for Human Rights Education and Action, Oct. 13, 2011.

177. Interview with the Executive Director, Shanghai AIDS Prevention Center, Oct. 20, 2011.

178. Interview with Advocacy Officer 1, ITPC, Eastern Europe and Central Asia, Sept. 24, 2011.

179. Interview with the former Communications Manager, AHRN, Dec. 2, 2011.

180. Interview with the Civil Society and Private Sector Partnerships Manager, Global Fund, June 26, 2012.

181. http://www.theglobalfund.org/en/terg/evaluations/5year [accessed Jan. 12, 2012].

182. http://www.huffingtonpost.com/2011/01/23/global-health-fund-fraud_n_812801 .html [accessed Jan. 12, 2012].

183. Interview with a Consultant, Aidspan, Mar. 27, 2012.

184. Ibid.

185. http://www.theglobalfund.org/en/highlevelpanel [accessed Jan. 12, 2012].

186. http://www.theglobalfund.org/en/board/meetings/twentyfifth [accessed Jan. 12, 2012].

187. Interview with a former Civil Society Team Officer, Global Fund, June 28, 2012.

188. http://keionline.org/node/1439 [accessed Jan. 12, 2012].

189. http://www.cptech.org/ip/health/who/hgapwhareport.html, qtd. in http://keion line.org/node/1439 [accessed Jan. 12, 2012].

190. http://keionline.org/node/1439 [accessed Feb. 12, 2012].

191. See http://lists.keionline.org/pipermail/ip-health_lists.keionline.org/2013-February /002802.html [accessed Apr. 30, 2014].

192. http://keionline.org/node/1648 [accessed Feb. 12, 2012].

193. Ibid.

194. http://www.ip-watch.org/2012/11/12/next-global-fund-director-to-be-chosen -from-four-candidates-this-week [accessed Jan. 12, 2012].

195. Ibid.

196. http://www.ip-watch.org/2012/11/15/global-fund-names-mark-dybul-executive -director [accessed Jan. 12, 2012].

197. Interview with the Civil Society and Private Sector Partnerships Manager, Global Fund, June 26, 2012.

198. Interview with a Consultant, Aidspan, Mar. 27, 2012.

199. Interview with a former Civil Society Team Officer, Global Fund, June 28, 2012.

200. Interview with the Director, International Harm Reduction Development Program, OSF, July 3, 2012.

201. Interview with the Executive Director, Aidspan, Mar. 26, 2012.

202. Interview with the Executive Director, UNITAID, June 25, 2012.

203. Interview with the Executive Director, Stop TB Partnership, June 26, 2012.

204. Interview with the Co-Founder, Health and Development Network, Aug. 15, 2012.

205. Interview with Advocacy Officer 2, ITPC, Eastern Europe and Central Asia, Sept. 26, 2011.

206. Interview with the Senior Program Officer, Global Campaign for Microbicides, Apr. 30, 2012.

207. Interview with the Advisor to the Executive Director, Global Health Workforce Alliance, June 29, 2012.

208. Interview with a Member of the PHM, Nov. 8, 2011.

209. Interview with the Executive Director, Stop TB Partnership, June 26, 2012.

210. Interview with the Associate Director, Global Fund Watch, China, Oct. 11, 2011.

211. Interview with the Director, International Harm Reduction Development Program, OSF, July 3, 2012.

212. Interview with the Advisor to the Executive Director, Global Health Workforce Alliance, June 29, 2012.

213. Interview with the Coordinator of Advocacy and Civil Society, Uganda AIDS Commission, Apr. 24, 2012.

214. Interview with the Senior Technical Advisor, ILO Programme on HIV/AIDS and the World of Work, June 29, 2012.

215. Ibid.

216. Interview with the Executive Director, Roll Back Malaria Partnership, June 29, 2012.

217. Interview with a Lawyer, GTPI/REBRIP, Feb. 24, 2012.

218. Interview with the Executive Director, Canadian HIV/AIDS Legal Network, July 9, 2012.

219. Interview with a Campaigner, KEI, June 27, 2012.

220. Interview with the Director, International Harm Reduction Development Program, OSF, July 3, 2012.

221. Interview with the Vice President and Regional Director, Global Business Coalition for Health, Sept. 6, 2011.

222. Ibid.

223. Interview with the Senior Program Officer, Global Campaign for Microbicides, Apr. 30, 2012.

224. Interview with a Member of the PHM, Nov. 8, 2011.

225. Interview with the Civil Society and Private Sector Partnerships Manager, Global Fund, June 26, 2012.

226. Interview with the External Relations Officer, UNAIDS, June 25, 2012.

227. Interview with a former Civil Society Team Officer, Global Fund, June 28, 2012.

228. Interview with the Executive Director, Stop TB Partnership, June 26, 2012.

229. Interview with the Executive Director, Roll Back Malaria Partnership, June 29, 2012.

230. Interview with the Senior Program Officer, Global Campaign for Microbicides, Apr. 30, 2012.

231. Interview with Advocacy Officer 1, ITPC, Eastern Europe and Central Asia, Sept. 24, 2011.

232. Interview with the Director, International Harm Reduction Development Program, OSF, July 3, 2012.

233. Ibid.

234. Ibid.

235. Interview with the Country Coordinator, UNAIDS-Egypt, May 29, 2012.

236. Interview with the Community Mobilization Chief, UNAIDS, June 28, 2012.

237. Interview with the Civil Society and Private Sector Partnerships Manager, Global Fund, June 26, 2012.

238. Interview with an External Relations Officer, UNAIDS, June 25, 2012.

239. Ibid.

240. Ibid.

241. Interview with the Executive Director, Stop TB Partnership, June 26, 2012.

242. Interview with the Civil Society and Private Sector Partnerships Manager, Global Fund, June 26, 2012.

243. Interview with the Executive Director, Friends of Life, June 4, 2012.

244. Ibid.

245. Interview with a Researcher, EATG, Aug. 6, 2012.

246. Interview with a former Civil Society Team Officer, Global Fund, June 28, 2012.

Chapter 5 · Against Community

Epigraphs. Carroll 1865: 41; interviews with the Global Campaigns Director, Health GAP, Mar. 26, 2012, and with a Member of the PHM, Nov. 8, 2011.

1. Interview with the Project Coordinator, Coalition for Children Affected by AIDS, July 9, 2012.

2. Interview with the Global Campaigns Director, Health GAP, Mar. 26, 2012.

3. Interview with the Regional Advocacy Team Leader and Advocacy Officer, ARASA, May 2, 2012.

4. For early AIDS activism in the United States, see the films *United in Anger* (2012) and *How to Survive a Plague* (2012).

5. http://www.apnplus.org/main/Index.php?module=aboutus [accessed Feb. 6, 2013].

6. Interview with the President, DNP+, Nov. 8, 2011.

7. Interview with the Executive Director, National Empowerment Network of People Living with HIV/AIDS, Mar. 30, 2012.

8. http://www.globaltimes.cn/features/metroshanghai/culture/2010-07/557894
.html [accessed Feb. 6, 2013].

9. Interview with the Executive Director, Friends of Life, June 4, 2012.

10. Interview with the Director, Tajik Network of Women Living with HIV/AIDS, Aug. 8, 2011.

11. Altman 1994.

12. Sedgwick 2008: 38–39, qtd. ibid.: 19.

13. Interview with the Executive Director, RedTraSex, Dec. 15, 2010.

14. Interview with the former Program Director, EHRN, July 29, 2011.

15. Interview with the Executive Director, CARAM, Nov. 18, 2011.

16. Interview with the former Program Director, EHRN, July 19, 2011.

17. Interview with the Co-Founder, GYCA, July 3, 2012.

18. Interview with the Project Coordinator, Coalition for Children Affected by AIDS, July 9, 2012.

19. http://www.redribbonaward.org/index.php?option=com_content&view=article
&id=356%3Apinitiative-ukraine&catid=56&Itemid=54&lang=en#.URNTnc3vRrY [accessed Feb. 8, 2013].

20. O'Malley, Nguyen, and Lee 1996.

21. http://www.aidsalliance.org/Pagedetails.aspx?id=166 [accessed Feb. 8, 2013].

22. Interview with the Executive Director, ITPC, Dec. 7, 2011.

23. Interview with the Global Campaigns Director, Health GAP, Mar. 26, 2012.

24. Interviews with an Activist, ACT UP, July 4, 2012, and the Co-Founder, Health and Development Network, Aug. 15, 2012.

25. Interview with an Activist, ACT UP, July 4, 2012.

26. Interview with Advocacy Officer 2, ITPC, Eastern Europe and Central Asia, Sept. 26, 2011.

27. Interview with the Co-Founder, ITPC, July 4, 2012.

28. Daniel and Parker 1993: 239, qtd. in Altman 1994: 166.

29. Interview with the Executive Director, ABIA, Feb. 24, 2012.

30. Interview with the Health and Discrimination Project Manager, Egyptian Initiative for Personal Rights, May 30, 2012.

31. Interview with the Co-Founder, Al Shehab Foundation, May 29, 2012.

32. Cai 2011.

33. Interview with the former Executive Director, Chain, China, Oct. 25, 2011.

34. Interview with the Executive Director, AIDS Access Foundation, Dec. 2, 2012.

35. Interview with a Researcher, EATG, Aug. 6, 2012.

36. Interview with the Co-Founder, Treatment Action Group, July 17, 2012.

37. Ibid.

38. Interview with the Executive Director, Asia Pacific Network of Sex Workers, Dec. 5, 2011.

39. Interview with the Executive Director, ANPUD, Dec. 3, 2011.

40. Interview with the former Communications Manager, AHRN, Dec. 2, 2011.

41. Ibid.

42. Interview with the Executive Director, CARAM, Nov. 18, 2011.

43. Interview with the Regional Program Coordinator, 7 Sisters, Dec. 6, 2011.

44. http://www.icw.org [accessed Feb. 8, 2013].

45. Interview with a Steering Committee Member, ICW, July 9, 2012.

46. Interview with the Co-Founder, GYCA, July 3, 2012.

47. http://www.gnpplus.net/resources/strategic-review-of-the-global-network-of-people -living-with-hiv [accessed Feb. 8, 2013].

48. Ibid.: 5.

49. Interview with the Technical Support Officer, GNP+, May 3, 2012.

50. Interview with the Executive Director, ITPC, Dec. 7, 2011.

51. Ibid.

52. Interview with a Member of the PHM, Nov. 8, 2011.

53. Ibid.

54. Interview with the Co-Founder, Treatment Action Group, July 17, 2012.

55. Interview with a Researcher, EATG, Aug. 6, 2012.

56. Interview with the Executive Director, Russian Harm Reduction Network, Sept. 5, 2011.

57. Interview with a Founding Member, APCOM, Dec. 8, 2011.

58. Interview with the Executive Director, TNP+, Dec. 2, 2011.

59. Interview with the Executive Director, RedTraSex, Dec. 15, 2010.

60. http://www.aids.gov.br/es/pagina/grupo-de-cooperacion-tecnica-horizontal [accessed Feb. 9, 2013].

61. http://www.actupny.org/documents/DA.html [accessed Feb. 9, 2013].

62. http://healthgap.org/about-health-gap [accessed Feb. 9, 2013].

63. http://www.itpcglobal.org/history [accessed Feb. 9, 2013].

64. http://www.gnpplus.net/resources/strategic-review-of-the-global-network-of -people-living-with-hiv [accessed Feb. 9, 2013].

65. Interview with the Co-Founder, Access to Medicines Research Group, China, Oct. 11, 2011.

66. Interview with an Activist, ACT UP, July 4, 2012.

67. Ibid.

68. Interview with the Executive Director, ITPC, Dec. 7, 2012.

69. Interview with the President, DNP+, Nov. 9, 2012.

70. Interview with a Consultant, UNAIDS, May 30, 2012.

71. Altman 1994: 19.

72. Interview with the Team Leader in Advocacy and Networking, TASO, Apr. 19, 2012.

73. Patton 1990: 140, qtd. in Altman 1994: 28.

74. Interview with a Researcher, EATG, Aug. 6, 2012.

75. Interview with the Regional Advocacy Team Leader, ARASA, May 2, 2013.

76. Interview with the Executive Director, ABIA, Feb. 24, 2012.

77. Interview with the External Relations Officer, UNAIDS, June 25, 2012.

78. Interview with the Director, UNDP HIV/AIDS Group, July 2, 2012.

79. Interview with Advocacy Officer 2, ITPC-Russia, Sept. 26, 2011.

80. Interview with the Vice President and Regional Director, Global Business Coalition for Health, Russia, Sept. 6, 2011.

81. Interview with the President, DNP+, Nov. 8, 2011.

82. Interview with a former Staff Member, MSF–Hong Kong, Oct. 25, 2011.

83. Interview with a Consultant, Aidspan, Mar. 27, 2012.

84. Murray 1993: 8, qtd. in Altman 1994: 144.

85. Interview with the Founder and Executive Director, Dongzhen Center for Human Rights Education and Action, Oct. 13, 2011.

86. http://stopaids.org.uk/our-work/consultancy/investing-in-communities-achieves-results-findings-from-the-evaluation-of-the-community-response-to-hiv-and-aids [accessed Feb. 11, 2013].

87. Interview with the Civil Society and Private Sector Partnerships Manager, Global Fund, June 26, 2012.

88. Interview with the former Program Director, EHRN, July 19, 2011.

89. Interview with Advocacy Officer 2, ITPC-Russia, Sept. 26, 2011.

90. International HIV/AIDS Alliance 1995: 2, qtd. in Gordenker et al. 1995: 107–108.

91. Ibid.

92. Epstein 1996: 261.

93. European AIDS Treatment Group 2012.

94. Interview with a Researcher, EATG, Aug. 6, 2012.

95. Interview with an Activist, ACT UP, July 4, 2012.

96. Epstein 1996: 342.

97. Qtd. ibid.

98. Ibid.: 55.

99. http://unaidspcbngo.org/?page_id=1189 [accessed Feb. 12, 2013].

100. http://unaidspcbngo.org/?page_id=1194 [accessed Feb. 12, 2013].

101. McCoy and Hilson 2009.

102. Interview with the External Relations Officer, UNAIDS, June 25, 2012.

103. Interview with the Co-Founder, Health and Development Network, Aug. 15, 2012.

104. http://www.unaids.org/en/media/unaids/contentassets/dataimport/pub/externaldocument/2007/review_ngo_participation_item_3.2_en.pdf [accessed Feb. 12, 2013].

105. http://unaidspcbngo.org/?page_id=1199 [accessed Feb. 12, 2013].

106. Interview with the Civil Society and Private Sector Partnerships Manager, Global Fund, June 26, 2012.

107. Interview with a Consultant, Aidspan, Mar. 27, 2012.

108. Buse and Harmer 2009.

109. http://www.gavialliance.org/about/partners/the-partnership-model [accessed Feb. 12, 2013].

110. Buse and Harmer 2009.

111. Transnational Research Action Centre 2000, qtd. in McCoy and Hilson 2009: 212.

112. Iboudo 1993: 10, qtd. in Altman 1994: 144.

113. Interview with the Executive Director, WAC, May 2, 2012.

114. Interview with Advocacy Officer 1, ITPC, Eastern Europe and Central Asia, Sept. 25, 2011.

115. Interview with the former Executive Director, Chain, China, Oct. 25, 2011.

116. Interviews with the Director of Global Campaigns, Health GAP, Mar. 26, 2012, and with Advocacy Officer 2, ITPC, Eastern Europe and Central Asia, Sept. 26, 2011.

117. Woolcock and Altman 1996.

118. Interview with the Vice President and Regional Director, Global Business Coalition for Health, Russia, Sept. 6, 2011.

119. Interview with an Activist, ACT UP, July 4, 2012.

120. Interview with the President, DNP+, Nov. 8, 2011.

121. Gordenker et al. 1995.

122. Ibid.: 97.

123. Altman 1994: 61.

124. Ibid.: 60.

125. O'Malley, Nguyen, and Lee 1996.

126. Interview with the Co-Founder, Health and Development Network, Aug. 15, 2012.

127. Interview with the President, DNP+, Nov. 8, 2011.

128. Interview with Advocacy Officer 1, ITPC, Eastern Europe and Central Asia, Sept. 25, 2011.

129. Interview with the Executive Director, ITPC, Dec. 7, 2011.

130. Gordenker et al. 1995.

131. Ibid.: 98.

132. Interview with the Co-Founder, Health and Development Network, Aug. 15, 2012.

133. Interview with the Executive Director, WAC, May 2, 2012.

134. Ibid.

135. Interview with a Member of the PHM, Nov. 8, 2011.

136. Altman 1994: 151.

137. Interview with the Executive Director, WAC, May 2, 2012.

138. Interview with the Founder and Executive Director, Dongzhen Center for Human Rights Education and Action, Oct. 13, 2011.

139. European AIDS Treatment Group 2012: 8.

140. Sabatier 1988.

141. Ibid.

142. http://www.cdc.gov/hiv/topics/aa [accessed Feb. 13, 2013].

143. http://www.actuporalhistory.org/interviews/interviews_01.html#agosto [accessed Feb. 13, 2013].

144. Ibid.

145. Altman 1994: 76.

146. Fassin 2007: 173.

147. Ibid.

148. http://www.princeton.edu/~ota/disk1/1992/9206/920603.PDF [accessed Feb. 13, 2013].

149. Ibid.

150. Interview with the Global Fund Grants Program Manager, UNDP-Kyrgyzstan, July 19, 2011.

151. Interview with a Member of the International Steering Committee, ICW, July 9, 2012.

152. www.theglobalfund.org [accessed Feb. 13, 2013].

153. www.cgfwatch.org/c9990/w10048916.asp [accessed Feb. 13, 2013].

154. Interview with the Coordinator, Youth Lead, Dec. 7, 2011.

155. Interview with the Co-Founder, GYCA, July 3, 2012.

156. Ibid.

157. Interview with the Coordinator, Youth Lead, Dec. 7, 2011.

158. Interview with the Project Coordinator, Coalition for Children Affected by AIDS, July 9, 2012.

159. Interview with the former Program Director, EHRN, July 19, 2011.

160. Interview with a Founding Member, APCOM, Dec. 8, 2011.

161. Interview with the former Program Director, EHRN, July 19, 2011.

162. Interview with a Founding Member, APCOM, Dec. 8, 2011.

163. Interview with Advocacy Officer 1, ITPC, Eastern Europe and Central Asia, Sept. 25, 2011.

164. Interview with the former Communications Manager, AHRN, Dec. 2, 2011.

165. Interview with the Executive Director, ITPC, Dec. 7, 2011.

166. Interview with the Senior Technical Advisor, HIV and Key Populations, UNFPA, July 3, 2012.

167. Interview with a Founding Member, APCOM, Dec. 8, 2011.

168. Interview with the Executive Director, Canadian HIV/AIDS Legal Network, July 9, 2012.

169. Interview with the Executive Director, RedTraSex, Dec. 15, 2010.

170. Interview with the Advocacy Manager, SWEAT, May 2, 2012.

171. Interview with the Co-Founder, Al Shehab Foundation, May 29, 2012.

172. Ibid.

173. O'Malley, Nguyen, and Lee 1996.

174. Interview with the Vice President and Regional Director, Global Business Coalition for Health, Russia, Sept. 6, 2011.

175. Interview with the former Communications Manager, AHRN, Dec. 2, 2011.

176. Interview with the Regional Program Coordinator, 7 Sisters, Dec. 6, 2011.

177. Interview with a Founding Member, APCOM, Dec. 8, 2011.

178. Interview with the Executive Director, CARAM, Nov. 18, 2011.

179. Interview with the Executive Director, Chi Heng Foundation, Mar. 25, 2013.

180. Interview with the Assistant Communications Manager, M2M, May 3, 2012.

181. Interview with the Executive Director, TNP+, Dec. 2, 2011.

182. Interview with the Co-Founder, Health and Development Network, Aug. 15, 2012.

183. Rau 2007.

184. Interview with the former Program Director, EHRN, July 29, 2011.

185. Interview with the Technical Support Officer, GNP+, May 3, 2012.

186. Interview with the Regional Program Coordinator, 7 Sisters, Dec. 6, 2011.

187. Interview with the Executive Director, ANPUD, Dec. 3, 2011.

188. Interview with the Executive Director, Asia Pacific Network of Sex Workers, Dec. 5, 2011.

189. Interview with the Executive Director, ITPC, Dec. 7, 2011.

190. Interview with the Information Manager, Andrey Rylkov Foundation, Russia, Sept. 2, 2011.

191. Interview with the Executive Director, Shanghai AIDS Prevention Center, Oct. 20, 2012.

192. Interview with a Representative, MSF–South Africa Access Campaign, May 2, 2012.

193. Interview with the Regional Advocacy Team Leader and Advocacy Officer, ARASA, May 2, 2012.

194. Interview with the Health and Discrimination Project Manager, Egyptian Initiative for Personal Rights, May 30, 2012.

195. Interview with the Information Manager, Andrey Rylkov Foundation, Russia, Sept. 2, 2011.

196. Interview with the Co-Founder, Health and Development Network, Aug. 15, 2012.

197. Interview with an Activist, ACT UP, July 4, 2012.

198. Interview with a Member, International Steering Committee, ICW, July 9, 2012.

199. Korten 1986: 325, qtd. in Altman 1994: 11.

200. Interview with Advocacy Officer 2, ITPC, Eastern Europe and Central Asia, Sept. 26, 2011.

201. Interview with the Executive Director, ABIA, Feb. 24, 2012.

202. Interview with the Executive Director, Israel AIDS Task Force, June 20, 2012.

203. http://keionline.org/about [accessed Feb. 15, 2013].

204. http://www.gnpplus.net/about-gnp/strategic-plan-2011-2015 [accessed Feb. 15, 2013].

205. Interview with the Advocacy Officer, MSF–New Delhi, Dec. 9, 2011.

206. Interview with an Activist, ACT UP, July 4, 2012.

207. Interview with the Global Fund Grants Program Manager, UNDP-Kyrgyzstan, July 19, 2011.

208. Interview with a former Staff Member, MSF–Hong Kong, Oct. 25, 2011.

209. Interview with the Social Mobilization Advisor, UNAIDS-China, Oct. 13, 2011.

210. Interview with the Civil Society and Private Sector Partnerships Manager, Global Fund, June 26, 2012.

211. Interview with Advocacy Officer 2, ITPC, Eastern Europe and Central Asia, Sept. 26, 2011.

212. Interview with the Executive Director, TNP+, Dec. 2, 2011.

213. Interview with a Member of the PHM, Nov. 8, 2011.

214. Interview with the Director, UNDP HIV/AIDS Group, July 2, 2012.

215. Interview with the former Executive Director, Chain, China, Oct. 25, 2011.

216. Interview with the Co-Founder, Health and Development Network, Aug. 15, 2012.

217. Interview with an Activist, ACT UP, July 4, 2012.

218. Interview with the Executive Director, TNP+, Dec. 2, 2011.

219. Interview with a Researcher, EATG, Aug. 6, 2012.

220. For analyses of international development NGOs' management effectiveness, see Edwards 2006; Hilhorst 2003; Edwards and Fowler 2002; and Fowler 1997.

221. Interview with the Co-Founder, ITPC, July 4, 2012.

222. Interview with the Social Mobilization Advisor, UNAIDS-China, Oct. 13, 2011.

223. Interview with the Technical Support Officer, GNP+, May 3, 2012.

224. Interview with the Regional Program Coordinator, 7 Sisters, Dec. 6, 2011.

225. Interview with an Activist, ACT UP, July 4, 2012.

226. Interview with a Representative, MSF–South Africa Access Campaign, May 2, 2012.

227. Ibid.

228. Interview with the Country Coordinator, UNAIDS-Egypt, May 30, 2012.

229. Interview with the Vice President and Regional Director, Russia, Global Business Coalition for Health, Sept. 6, 2011.

230. Interview with an Activist, ACT UP, July 4, 2012.

Chapter 6 · *Conclusion*

Epigraphs. Bhabha 1994, qtd. in Young 2003: 83; interview with the General Secretary, TAC, May 4, 2012; interview with a Senior Researcher, AIDS Accountability International, May 4, 2013.

1. Epstein 1996.
2. Ibid.
3. See Nader et al. 1993.
4. Interview with the Executive Director, Canadian HIV/AIDS Legal Network, July 10, 2012.
5. http://www.oecd.org/dac/effectiveness/parisdeclarationandaccraagendaforaction .htm [accessed Mar. 8, 2013].
6. Low-Beer 2012.
7. Epstein 2007.
8. Richter 2004.
9. Agamben 1998.
10. Young 2003.
11. Boler and Archer 2008: 107.
12. http://www.msfaccess.org/content/msf-review-july-2011-gilead-licences-medicines -patent-pool [accessed Mar. 8, 2013].
13. http://www.who.int/phi/CEWG_Report_5_April_2012.pdf [accessed Mar. 8, 2013].
14. Ibid.
15. http://www.ip-watch.org/weblog/wp-content/uploads/2009/07/appg-policy -report.pdf [accessed Mar. 8, 2013].
16. Maathai 2009: 34, 39–40.
17. Ibid.: 77.
18. Global HIV Prevention Working Group 2007, qtd. in Boler and Archer 2008: 46.
19. Paisan Suwannawong, Treatment Action Group, Thailand, speaking at the March 2003 International Treatment Preparedness Summit, http://www.who.int/3by5/partners /en/factsheet.pdf [accessed Mar. 9, 2013].
20. Interview with a Member of the PHM, Nov. 8, 2011.
21. Lyotard 1984: 46.
22. Bourdieu 1993: 944, qtd. in Farmer 2003: 224.

Abel, Gillian, Lisa Fitzgerald, Catherine Healy, and Aline Taylor, eds. 2010. *Taking the Crime out of Sex Work: New Zealand Sex Workers' Fight for Decriminalisation*. Bristol, England: Policy Press.

Agamben, Giorgio. 1998. *Homo Sacer: Sovereign Power and Bare Life*. Stanford, CA: Stanford University Press.

All-Parliamentary Group on AIDS. 2003. *Migration and HIV: Improving Lives in Britain: An Enquiry into the Impact of the UK Nationality and Immigration System on People Living with HIV*. London: All-Parliamentary Group on AIDS.

Altman, Dennis. 1994. *Power and Community: Organizational and Cultural Responses to AIDS*. London: Taylor and Francis.

Balzano, John, and Jia Ping. 2006. "Coming Out of Denial: An Analysis of AIDS Law and Policy in China (1987–2006)." *Loyola University Chicago International Law Review* 3(2): 187–212.

Bartky, Sandra Lee. 1990. *Femininity and Domination: Studies in the Phenomenology of Oppression*. New York: Routledge.

Beyrer, Chris. 1998. *War in the Blood: Sex, Politics and AIDS in Southeast Asia*. London: Zed.

Bhabha, Homi. 1994. *The Location of Culture*. New York: Routledge.

Biehl, João. 2007. *Will to Live: AIDS Therapies and the Politics of Survival*. Princeton, NJ: Princeton University Press.

Boler, Tania, and David Archer. 2008. *The Politics of Prevention: A Global Crisis in AIDS and Education*. London: Pluto.

Bourdieu, Pierre. 1993. *La Misère du Monde*. Paris: Seuil.

Braithwaite, John, and Peter Drahos. 2000. *Global Business Regulation*. Cambridge: Cambridge University Press.

Briggs, Charles, and Clara Mantini-Briggs. 2003. *Stories in the Time of Cholera: Racial Profiling during a Medical Nightmare*. Berkeley: University of California Press.

Buchanan, Allen, and Robert O. Keohane. 2006. "The Legitimacy of Global Governance Institutions." *Ethics and International Affairs* 20(4): 405–437.

Buse, Kent, and Andrew Harmer. 2009. "Global Health Partnerships: The Mosh Pit of Global Health Governance." In *Making Sense of Global Health Governance*, edited by Kent Buse, Wolfgang Hein, and Nick Drager. New York: Palgrave Macmillan.

Buse, Kent, Wolfgang Hein, and Nick Drager, eds. 2009. *Making Sense of Global Health Governance*. New York: Palgrave Macmillan.

Cai, Rui. 2011. "Global Fund Pressures China to Engage with Civil Society Groups." *BMJ*, http://www.bmj.com/rapid-response/2011/11/03/global-funds-freeze-china-time-con sider-role-ngos-country [accessed Feb. 7, 2013].

Cakmak, Cenap. 2008. "Civil Society Actors in International Law and World Politics: Definition, Conceptual Framework, Problems." *International Journal of Civil Society Law* 6(1): 7–35.

Cameron, Edwin, Scott Burris, and Michaela Clayton. 2008. "HIV Is a Virus, Not a Crime: Ten Reasons against Criminal Statutes and Criminal Prosecutions." *Journal of the International AIDS Society* 13(2–3): 64–70.

Canadian HIV/AIDS Legal Network. 1999. *Summary: R. v. Cuerrier.* Toronto: Canadian HIV/AIDS Legal Network. http://www.aidslaw.ca/EN/lawyers-kit/documents/2.Cuer rier1998summary.pdf [accessed Jan. 6, 2013].

———. 2002. *Action on HIV/AIDS in Prisons: Too Little, Too Late—A Report Card.* Toronto: Canadian HIV/AIDS Legal Network.

———. 2005a. *Aboriginal People and HIV/AIDS: Legal Issues.* Toronto: Canadian HIV/ AIDS Legal Network.

———. 2005b. *Nothing about Us without Us—Greater Meaningful Involvement of People Who Use Illegal Drugs: A Public Health, Ethical, and Human Rights Imperative.* Toronto: Canadian HIV/AIDS Legal Network.

———. 2005c. *Sex, Work, Rights: Changing Canada's Criminal Laws to Protect Sex Workers' Health and Human Rights.* Toronto: Canadian HIV/AIDS Legal Network.

———. 2007. *Hard Time: HIV and Hepatitis C Prevention Programming for Prisoners in Canada.* Toronto: Canadian HIV/AIDS Legal Network.

———. 2008. *Nothing about Us without Us—A Manifesto by People Who Use Illegal Drugs.* Toronto: Canadian HIV/AIDS Legal Network.

———. 2010. *Summary: Court of Appeal of Manitoba: R. v. Mabior 2010 MBCA 93.* Toronto: Canadian HIV/AIDS Legal Network. http://www.aidslaw.ca/publications/interfaces /downloadFile.php?ref=1794 [accessed Jan. 6, 2013].

Carroll, Lewis. 1865. *Alice in Wonderland.* London: Medisat Group.

Castells, Manuel. 2010. *The Power of Identity.* Malden, MA: Wiley-Blackwell.

———. 2012. *Networks of Outrage and Hope: Social Movements in the Internet Age.* Cambridge: Polity.

Cerny, Philip. 2005. "Power, Markets and Authority: The Development of Multi-level Governance in International Finance." In *Governing Financial Globalization*, edited by Andrew Baker, Alan Hudson, and Richard Woodward. New York: Routledge.

Chen, Jiwen. 2001. "Better Patent Law for International Commitment: The Amendment of Chinese Patent Law." *Richmond Journal of Global Law and Business* 2(1): 61–73.

Chin, James. 2007. *The AIDS Pandemic: The Collision of Epidemiology with Political Correctness.* London: Radcliffe.

Conway, Janet. 2004. *Identity, Place, Knowledge: Social Movements Contesting Globalization.* Black Point, NS: Fernwood.

Crimp, Douglas. 2004. *Melancholia and Moralism: Essays on AIDS and Queer Politics.* Cambridge, MA: MIT Press.

D'Adesky, Anne-Christine. 2004. *Moving Mountains: The Race to Treat Global AIDS.* London: Verso.

Dallas Buyers Club. 2013. Dir. Jean-Marc Vallée. Focus Features.

Daniel, Herbert, and Richard Parker. 1993. *Sexuality, Politics and AIDS in Brazil.* London: Falmer.

de Carvalho, Felipe. 2012. "Success Story: The Case of TDF in Brazil." http://patentoppositions.org/case_studies/4f106d0504a7f92f5b000003 [accessed Jan. 8, 2013].

Derrida, Jacques. 1981. *Positions.* Chicago: University of Chicago Press.

Desmond Tutu HIV Foundation and Joint UN Team on HIV/AIDS. 2011. *Key Populations, Key Solutions: A Gap Analysis and Recommendations for Key Populations in South Africa, and Recommendations for the National Strategic Plan for HIV/AIDS, STIs and TB (2012–2016).* Cape Town, South Africa: Desmond Tutu HIV Foundation.

Desphande, Rohit, Sandra Sucher, and Laura Winig. 2011. *Cipla.* Cambridge, MA: Harvard Business School.

Dreifus, Claudia. 1994. "Joycelyn Elders." *New York Times* (Jan. 30), http://www.nytimes.com/1994/01/30/magazine/joycelyn-elders.html?pagewanted=all&src=pm [accessed Jan. 6, 2013].

Dunkley, Graham. 2004. *Free Trade: Myth, Reality and Alternatives.* London: Zed.

Edwards, Michael. 2006. *Future Positive: International Cooperation in the 21st Century.* London: Routledge/Earthscan.

Edwards, Michael, and Alan Fowler. 2002. *Earthscan Reader on NGO Management.* London: Routledge/Earthscan.

Engel, Jonathan. 2006. *The Epidemic: A Global History of AIDS.* Washington, DC: Smithsonian Institution Press.

Epstein, Steven. 1996. *Impure Science: AIDS, Activism, and the Politics of Knowledge.* Berkeley: University of California Press.

———. 2007. *Inclusion: The Politics of Difference in Medical Research.* Chicago: University of Chicago Press.

European AIDS Treatment Group. 2012. *Twenty Years of Treatment Activism.* http://www.eatg.org/gallery/6/EATG_20%20years%20report.pdf [accessed Feb. 11, 2013].

Eyerman, Ron, and Andrew Jamison. 1991. *Social Movements: A Cognitive Approach.* Philadelphia: University of Pennsylvania Press.

Farmer, Paul. 1992. *AIDS and Accusation: Haiti and the Geography of Blame.* Berkeley: University of California Press.

———. 2003. *Pathologies of Power: Health, Human Rights, and the New War on the Poor.* Berkeley: University of California Press.

Fassin, Didier. 2007. *When Bodies Remember: Experiences and Politics of AIDS in South Africa.* Berkeley: University of California Press.

Fight Back, Fight AIDS: 15 Years of ACT UP. 2004. Dir. James Wentzy. Frameline.

Foller, Maj-Lis, and Hakan Thorn, eds. 2008. *The Politics of AIDS: Globalization, the State, and Civil Society.* New York: Palgrave Macmillan.

Fort, Meredith, Mary Ann Mercer, Oscar Gish, and Steve Gloyd, eds. 2004. *Sickness and Wealth: The Corporate Assault on Global Health.* Boston: South End.

Foucault, Michel. 1972. "Truth and Power." In *Power/Knowledge: Selected Interviews and Other Writings 1972–1977,* edited by Colin Gordon. New York: Vintage.

———. 1978. *History of Sexuality,* vol. 1: *An Introduction.* New York: Pantheon.

Fowler, Alan. 1997. *Striking a Balance: A Guide to Enhancing the Effectiveness of Non-Governmental Organisations in International Development.* London: Routledge.

Fraser, Nancy. 2003. "Social Justice in the Age of Identity Politics: Redistribution, Recognition, and Participation." In *Redistribution or Recognition: A Political-Philosophical Exchange*, edited by Nancy Fraser and Axel Honneth. London: Verso.

Gallahue, Patrick, and Rick Lines. 2010. *The Death Penalty for Drug Offences: Global Overview 2010*. London: International Harm Reduction Association. http://www.ihra.net/files/2010/06/16/IHRA_DeathPenaltyReport_Web1.pdf [accessed Jan. 6, 2013].

Garnier, Jean-Pierre. 2003. "He Will Drop the Prices of His Drugs to the Poorest Countries." *Guardian* (Feb. 18).

Gaucher, Bob. 2002. *Writing as Resistance*. Toronto: Canadian Scholars' Press.

George, Julie, Ramya Sheshadri, and Anand Grover. 2009. "Intellectual Property and Access to Medicines: Development and Civil Society Initiatives in India." In *Intellectual Property Rights and Access to ARV Medicines: Civil Society Resistance in the Global South*, edited by Veriano Terto, Renata Reis, and Cristina Pimenta. Rio de Janeiro: ABIA.

Global Commission on HIV and the Law. 2012. *HIV and the Law: Risks, Rights, and Health*. New York: Global Commission on HIV and the Law. http://www.hivlawcommission.org/index.php/report [accessed Jan. 8, 2013].

Global Fund. 2008. *Listening to the Voices: Recommendations from the Global Fund Partnership Forum, Dakar, Senegal, 8–10 December 2008*. http://www.theglobalfund.org/documents/partnershipforum/2008/PF2008_Recommendations.pdf [accessed Jan. 8, 2012].

Global HIV Prevention Working Group. 2007. *Bringing HIV Prevention to Scale: An Urgent Global Priority*. http://www.globalhivprevention.org/pdfs/PWG-HIV_prevention_report_FINAL.pdf [accessed Mar. 10, 2013].

Global Network of People Living with HIV/AIDS. 2011. *Strategic Plan 2011–2015*. http://www.gnpplus.net/images/stories/About_GNP/GNP_StrategicPlan_EN_web.pdf [accessed Feb. 15, 2013].

Gonsalves, Gregg, and Mark Harrington. 1992. *AIDS Research at the NIH: A Critical Review*. http://www.treatmentactiongroup.org/sites/g/files/g450272/f/AIDS%20Research%20at%20the%20NIH%20Part%20I%20Jul%201992.pdf [accessed Apr. 4, 2014].

Gordenker, Leon, Roger Coate, Christer Jonsson, and Peter Soderholm, eds. 1995. *International Cooperation in Response to AIDS*. London: Pinter.

Gorman, Christine. 2012. "Timeline: A Few Landmarks in the Effort to Treat AIDS." *Scientific American* (Mar.), http://www.scientificamerican.com/article.cfm?id=hiv-timeline-landmarks-aids-treatment-effort [accessed Mar. 10, 2013].

Green, Edward. 2003. *Rethinking AIDS Prevention: Learning from Successes in Developing Countries*. Westport, CT: Praeger.

Griffin, Gabriele. 2000. *Representations of HIV and AIDS: Visibility Blue/s*. Manchester, England: Manchester University Press.

Grover, Anand. 2008. *TRIPS Patent Law and Access to Medicines*. http://www.3dthree.org/pdf_3D/GroverTRIPSMeds.pdf [accessed Jan. 8, 2013].

Guest, Emma. 2003. *Children of AIDS: Africa's Orphan Crisis*. London: Pluto.

Hamied, Yusuf. 2005a. "The Cipla Story on HIV and AIDS." Presentation at Tufts University, India, Nov. 9.

———. 2005b. *Indian Pharma Industry: Decades of Struggle and Achievements*. Mumbai: Cipla.

Harden, Victoria. 2012. *AIDS at 30: A History*. Dulles, VA: Potomac Books.

Hein, Wolfgang, Sonja Bartsch, and Lars Kohlmorgen. 2007. *Global Health Governance and the Fight against HIV/AIDS*. New York: Palgrave Macmillan.

Hein, Wolfgang, Scott Burris, and Clifford Shearing. 2009. "Conceptual Models for Global Health Governance." In *Making Sense of Global Health Governance*, edited by Kent Buse, Wolfgang Hein, and Nick Drager. New York: Palgrave Macmillan.

Hekman, Susan. 1996. *Feminist Interpretations of Michel Foucault*. Philadelphia: University of Pennsylvania Press.

Held, David. 2003. "From Executive to Cosmopolitan Multilateralism." In *Taming Globalization*, edited by David Held and Mathias Koenig-Archibugi. Cambridge: Polity.

Hilhorst, Dorothea. 2003. *The Real World of NGOs: Discourses, Diversity and Development*. London: Zed.

Hood, Joanna. 2011. *HIV/AIDS, Health and the Media in China: Imagined Immunity through Racialized Disease*. New York: Routledge.

How to Survive a Plague. 2012. Dir. David France. Sundance Selects.

Hrdy, Daniel. 1987. "Cultural Practices Contributing to the Transmission of Human Immunodeficiency Virus in Africa." *Reviews of Infectious Diseases* 9(6): 1109–1119, http://www.msfaccess.org/content/acta-and-its-impact-access-medicines [accessed Jan. 8, 2013].

Hu, Yuan Qion. 2011. *Access to Medicines and IPR Advocacy in China: Review and Initial SWOT Discussion*. http://health.accel-it.lt/en/seminar/civil_society_strategy_meeting_on_the_future_of_access_to_medicines/presentation [accessed Jan. 8, 2013].

Human Rights Watch. 2005. *The Less They Know, the Better*. New York: Human Rights Watch. http://www.hrw.org/reports/2005/03/29/less-they-know-better [accessed Jan. 8, 2012].

———. 2013. *Laws of Attrition: Crackdown on Russia's Civil Society after Putin's Return to the Presidency*. New York: Human Rights Watch.

Hunter, Susan. 2003. *Black Death: AIDS in Africa*. New York: Palgrave Macmillan.

———. 2005. *AIDS in Asia: A Continent in Peril*. New York: Palgrave Macmillan.

Iboudo, A.-E. 1993. "A Message for the Development Community." *AIDSLink*, NCIH Washington (Mar. 10).

International HIV/AIDS Alliance. 1995. "Mission, Vision and Values Statements." In *International Cooperation in Response to AIDS*, edited by Leon Gordenker, Roger Coate, Christer Jonsson, and Peter Soderholm. London: Pinter.

International Treatment Preparedness Coalition and Initiative for Medicines, Access, and Knowledge. 2011. *Measuring the Impact of Medicines Patent Pool Licenses: A Civil Society Assessment*. http://www.i-mak.org/publications [accessed Dec. 22, 2012].

Jambert, Elodie. 2004. *MSF Experiences in China: Challenges in Procurement*. apps.who.int/hiv/amds/capacity/khm16.pdf [accessed Jan. 8, 2013].

Johnson, Harry. 1967. *Economic Policies for the Less Developed Countries*. New York: Praeger.

Jones, Kent. 2004. *Who's Afraid of the WTO?* Oxford: Oxford University Press.

Kickbush, Ilona. 2007. "Foreword: Governing Interdependence." In *Global Health Governance and the Fight against HIV/AIDS*, edited by Wolfgang Hein, Sonja Bartsch, and Lars Kohlmorgen. New York: Palgrave Macmillan.

Kijtiwatchakul, Kannikar. 2009. *The Rights to Life: Advocacy Experience of Access to ARVS in Thailand*. Beijing: Third World Network; China Access to Medicines Research Group; and China Global Fund Watch.

Kirby, Michael. 1988. "The New AIDS Virus—Ineffective and Unjust Laws." *Journal of Acquired Immunodeficiency Syndrome* 1(3): 304–312.

Korten, David. 1986. "Community Management and Social Transformation." In *Community Management: Asian Experience and Perspectives*, edited by David Korten. West Hartford, CT: Kumarian.

Lancet. 2009. "What Has the Gates Foundation Done for Global Health?" *Lancet* 373 (9675): 1577. http://www.thelancet.com/journals/lancet/article/PIIS01406736096088 50/fulltext?rss=yes [accessed Jan. 8, 2012].

Lawson, Gary, Ann Lawson, and Clayton Rivers. 2001. *Essentials of Clinical Dependency Counseling.* New York: Aspen.

Limpananont, Jiraporn, Achara Eksaengsri, Kannikar Kijtiwatchakul, and Noah Metheny. 2009. "Thailand: Access to AIDS Treatment and Intellectual Property Rights Protection in Thailand." In *Intellectual Property Rights and Access to ARV Medicines: Civil Society Resistance in the Global South*, edited by Veriano Terto, Renata Reis, and Cristina Pimenta. Rio de Janeiro: ABIA.

Low-Beer, Daniel, ed. 2012. *Innovative Health Partnerships: The Diplomacy of Diversity.* Singapore: World Scientific.

Lyotard, Jean-François. 1984. *The Postmodern Condition: A Report on Knowledge.* Minneapolis: University of Minnesota Press.

Lyttleton, Chris. 2008. *Mekong Erotics: Men Loving/Pleasuring/Using Men in Lao PDR.* Bangkok: UNESCO Bangkok. http://unesdoc.unesco.org/images/0017/001798 /179862e.pdf [accessed Jan. 6, 2013].

Maathai, Wangari. 2009. *The Challenge for Africa.* London: Arrow Books.

Mann, Jonathan. 1999. "Human Rights and AIDS: The Future of the Epidemic." In *Health and Human Rights*, edited by Jonathan Mann, Sofia Gruskin, Michael Grodin, and George Annas. New York: Routledge.

McCoy, D., and M. Hilson. 2009. "Civil Society, Its Organizations, and Global Health Governance." In *Making Sense of Global Health Governance*, edited by Kent Buse, Wolfgang Hein, and Nick Drager. New York: Palgrave Macmillan.

McCoy, David, Gayatri Kembhavi, Jinesh Patel, and Akish Luintel. 2009. "The Bill and Melinda Gates Foundation's Grant-Making Programme for Global Health." *Lancet* 373(9675): 1645–1653. http://www.thelancet.com/journals/lancet/article/PIIS0140-6736 %2809%2960571-7/abstract [accessed Jan. 8, 2012].

McDonnell, Margaret Reilly. 2007. *Case Study of the Campaigns Leading to the President's Emergency Plan for AIDS Relief.* Arlington, VA: US Coalition for Child Survival.

McSherry, Corynne. 2001. *Who Owns Academic Work: Battling for Control of Intellectual Property.* Cambridge, MA: Harvard University Press.

Melucci, Alberto. 1996. *Challenging Codes: Collective Action in the Information Age.* Cambridge: Cambridge University Press.

Millen, Joyce, Dorothy Fallows, and Alexander Irwin. 2003. *Global AIDS: Myths and Facts.* Cambridge, MA: South End.

Miller, James. 2005. "African Immigrant Damnation Syndrome: The Case of Charles Ssenyonga." *Sexuality Research and Social Policy* 2(2): 31–50.

Moore, Mike. 2004. *Doha and Beyond: The Future of the Multilateral Trading System.* Cambridge: Cambridge University Press.

MSF. 2007. *Help Wanted: Confronting the Health Care Worker Crisis to Expand Access to HIV /AIDS Treatment.* http://www.doctorswithoutborders.org/publications/reports/2007 /healthcare_worker_report_05-2007.pdf [accessed Jan. 11, 2013].

———. 2010. *No Time to Quit: HIV/AIDS Treatment Gap Widening in Africa.* http://www .doctorswithoutborders.org/publications/reports/2010/MSF-No-Time-to-Quit-HIV -AIDS.pdf [accessed Jan. 8, 2013].

———. 2011. *MSF Review of the July 2011 Gilead Licences to the Medicines Patent Pool.* http://www.msfaccess.org/content/msf-review-july-2011-gilead-licences-medicines -patent-pool [accessed Jan. 8, 2013].

———. 2012a. *Untangling the Web of Antiretroviral Price Reductions.* http://d2pd3b5abq7 5bb.cloudfront.net/2012/11/27/10/34/06/884/MSF_Access_UTW_15th_Edition_2012 _updatedOct2012.pdf [accessed Jan. 8, 2013].

———. 2012b. *Blank Cheque for Abuse: ACTA and Its Impact on Access to Medicines.* http://www.msfaccess.org/sites/default/files/MSF_assets/Access/Docs/Access_ Briefing_ACTABlankCheque_ENG_2012.pdf [accessed Jan. 8, 2013].

Murray, Alison. 1993. "Dying for a Fuck: Implications for HIV/AIDS in Indonesia." Paper presented at the Gender Relations Conference, Australian National University, Canberra.

Nader, Ralph, et al. 1993. *The Case against "Free Trade": GATT, NAFTA, and the Globalization of Corporate Power.* San Francisco, CA: Earth Island.

Nattrass, Nicoli. 2004. *The Moral Economy of AIDS in South Africa.* Cambridge: Cambridge University Press.

Nunn, Amy. 2009. *The Politics and History of AIDS Treatment in Brazil.* New York: Springer.

Okie, Susan. 2006. "Global Health: The Gates-Buffett Effect." *New England Journal of Medicine* 355: 1084–1088.

O'Malley, Jeff, Vinh Kim Nguyen, and Sarah Lee. 1996. "Nongovernmental Organizations." In *AIDS in the World II*, edited by Jonathan Mann and Daniel Tarantola. Oxford: Oxford University Press.

Oppenheimer, Gerald. 1988. "In the Eye of the Storm: The Epidemiological Construction of AIDS." In *AIDS: The Burdens of History*, edited by Elizabeth Fee and Daniel Fox. Berkeley: University of California Press.

Orubuloye, I. O., John Caldwell, Pat Caldwell, and Gigi Santow. 1994. *Sexual Networking and AIDS in Sub-Saharan Africa: Behavioral Research and the Social Context.* Canberra: Australian National University.

Patterson, Amy. 2010. *The Church and AIDS in Africa: The Politics of Ambiguity.* Boulder, CO: Lynne Rienner.

Patton, Cindy. 1990. *Inventing AIDS.* New York: Routledge.

———. 1996. *Fatal Advice: How Safe-Sex Education Went Wrong.* Durham, NC: Duke University Press.

———. 2002. *Globalizing AIDS.* Minneapolis: University of Minnesota Press.

Pearshouse, Richard. 2007. "Legislation Contagion: The Spread of Problematic New HIV Laws in Western Africa." *HIV/AIDS Policy and Law Review* 12(2–3): 1–11. http://www .aidslaw.ca/publications/interfaces/downloadFile.php?ref=1275 [accessed Jan. 6, 2013].

People's Health Movement, Medact, Health Action International, and Medico International. 2011. *Global Health Watch: An Alternative World Health Report.* London: Zed.

Pepin, Jacques. 2011. *The Origins of AIDS.* Cambridge: Cambridge University Press.

Pisani, Elizabeth. 2008. *The Wisdom of Whores: Bureaucrats, Brothels and the Business of AIDS*. New York: Norton.

Rabinow, Paul, ed. 1984. *The Foucault Reader*. New York: Pantheon.

Rajagopal, Balakrishnan. 2003. *International Law from Below: Development, Social Movements and Third World Resistance*. Cambridge: Cambridge University Press.

Ramazanoglu, Caroline. 1993. *Up against Foucault: Explorations of Some Tensions between Foucault and Feminism*. New York: Routledge.

Rao, Prasada J. V. R. 2010. "Avahan: The Transition to a Publicly Funded Programme as a Next Stage." *Sexually Transmitted Infections* 86: i7–i8, http://sti.bmj.com/content/86/Suppl_1/i7.full.pdf [accessed Jan. 8, 2012].

Rau, Bill. 2007. "The Politics of Civil Society in Confronting HIV/AIDS." In *AIDS and Governance*, edited by Nana Poku, Alan Whiteside, and Bjorg Sandkjaer. Hampshire, England: Ashgate.

Reis, Renata, Marcela Vieira, and Gabriela Chaves. 2009. "Access to Medicines and Intellectual Property in Brazil: A Civil Society Experience." In *Intellectual Property Rights and Access to ARV Medicines: Civil Society Resistance in the Global South*, edited by Veriano Terto, Renata Reis, and Cristina Pimenta. Rio de Janeiro: ABIA.

Richter, Judith. 2004. "Public-Private Partnerships for Health: A Trend with No Alternatives?" *Development* 47(2): 43–48. http://www.haiweb.org/pdf/JRichter%20SID%20Article%202004.pdf [accessed Mar. 8 2013].

Rushton, Philippe, and Anthony Bogaert. 1989. "Population Differences in Susceptibility to AIDS: An Evolutionary Analysis." *Social Science and Medicine* 28(12): 1211–1220.

Sabatier, Renée. 1988. *Blaming Others: Prejudice, Race and Worldwide AIDS*. Philadelphia: New Society.

Safreed-Harmon, Kelly. 2008. "GMHC Treatment Issues: Human Rights and HIV/AIDS in Brazil." *GMHC Treatment Issues* (Apr.). http://www.gmhc.org/files/editor/file/ti_poz_0408.pdf [accessed Dec. 10, 2012].

Seale, Andy, Anurita Bains, and Sam Avrett. 2010. "Partnership, Sex, and Marginalization: Moving the Global Fund Sexual Orientation and Gender Identities Agenda." *Health and Human Rights: An International Journal* 12(1): 123–135.

Sedgwick, Eve. 2008. *Epistemology of the Closet*. Berkeley: University of California Press.

Sell, Susan. 2003. *Private Power, Public Law: The Globalization of Intellectual Property Rights*. Cambridge: Cambridge University Press.

Sellman, Doug. 2010. "The 10 Most Important Things to Know about Addiction." *Addiction* 105(1): 6–13.

Shilts, Randy. 1987. *And the Band Played On*. New York: St. Martin's.

Silversides, Ann. 2003. *AIDS Activist: Michael Lynch and the Politics of Community*. Toronto: Between the Lines.

Slaughter, Marie. 2005. *A New World Order*. Princeton, NJ: Princeton University Press.

Smith, Raymond, and Patricia Siplon. 2006. *Drugs into Bodies: Global AIDS Treatment Activism*. Santa Barbara, CA: Praeger.

Sontag, Susan. 1990. *Illness as Metaphor and AIDS and Its Metaphors*. New York: Picador.

Stanton, Donna. 1993. *Discourses of Sexuality: From Aristotle to AIDS*. Ann Arbor: University of Michigan Press.

Stillwaggon, Eileen. 2003. "Racial Metaphors: Interpreting Sex and AIDS in Africa." *Development and Change* 34(5): 809–832.

Stockdill, Brett. 2002. *Activism against AIDS: At the Intersections of Sexuality, Race, Gender and Class.* Boulder, CO: Lynne Rienner.

Stoler, Ann Laura. 1995. *Race and the Education of Desire: Foucault's History of Sexuality and the Colonial Order of Things.* Durham, NC: Duke University Press.

Sutherland, Dylan, and Jennifer Hsu. 2012. *HIV/AIDS in China: The Economic and Social Determinants.* New York: Routledge.

Terto, Veriano, Renata Reis, and Cristina Pimenta, eds. 2009. *Intellectual Property Rights and Access to ARV Medicines: Civil Society Resistance in the Global South.* Rio de Janeiro: ABIA. http://www.abiaids.org.br/_img/media/Intellectual_Property_internet.pdf [accessed Jan. 8, 2013].

Transnational Research Action Centre. 2000. *Tangled Up in Blue: Corporate Partnerships at the United Nations.* http://s3.amazonaws.com/corpwatch.org/downloads/tangled.pdf [accessed Feb. 11, 2013].

Treichler, Paula. 1999. *How to Have Theory in an Epidemic: Cultural Chronicles of AIDS.* Durham, NC: Duke University Press.

UGANET. 2010. *Civil Society Coalition Memoranda on the HIV/AIDS Prevention and Control Bill Submitted to the Members of Parliament.* Kampala: UGANET.

UNAIDS. 2002. *HIV/AIDS: China's Titanic Peril.* Geneva: UNAIDS. http://www.hivpolicy.org/Library/HPP000056.pdf [accessed Apr. 30, 2014].

———. 2007. *Handbook on HIV and Human Rights for National Human Rights Institutions.* Geneva: UNAIDS. http://data.unaids.org/pub/Report/2007/jc1367-handbookhiv_en.pdf [accessed Jan. 6, 2013].

———. 2008. *Report of the International Task Team on HIV-Related Travel Restrictions: Findings and Recommendations.* Geneva: UNAIDS. http://data.unaids.org/pub/Report/2009/jc1715_report_inter_task_team_hiv_en.pdf [accessed Jan. 6, 2013].

———. 2010. *UNAIDS Division of Labor: Consolidated Guidance Notes.* Geneva: UNAIDS. http://www.unaids.org/en/media/unaids/contentassets/documents/unaidspublication/2011/JC2063_DivisionOfLabour_en.pdf [accessed Jan. 11, 2013].

———. 2011a. *Global AIDS Response Progress Reporting 2012: Guidelines.* Geneva: UNAIDS. http://www.unaids.org/en/media/unaids/contentassets/documents/document/2011/JC2215_Global_AIDS_Response_Progress_Reporting_en.pdf [accessed Jan. 6, 2013].

———. 2011b. *UNAIDS Terminology Guidelines.* Geneva: UNAIDS. http://www.unaids.org/en/media/unaids/contentassets/documents/unaidspublication/2011/JC2118_terminology-guidelines_en.pdf [accessed Jan. 6, 2013].

———. 2011c. *Outlook 30.* Geneva: UNAIDS. http://www.unaids.org/en/media/unaids/contentassets/documents/unaidspublication/2011/20110607_jc2069_30outlook_en.pdf [accessed Jan. 6, 2013].

UNAIDS Reference Group on HIV and Human Rights. 2011. *Staying the Rights Course: Statement to the 2011 UN High-Level Meeting on AIDS.* Geneva: UNAIDS. http://unaidspcbngo.org/wp-content/uploads/2011/04/HRRefGrp-RightsCourse-ENG.pdf [accessed Jan. 6, 2013].

UNAIDS, UNICEF, and USAID. 2004. *Children on the Brink: A New Report on Orphan Estimates and a Framework for Action.* Geneva: UNAIDS. http://www.unicef.org/publications/cob_layout6-013.pdf [accessed Jan. 6, 2013].

UNICEF. 2002. *Young People and HIV/AIDS: Opportunity In Crisis.* New York: UNICEF.

————. 2008. *Scaling Up the Response for Children: Background Paper for East Asia and Regional Partnership Forum on Children and HIV and AIDS.* New York: UNICEF.

————. 2009. *Consultation on Strategic Information and HIV Prevention among Most-at-Risk Adolescents.* New York: UNICEF. http://www.unfpa.org/webdav/site/global/shared /iattyp/docs/MARA_Consultation_Final_v3.pdf [accessed Jan. 6, 2013].

UNICEF, UNAIDS, and WHO. 2002. *Young People and HIV/AIDS: Opportunity in Crisis.* New York: UNICEF. http://www.unaids.org/en/media/unaids/contentassets/dataim port/topics/young-people/youngpeoplehivaids_en.pdf [accessed Feb. 28, 2013].

UNICEF and WHO. 2008. *More Positive Living: Strengthening the Health Sector Response to Young People Living with HIV.* New York: UNICEF. http://whqlibdoc.who.int/publi cations/2008/9789241597098_eng.pdf [accessed Jan. 6, 2013].

UNIFEM. 2010. *Transforming the National AIDS Response: Advancing Women's Leadership and Participation.* New York: UNIFEM.

United in Anger. 2012. Dir. Jim Hubbard. Film Collaborative.

Waldby, Catherine. 1996. *AIDS and the Body Politic: Biomedicine and Sexual Difference.* London: Routledge.

Wang, Xian Gyu, Hu Yuan Qion, and Jia Ping. 2009. "Multi-Sector Approaches on Improving Access to ARVs in China." In *Intellectual Property Rights and Access to ARV Medicines: Civil Society Resistance in the Global South,* edited by Veriano Terto, Renata Reis, and Cristina Pimenta. Rio de Janeiro: ABIA.

Wetzler, Jennryn. 2007. *Timeline on Brazil's Compulsory Licensing.* http://search.wcl.amer ican.edu/search?q=cache:JeJB6DO2NlIJ:www.wcl.american.edu/pijip/download.cfm %3Fdownloadfile%3D9C0107B5-DE2F-4E48-6CE8D03F4933FCD4%26typename %3DdmFile%26fieldname%3Dfilename+Timeline+on+Brazil%27s&site=default _collection&client=default_frontend&output=xml_no_dtd&proxystylesheet=default _frontend&ie=UTF-8&access=p&oe=UTF-8 [accessed Jan. 8, 2013].

WHO. 2008. *Closing the Gap in a Generation: Health Equity through Action on the Social Determinants of Health.* http://whqlibdoc.who.int/publications/2008/9789241563703 _eng.pdf [accessed Jan. 9, 2012].

WHO, UNAIDS, and UNICEF. 2011. *Global HIV/AIDS Response: Epidemic Update and Health Sector Progress towards Universal Access.* Geneva: WHO.

WHO, UNAIDS, and UNODC. 2008. *HIV and AIDS in Places of Detention: A Toolkit.* Geneva: WHO. http://www.unodc.org/documents/hiv-aids/HIV-toolkit-Dec08.pdf [accessed Jan. 6, 2013].

WIPO. 2004. *WIPO Intellectual Property Handbook: Policy, Law and Use.* Geneva: WIPO.

Woolcock, Geoffrey, and Dennis Altman. 1996. "Empowerment and Gay Community in Australia." In *AIDS in the World II,* edited by Jonathan Mann and Daniel Tarantola. Oxford: Oxford University Press.

Yang, Wei Ning, and Andrew Yen. 2009. "The Dragon Gets New IP Claws: The Latest Amendments to the Chinese Patent Law." *Intellectual Property and Technology Law Journal* 21(5): 18–27.

Young, Robert. 2003. *Postcolonialism: A Very Short Introduction.* Oxford: Oxford University Press.